BREAST HEALTH

CHARLES B. SIMONE, MD

Avery Publishing Group
Garden City Park, New York

Cover Design: Bill Gonzalez
In-House Editor: Linda Comac
Typesetter: Bonnie Freid
Printer: Paragon Press, Honesdale, PA

Library of Congress Cataloging-in-Publication Data

Simone, Charles B.
   Breast health : what you need to know / by Charles B. Simone.
      p. cm.
   Includes bibliographical references and index.
   ISBN 0-89529-660-8 (pbk.)
      1. Breast—Cancer—Popular works. 2. Breast—Diseases—Popular
   works. I. Title.
   RC280.B8S499 1995
   616.99'499—dc20   95-14177
                                                          CIP

Printed in the United States of America

10 9 8 7 6 5 4 3 2 1

Contents

To my family.

Acknowledgments

Heartfelt thanks go to Nicole L. Simone, who wrote the section on breast feeding beginning on page 148.

Thanks to photographers Leona Law and Sally Davidson.

Thanks go, too, to Rudy Shur, publisher, for his understanding of the need for this book, and to all the people at Avery Publishing Group for their role in getting this book to the public.

Introduction

All women should strive to attain optimum breast health because the incidence of benign lumpy breast disease and breast cancer is rising at alarming rates. Eight of ten women develop benign lumpy breast disease; one in every eight women in the United States will develop breast cancer, and the odds are getting worse.

Cancer is the most feared of all diseases. People immediately associate cancer with dying. Unlike some other killer diseases, cancer usually causes a slow death involving pain, suffering, mental anguish, and a feeling of hopelessness. It now affects one out of every three Americans. By the year 2000, two of every five Americans will be affected. The number of new cancer cases has been increasing over the past nine decades; the accelerated rise in lung cancer, for example, is alarming. According to the U.S. Bureau of the Census, 47 people out of every 100,000 died of cancer in 1900, making it the sixth leading cause of death. Today, 173 people out of every 100,000 will die of cancer, ranking it second.

In 1971, the United States declared war on cancer with the following statement from President Nixon: "The time has come in America when the same kind of concentrated effort that split the atom and took man to the moon should be turned toward conquering this dread disease." In that year, 337,000 people died of cancer, and about $250 million was spent on cancer research.

Since then, tens of billions of dollars has been invested in cancer research. Approximately $104 billion is spent on cancer treatment each year: about $35 billion for direct health care, $12 billion in lost productivity due to treatment or disability, and $57 billion in lost productivity due to premature death.[1] Each month, it seems, new therapies are trumpeted. Some show promise, others fizzle quickly. So intense is the concern to find "the cure for cancer" that more money is collected each year than can actually be spent responsibly on meaningful research. More of these funds should be directed to cancer prevention than the National Cancer Institute's current allocation of less than 5 to 7 percent.

Despite the enormous effort to combat cancer, the number of new cases of nearly every form of cancer has increased annually over the last century as shown in Table 1 and Figure 1. From 1930 to the present—despite the introduction of radiation therapy, chemotherapy, and immunotherapy with biologic response modifiers, despite CT scans, MRI scans, and all the other new medical technology—lifespans for victims of almost every form of cancer except cervical cancer and lung cancer have remained constant, which means that there has been no significant progress in treatment for cancer including breast cancer (see Figure 2).[2] The incidence of stomach cancer has gone down probably due to the advent of refrigeration in the 1930s and the consequent removal of carcinogenic chemicals as food preservatives. And we are faced with the unrealistic—perhaps even deceptive—goal set by the National Cancer Institute and American Cancer Society of a 50 percent reduction in cancer mortality by the year 2000.[3-9] Looking at the almost vertical rise in Figure 1 in the number of new cancer cases each year, I am convinced that the goal cannot be attained.

Table 1   United States Cancer Incidence

	1900	1962	1971*	1995
Total Cases	25,000	520,000	635,000	1,252,000
Leading Cancers				
Prostate	N/A	31,000	35,000	244,000
Lung	N/A	45,000	80,000	186,000
Breast	N/A	63,000	69,600	185,000
Colon/Rectum	N/A	72,000	75,000	158,500
Uterus	N/A	N/A	N/A	48,600

* The year Nixon declared war on cancer.
N/A=Not available.
Data from U.S. Bureau of Vital Statistics and *CA—A Cancer Journal for Clinicians*. See References 14 and 15.

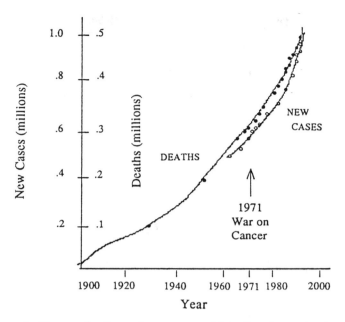

Figure 1 Cancer deaths and new cases. Note the sharp rise in new cancer cases and cancer-related deaths despite billions of dollars in research.

The chilling prospect remains: one out of three Americans alive today will develop cancer, and the majority of them will die from it. By the year 2000, two of every five will develop cancer.

Cancer research and treatment are extremely complex fields of study because the exact nature of the single cancer cell is so elusive. Cancer is many diseases with many different causes. We cannot expect miracle cures just because so much money has been poured into cancer research. At the same time, we should not expect miracles from "cancer-cure" facilities that take money from cancer victims desperate to try any treatment in hope of another chance at life.

After collating the existing cancer data, I found that 80–90 percent of all cancers are produced as a result of dietary and nutritional factors, lifestyle (smoking, alcohol consumption, lack of exercise, etc.), chemicals, and other environmental factors.[10] This information has now been corroborated by major agencies: the National Academy of Sciences,[11] the U.S. Department of Health and Human Services,[12] the National Cancer Institute,[13] and the American Cancer Society.

Since nutrition, lifestyle, and the environment are the most common risk factors for cancer, many of these cancers can be eliminated

BREAST CANCER DEATH RATE: 1930-1990

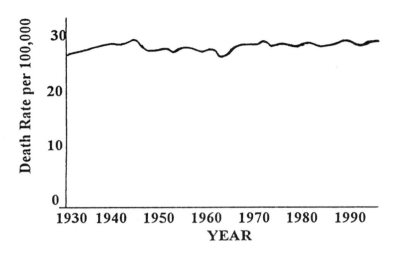

Figure 2 Breast Cancer Death Rate 1930–1990.
Source: 1995 *Ca-A Cancer Journal for Clinicians*, 45:22.
Data source: NCI, SEER data bank.

or substantially reduced in number if you can identify the risk factors pertinent to you and modify them accordingly. Many people have the fatalistic attitude that anything and everything can cause cancer, and believe there is no use in trying to do anything about it. That attitude is unwarranted and fosters even more apathy. Everything does not cause cancer.

The public's perception of cancer causes and cancer "cures" comes mainly from the news media. A study finally has been done that shows serious discrepancies between media people's beliefs about what constitutes cancer risks and what scientists have actually shown to be cancer risks.[16] By reviewing over 1,100 newspaper, magazine, and television news stories between 1972 and 1992, media representatives cited the risks they believed to be the leading factors in causing cancer: manmade chemicals such as food additives and pesticides, pollution, hormone treatments, and radiation. When members of the American Association for Cancer Research were asked the same question, they cited the following as the major risk factors for causing cancer: tobacco, diet, and sunlight. Here again, it is easier for people to complain about risk factors perceived to be important and over which they have no control, rather than take on the responsibility to modify risk factors over which they have total control. People do, in fact, have total control over the leading causes of cancer.

The type of diet we eat today and its preparation are proving to be major risk factors in the development of certain cancers, risk factors that can definitely be modified. Nutrition is a very complex topic— one that is not well understood by the public or even by some physicians. Americans need to know the role that nutrition plays in major diseases.

Diet and nutrition appear to be factors in 60 percent of women's cancers and 40 percent of men's cancers as well as about 75 percent of cardiovascular disease cases. Tobacco is a factor in about 30 percent of human cancers. Other known risk factors associated with the development of cancer include alcohol, age, immune system deficiencies, chemicals, and drugs. You have total control over most of these risk factors, including the major two: diet and tobacco. The cancers most closely associated with nutritional factors are cancers of the breast, colon, rectum, prostate, and endometrium.

Exposure to one or more of the risk factors does not mean that cancer will necessarily develop. It simply means that a person exposed to risk factors has a greater than normal chance of developing cancer.

Physicians in our country too often wind up treating the cancer rather than the whole cancer patient. Much has been learned since 1981 about the role of nutrition, the immune system, and the patient's mental state in the healing process. Because these issues are not addressed properly by the medical community at large, many patients with advanced tumors seek alternative treatment. At great financial and emotional cost to themselves and their families, they resort to quack remedies, get-healthy-quick schemes, and practitioners and "health" centers that claim to reverse or eliminate chronic diseases easily and quickly.

It is *your* responsibility to learn about the risk factors involved in cancer development, and specifically breast cancer, and then modify those risk factors accordingly. In order to prevent cancer, you should devise your own anticancer plan based on risk factor modification. In addition, your family, and particularly your children, should be taught about risk factor modification. If nutritional and other risk factors are modified, the benefit will be evident in all people, but especially in the young and in the succeeding generations. Obviously, there are some risk factors, like air and water, that you cannot control; therefore, your community must also devise a plan to modify environmental risk factors.

We must eliminate or modify all known risk factors so that we will eventually be able to prevent cancer and heart disease more effectively. Nutritional factors and tobacco smoking, for example, are major risk factors, which, if modified or eliminated, can dramatically reduce the number of cancer as well as heart disease patients. Our health-care system emphasizes expensive medical technology and hospital care. It does not emphasize preventive medicine and health education. *It is your responsibility to learn about risk factors and then modify them.* Good health does not come easily—you must work for it.

You have almost total control over the destiny of your health and the health of your family! Do something about it.

PART ONE

Breast Disease Today

1
The Scope of Breast Disease

One woman in eight will develop breast cancer during her lifetime. In the United States, it is the second leading cause of death in women with cancer; 29 percent of the cancers that women develop are breast cancers. In 1994, the number of new cases of breast cancer in the United States was about 183,400; 182,000 in women and 1,400 in men.[1] Total deaths from breast cancer in 1995 are estimated to be 46,300; 46,000 females and 300 males. Black women are less likely to develop breast cancer than white women. However, black women have not done as well as white women once breast cancer had developed. This may be related to the extent of spread of the cancer (known as stage); breast cancer is usually more advanced in blacks than in whites at the time of diagnosis. Physicians use the term "stage of disease" to denote the extent to which a cancer has spread. The stage of breast cancer at diagnosis profoundly influences survival. There are three general terms to describe the stage:

Localized—cancer is in its primary site of the breast.
Regional—cancer has spread to lymph nodes in the region
of the breast.
Distant—cancer has spread to other parts of the body.

The prognosis worsens with each higher stage.

Breast cancer is more often fatal in white men than in white women. Of all those who survive for five years after the diagnosis has been made, 65 percent are women and 53 percent are men. Because most people think that breast cancer is a woman's disease, when men get lumps in their breasts or other symptoms related to their breasts, they tend to ignore or dismiss them as not possibly being cancer. For all white breast cancer patients (both male and female) from 1960 to 1973, the length of time that most people survived after initial diagnosis was six years and seven months, compared to three years and eight months for blacks. While survival rates of several cancers—such as cancers of the uterus, stomach, and liver—improved in women from 1930 to the present, there has been little or no change in lifespan (survival rate) for breast cancer patients. Breast cancers appear also to have a seasonal variation. More breast cancer cases are reported in the spring, and fewer in the autumn.[2]

For this very reason, it is important to understand the role nutrition and other risk factors play in the development of breast cancer so that you can modify them wherever possible. For example, a diet that is high in fat is a risk factor that can be modified. Simply reduce the amount of fat in your diet. An example of a risk factor that cannot be modified is your genetic makeup (inherited risk factors contribute to the development of breast cancer in a small percentage of patients). Age is another risk factor that cannot be modified. Most risk factors for breast cancer and benign breast disease can be modified.

In 1960, one in twenty women developed breast cancer; and in 1974, one in seventeen. Those odds have gotten worse with every succeeding year as seen in Figure 1.1. By 1990, the rate had risen astronomically to one in ten and kept zooming: in 1991, one in nine and in 1994, one in eight women developed breast cancer. This alarming rise is depicted in Figure 1.1. Breast cancer is the second most prevalent cancer in the United States. Table 1.1 shows new breast cancer cases and breast cancer mortality in each state.

These statistics should be no surprise because we know that one in every three Americans will develop cancer. Second only to cardiovascular disease as the leading cause of death in the United States, cancer accounts for 23 percent of all deaths with 526,000 mortalities. By the year 2000, two of every five people will develop cancer and one-third of the deaths in the United States will be caused by cancer. These figures do not even include an estimated 400,000 patients with non-melanomas skin cancers. The leading cancers in the United States include lung cancer, breast cancer, colon-rectal cancer, prostate cancer, and cancer of the uterus; the latter four are all associated with nutritional factors.

**Table 1.1.   Estimated New Breast Cancer Cases
and Mortality by State—1995**

State	New Cases	Mortality	State	New Cases	Mortality
Alabama	3,000	710	Nebraska	1,200	320
Alaska	130	40	Nevada	780	190
Arizona	2,500	630	New Hampshire	880	230
Arkansas	1,800	480	New Jersey	7,000	1,800
California	17,800	4,400	New Mexico	800	210
Colorado	2,100	560	New York	14,500	3,700
Connecticut	2,300	580	North Carolina	4,600	1,200
Delaware	570	150	North Dakota	480	130
Dist. of Columbia	620	160	Ohio	8,400	2,100
Florida	11,800	2,900	Oklahoma	2,100	500
Georgia	3,900	970	Oregon	2,000	480
Hawaii	440	110	Pennsylvania	11,200	2,800
Idaho	700	190	Rhode Island	880	240
Illinois	9,200	2,400	South Carolina	2,700	690
Indiana	4,100	1,000	South Dakota	420	120
Iowa	2,200	590	Tennessee	3,600	880
Kansas	1,800	480	Texas	9,800	2,600
Kentucky	2,400	610	Utah	850	220
Louisiana	3,200	810	Vermont	390	110
Maine	910	250	Virginia	4,500	1,200
Maryland	3,500	870	Washington	3,400	850
Massachusetts	5,000	1,200	West Virginia	1,300	330
Michigan	6,800	1,600	Wisconsin	3,800	950
Minnesota	3,100	780	Wyoming	290	80
Mississippi	1,700	470	Puerto Rico	1,100	330
Missouri	4,200	1,000	United States	183,400	46,220
Montana	560	130			

Even though many cancer organizations have been saying there is an improvement for breast cancer statistics, the numbers keep getting worse. The number of new cases of breast cancer went from 73,000 in 1973 to over 190,000 in 1994. The population in the United States did increase during those years but even controlling for the increased population, the number of new breast cancer cases went from 82 per 100,000 women in 1973 to 127 per 100,000 in 1994. And the annual percentage increase is roughly 2 percent every year. Table 1.2 reveals the risk for developing breast cancer at various ages.

When mortality figures are examined from 1930 onward, however, no change is seen in survival for women with breast cancer, which means there has been no change in the life span of women affected with breast cancer since 1930. And the number of breast cancer deaths goes up every year.

At the request of the Congress in December 1991, the Government Accounting Office released its findings concerning breast cancer—

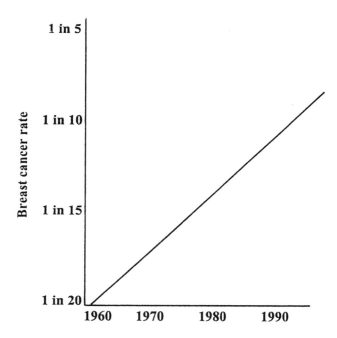

Figure 1.1   Odds of a woman's developing breast cancer in the United States.

Breast Cancer, 1971–1991: Prevention, Treatment, and Research. The report states that there has been no progress in the prevention of breast cancer or in the reduction of breast cancer mortality. In the last two decades, the National Cancer Institute has spent over $1 billion on breast cancer alone, touting spectacular progress at the research level with almost no change in reducing mortality or changing life spans. The trend of mortality rates is upward.

Treatment has improved survival only slightly. The five-year survival rate for breast cancer in 1976 was 75 percent; in 1983, 77 percent; and, in 1989, 78 percent. Most scientists/physicians are convinced, however, that the slight increase in time of survival or life span is due largely to earlier detection of breast cancer by improved mammographic technology. But let us not forget what five-year survival means as defined by the oncologist. If a patient lives five years and one day, that woman is counted as a cure or survivor even though she has died. If, however, she lives one day less than five years, she is counted as a nonsurvivor.

Currently, the incidence of breast cancer is lower in developing countries than elsewhere, but almost half of all the world's breast

Table 1.2. Risk of Developing Breast Cancer

By age 25: 1 in 19,608	By age 60: 1 in 24
By age 30: 1 in 2,525	By age 65: 1 in 17
By age 35: 1 in 622	By age 70: 1 in 14
By age 40: 1 in 217	By age 75: 1 in 11
By age 45: 1 in 93	By age 80: 1 in 10
By age 50: 1 in 50	By age 85: 1 in 9
By age 55: 1 in 33	Ever: 1 in 8

cancer deaths will be in these developing countries.[3] The women will face all the same risk factors, and their immune systems are poor due, in part, to poor food. Breast cancer is likely to become the number one cause of death for cancer patients in the Third World. Most breast cancers in these countries will be in premenopausal women. And even if mammography were available in these countries, studies now show that mammography has little impact on the survival of young women. Breast self-examination is obviously inexpensive and available if taught, however, women in developing countries don't recognize that breast cancer is a hazard, nor do they have time to think about breast cancer given the fact that they face so many other problems simply to exist on a daily basis.

The five-year mortality for patients having a three centimeter breast cancer lesion was studied in patients in Bombay, India, and the United States.[4] Only 25 percent of the patients in the United States die at five years compared with 41 percent of breast cancer patients who die in Bombay, India, at the end of five years. Within the first year of breast cancer detection, 21 percent of the people in Bombay, India, died, compared to only 5 percent of United States breast cancer patients in the first year. This shows that over half of the women who were going to die in the first five years, did so within the first year of diagnosis in Bombay, India.

As countries around the world have become more westernized especially in their dietary habits, the number of deaths from diet-related tumors has increased. For example, Table 1.3 shows the death rate of breast cancer cases per 100,000 people in various countries. When you examine the mortality from cancers in Japan, you find that tumors related to dietary/nutritional factors have increased dramatically in the last twenty-five years. Cancers of the colon and rectum, cancers of the breast, and prostate cancer all have increased dramatically. Previously, Japanese women enjoyed a very low rate of breast cancer. It affected only 3.9 women per 100,000 between the years 1955 and 1959. It rose to 6.1 women per 100,000 during the years 1985 to 1989. This trend is mainly seen in younger Japanese

Table 1.3.   Worldwide Death Rate of Breast Cancer Per 100,000 in 1991

Country	Number/100,000	Country	Number/100,000
1. England & Wales	29	21. Australia	21
2. Malta	28	22. Czechoslovakia	20
3. Ireland	28	23. France	20
4. Denmark	28	24. Norway	19
5. Scotland	27	25. Sweden	18
6. New Zealand	27	26. Portugal	18
7. Netherlands	27	27. Spain	17
8. Northern Ireland	27	28. Finland	17
9. Uruguay	26	29. Yugoslavia	16
10. Luxembourg	25	30. Poland	16
11. Switzerland	24	31. Bulgaria	16
12. Canada	24	32. Greece	15
13. Iceland	24	33. Cuba	15
14. Israel	23	34. Romania	15
15. Hungary	23	35. Puerto Rico	14
16. United States	22	36. Russia	14
17. Austria	22	37. Singapore	13
18. Germany	22	38. Costa Rica	13
19. Argentina	21	39. Chile	13
20. Italy	21		

women who are more likely to have adopted Western ideas and habits, especially dietary habits.[5]

We still hear that if more money were given for the war on cancer and specifically breast cancer, the magic bullet would be found. The major finding of the Government Accounting Office report showed that *prevention* of cancer is paramount in the battle against cancer since there is no clear strategy for improving survival. And even though the medical management of the disease has improved, life span has not, and that is the primary objective of any treatment—to make the life span longer, improve survival. Two advances have come about, however: 1) minimizing pain and suffering, and 2) less mutilating surgery to achieve the same survival. Even though this information is well-known to all scientists and physicians, the great majority of all breast cancers are still handled in the same way, i.e., modified radical mastectomy rather than lumpectomy, axillary node dissection, and radiation therapy.

The *prevention* of all cancers, including breast cancer, should be of primary importance. Less than 5 percent of the National Cancer Institute's budget currently is earmarked for prevention and of these studies, true prevention studies, unencumbered with other agenda, account for well under 2 percent. We are not winning the war against breast cancer with the current conventional approach; therefore, we must prevent the disease.

Breast diseases other than cancer also afflict many women today. It is estimated that 60 percent to 80 percent of all women develop benign breast disease. Some men also develop benign breast disease. We will consider benign breast diseases at length in the next chapter.

2
Benign Breast Syndromes

The term "benign breast syndromes" embodies many benign breast disorders. There have been numerous terms ascribed to these disorders including fibrocystic breast disease, lumpy breast disease, chronic mastitis, mammary dysplasia, cysts, and many others. Many physicians inappropriately label all the disorders that we will discuss as "fibrocystic disease."

About 60 to 80 percent of all women will develop some benign breast disorder. Most benign breast disorder symptoms occur predominantly in women who menstruate and these symptoms are relatively rare in post-menopausal women. Young women tend to have *fibroadenomas*, middle-aged women or perimenopausal women commonly have *cysts*, and only 15 percent of post-menopausal women have gross cysts.

There are some racial differences with regard to benign breast syndromes. There is a decreased incidence in rural Africans, first-generation Chinese immigrants, and Native Americans. Japanese women have half as many biopsy-proven changes as American women. Lumpy breasts are more commonly seen in white women than in black women and more black women than white women have fibroadenomas.

There are many risk factors that contribute to the development of benign breast symptoms and physical changes. Each of these risk factors influences all of the others. The most important include:

1. High-fat diet.[1]
2. Lack of certain vitamins and minerals.[2]
3. Caffeine from any source—coffee, tea, colas, chocolate, etc.[3,4]
4. Nicotine, whether you smoke or inhale other people's smoke.
5. Alcohol consumption.
6. Hormonal factors.

Hormonal changes are very important because estrogen and progesterone influence different anatomical parts of the breast. Estrogen influences the cells that make up the ducts of the breasts. Progesterone influences the lobules that manufacture breast secretions.

There are two ways of classifying benign breast problems. The first and most common is based upon the clinical presentation of symptoms and physical characteristics. The second is based upon the pathologist's opinion after seeing a biopsied specimen under the microscope.

SYMPTOMS AND PHYSICAL CHARACTERISTICS OF BENIGN BREAST SYNDROMES

Since the majority of lumps do not get biopsied, a clinical classification system for benign breast syndromes was developed and is based upon symptoms and physical characteristics.

Lumpiness or the feeling of grape-like structures is not the same as a single, large, dominating mass in the breast. Lumpiness is generally diffuse and located particularly in the upper outer quadrants of each breast. A dominant mass or lump does not change with the menstrual cycle, however, lumpiness does. Sometimes the difference between a dominant lump and generalized lumpiness is not very distinct.

Cyclical Swelling Without Tenderness

There is swelling *without* tenderness that starts at ovulation and continues to increase up through menstruation.

Cyclical Swelling and Tenderness

There is swelling and tenderness that starts at ovulation, which is midcycle, and continues to increase up through menstruation.

Breast Pain Both Cyclical and Noncyclical

More than half of all women complain of breast pain at some time in their cycles and lives. Women generally seek the attention of a physician because they have breast pain and are not sure whether the pain is due to a cancer or not. They simply want reassurance. There are five conditions that cause breast pain:

- cyclical hormonal changes of menstrual cycle;
- pain that is continuous or aching and unrelated to cycle changes (sclerosing adenosis);
- infection of ducts;
- inflammation of the joint in which the rib joins the sternum; and
- cancer.

Dominant Lumps—Cysts and Fibroadenomas

Dominant lumps are important because they must be distinguished from cancers. Cysts, galactoceles (milk-filled cysts), and fibroadenomas usually form dominant lumps.

- Cysts and galactoceles are fluid-filled and the fluid can be aspirated with a needle and syringe.
- Fibroadenomas, on the other hand, are solid breast tumors that are benign. Needle aspiration will yield no fluid. Fibroadenomas are usually seen in young women under the age of 25. Fibroadenomas may increase in size near the end of each menstrual cycle and are generally painless. Because they are solid masses and do not get smaller on their own, they must be removed surgically to determine with certainty that the mass is not a cancer. Fibroadenoma is a real risk factor for future breast cancer.[5]

Discharge From Nipple—Papilloma and Duct Problems

A mature woman or a newborn baby may secrete fluid from the nipple. Most hormones, including growth hormone, insulin, adrenal hormones, estrogen, progesterone, and prolactin may cause the breast to secrete fluid.

Prolactin, a hormone that is secreted from the pituitary in the brain, can cause a milky discharge from the nipple or menstrual irregularities. A blood test will determine the prolactin level and, if elevated, the cause of this elevation should be determined. Many things may cause the elevation of prolactin: thyroid disorder, drugs that are used for sedation or tranquilization, oral contraceptives, breast or chest stimulation, and tumors located in the brain such as a pituitary tumor or craniopharyngiomas.

If the fluid secreted from the nipple is other than milky white, that is, if it is grossly bloody, then further investigation should be conducted. A smear may be done using the fluid put onto a slide and sent for microscopic evaluation. A mammogram should be done—and in some instances, a contrast ductographic mammogram—to determine the origin of the discharge.

The following are the most common causes of bloody nipple discharge:

* Intraductal papilloma (45 percent of all cases);
* "Fibrocystic" duct ectasia (35 percent—this condition affects mainly elderly females in whom the ends of the ducts are dilated and filled with debris);
* Infection (8 percent); and
* Cancer (7 percent).

A bloody discharge must be evaluated. In some cases, surgical removal of the area causing the discharge is indicated.

Infections

Most infections of the breast occur during lactation or shortly thereafter. Treatment is with antibiotics or surgical intervention.

A woman may have any or all of these clinical characteristics in any combination. Lumps may occur in one breast or both, but one breast is more often involved.

MICROSCOPIC PATHOLOGICAL CLASSIFICATION OF BENIGN BREAST LESIONS

The following classifications are based on biopsies. A breast lesion can only be classified in this way after a pathologist has examined tissue samples with a microscope. Some of the benign pathological categories of breast disease are precursors of future cancer and some are not. Some cause symptoms and lumps, others do not. Some grow larger and larger, others do not.

Those benign conditions that do grow larger and larger are termed *proliferative* lesions, i.e., they proliferate. Those that do not grow are termed *non-proliferative* lesions. Proliferative lesions may have either atypical cells, that is cells that do not look normal, or typical or normal-looking cells. Any benign-looking lesion that has atypical cells brings with it a much higher risk of developing cancer. The more abnormal the cells look, the higher the risk.

Non-Proliferative Lesions (Non-Growers)

Cyst

A breast cyst is an example of a non-proliferative lesion. Once the walls of the cyst are formed, the walls do not increase but they can stretch like a balloon being filled with water; hence, the size varies during the menstrual cycle. There are small cysts less than 3 mm in diameter that pose little or no risk to future cancer development. And there are very large cysts that are clinically evident by palpation of the breast. They are greater than 3 mm in diameter and can be felt when they reach 10 mm or more. The larger cysts are the ones that do, in fact, predispose to subsequent cancer development. The more atypical the cells that line the chamber of the cyst, the higher the risk of developing cancer.

Apocrine Cells

The breast is classified as a sweat gland and as such may have atypical apocrine cells. Apocrine cells generally make up all sweat glands, and in some patients, these cells may become atypical, not normal. Generally, however, this poses no subsequent risk for developing cancer.

Fibroadenoma

It is solid and generally occurs in very young women. It must be removed to differentiate it from a cancer.

Hyperplastic Cells

This simply means that there are more than the usual number of cells in one area of the breast. Hyperplastic cells are normal in appearance when viewed with a microscope.

Proliferative Lesions With Normal Cells

Sclerosing adenosis

This lesion is not a cancer but may look like a cancer under the microscope. It can be small or large and palpable and is usually located in one area of the breast. Microcalcifications on a mammogram are typical for an adenosis, which must then be distinguished from a cancer since some cancers also present with microcalcifications on a mammogram.

Proliferative Lesions With Abnormal or Atypical Cells

Hyperplasia—high degree

A much larger number of cells are seen, much more than normal. Some of these cells may look abnormal or atypical and, hence, may have a higher malignant potential.

Lobular Neoplasia

An abnormal growth of cells that line the ducts and lobules, lobular neoplasia, misnamed lobular carcinoma *in situ*, usually does not form a palpable tumor. It does predispose to the development of frank outright cancer.

Intraductal Papilloma

Multiple intraductal papillomas involve a number of ducts, and generally do form palpable masses in the breast. These also predispose to the development of cancer.

The above lesions and categories represent the majority of benign breast conditions typically seen. By no means, however, are all of them represented.

RELATIONSHIP BETWEEN BENIGN ENTITIES AND CANCER

Numerous studies have examined the relationship between the above benign conditions and future risk of cancer. The bottom line with all these is a single important factor: the more abnormal the cells look under the microscope, i.e., the more atypical they are, the higher the chance for developing cancer. The less atypical or abnormal, the less is the risk for future cancer. Hence, any pathologically benign disorder of the breast should be treated aggressively because all cells are on a continuum starting with normal cells that can transform to various degrees of abnormality or atypia, and proceeding onward to an outright cancer cell. Once a benign condition is diagnosed, tremendous effort should be made to change the lifestyle factors that produced this condition. If those lifestyle factors are not changed, that so-called benign condition may transform ultimately into a higher form of atypical cells or abnormal cells, and then into a cancer.

Table 2.1 represents an updated consensus statement issued in 1992 by the Cancer Committee, College of American Pathologists, Relative Risk of Invasive Breast Cancer based on pathological examination of benign breast tissue.[6] About 25 percent of all women with benign breast conditions have pathology that puts them into the

**Table 2.1. Risk of Developing Cancer Based on
Pathological Examination of Benign Breast Tissue**

No Increased Risk
  Adenosis
  Apocrine cellular changes
  Small cysts
  Mild hyperplasia
  Duct ectasia
  Fibrosis
  Inflammation/infection (mastitis)
  Squamous cellular changes

Slightly Increased Risk (1.5 to 2 times)
  Large cysts and a first-degree relative with breast cancer
  Fibroadenoma—moderate to extensive hyperplasia
  Papilloma
  Sclerosing adenosis, well developed

Moderately Increased Risk (4 to 5 times)
  Hyperplasia with abnormal or atypical cells

High Risk
  Comedo (a pathological cell type) or non-comedo carcinoma *in situ*

"slightly increased risk" category. However, for women with atypical
or abnormal hyperplasia (borderline lesions) who also have a first-
degree relative with breast cancer, the risk for developing breast
cancer is 20 percent in the next 10 to 15 years.

GYNECOMASTIA

Gynecomastia is the condition in which the male breast enlarges. This
male breast condition occurs when the influence of estrogen or estrogen-
like chemicals is greater than the influence of testosterone. Gynecomastia generally affects the left breast more often than the right.[7,8] This
condition may affect as much as one-third of the male population of all
ages from puberty to old age and is seen in 57 percent of men over age
44.[9,10,11,12,13] Gynecomastia is associated with four main causes:

  1. Hormonal Changes
      Normal changes in:
        Neonatal period
        Puberty
        Elderly

Abnormal disease conditions:
 Testicle fails to work
 Puberty
 Postpuberty
 Klinefelter's syndrome
 Testicle fails to work secondary to:
  Radiation
  Infection: orchitis, tuberculosis, leprosy
  Cryptorchidism
  Trauma
  Hydrocele
  Varicocele
  Spermatocele
 Thyroid underactivity or overactivity
 Hormone produced from cancers of:
  Testicle
   Seminoma, teratoma
   Choriocarcinoma
   Interstitial (Leydig) cell
   Androblastoma
   Embryonal cell carcinoma
  Adrenal—Hyperplasia, carcinoma
  Pituitary—Adenoma
  Bronchogenic carcinoma
  Hepatoma

2. Drugs

Amiloride	Fluphenazine	Prochlorperazine
Amphetamines	Flutamide	Propranolol
Anabolic steroids	Guanabenz	Ranitidine
Busulfan	Heroin	Reserpine
Chlorpromazine	Isoniazid	Spironolactone
Cimetidine	Ketocanazole	Sulindac
Clomiphene	Leuprolide	Tamoxifen
Diazepam	Marijuana	Theophylline
Diethylstilbestrol	Methadone	Thiazide
Digoxin	Methyldopa	Thiethylperazine
Diphenylhydantoin	Metronidazole	Thioridazine
D-penicillamine	Neuroleptic drugs	Trifluoperazine
Ergotamine tartrate	Perphenazine	Tricyclics
Estramustine	Phenothiazines	Vincristine
Estrogen	Procarbazine	

3. Systemic Disorders
    Chronic disease of the: liver, kidney, lung, central nervous
       system
    Malnutrition or starvation
    Cancer of the colon or prostate, or lymphoma
    Ulcerative colitis
    Rheumatic fever

4. Idiopathic
    Cause unknown

EXAMINATION AND FOLLOW-UP OF BENIGN BREAST SYNDROMES

Patients who have benign breast syndromes are difficult to physically examine. No matter how thorough a physician is in examining lumpy breasts, he/she can never be absolutely sure that there is not something evil like a cancer lurking within the nodularity or lumpiness or, in fact, behind them. The same caveat holds true for mammogram interpretation because the nodularity and fibrous tissue may mask areas that can also harbor a cancer. In addition, there are no good blood tests that can detect an early breast cancer. So the best course is to practice self-examination and "memorize" your breasts as much as possible, noting the location of the nodularities. Notify your physician if any *new* nodules develop, persist, or become hard.

Before a physician examines your breasts, he/she should know your risk factors for developing breast cancer. These risk factors should include those from Chapter 1 and, if you had a previous breast biopsy, the assigned risk from Table 2.1. This overall risk assessment will enable the physician to mentally assign a certain degree of suspicion of possible cancer to your breast examination. If you have a high malignant potential as determined by your overall risk assessment, then minor changes in your breast should be viewed as highly suspicious. If your risk assessment is low, then minor breast changes would not be as suspicious.

For instance, if you are in a high risk category on the self-assessment test in Chapter 3 and also had a breast biopsy that was "hyperplasia with abnormal or atypical cells" (see Table 2.1), I would examine you with a high degree of suspicion, looking for even subtle changes. If, on the other hand, you are in a low-risk category and had a biopsy that also conferred low-risk, like adenosis (see Table 2.1), I would feel more relaxed about any minor breast changes. If you never had a breast biopsy, then the examiner's degree of suspicion should be linked to the level of risk as determined by the self-assessment test alone.

How Often Should You Be Examined?

If you have lumpy breasts, you should be examined three to four times a year by a physician who has extensive clinical experience in breast diseases. OB-GYN physicians who do the majority of all breast examinations did not find as many breast masses when compared to the number of breast masses detected by other physicians.[14] Physicians, like internists or family physicians, who spend the most amount of time doing a breast examination, find the most abnormalities.

TREATMENT OF BENIGN BREAST DISORDERS

The most important thing a physician can do for a patient who comes into the office complaining of a lump is to make sure that the lump is not a cancer. A full discussion of the proper work-up of a lump begins on page 226. Needle aspiration, ultrasound, and mammogram are all part of the evaluation process. Cyclical pain and generalized lumps have been handled in many different ways:

- Hormonal manipulation using progesterone, thyroid hormones, human chronic gonadotropin hormone, tamoxifen, bromocriptine, danazol;
- Diuretics;
- Surgical maneuvers;
- Caffeine restriction;
- Vitamin E;
- Oral contraceptives;
- Evening primrose oil;
- Steroids injected directly into the breast.

Although some of these have provided relief for women, many of these drugs are too expensive or have too many side effects that most women are not willing to tolerate. And some of the treatments also bring with them a risk for future cancer; for instance, there is a 400 percent increased risk of developing breast cancer for women who used oral contraceptives for four years or more before the age of twenty-five.

PREMENSTRUAL SYNDROME

Premenstrual syndrome, or PMS, is a syndrome caused by the changes of estrogen and progesterone and other hormones during ovulation and, ultimately, premenstrually and menstrually. These hormonal changes are necessary if ovulation (the release of an egg from the ovary into the uterus) is to proceed. However, the hormonal changes lead to a combination of cyclical and distressing physical, psychological, and/or behavioral changes in many women. Some of these changes include acne, cravings for sweets, bloating, breast tenderness as already discussed, constipation, depression, anxiety, irritability, fatigue, insomnia, and headaches. Premenstrual syndrome even has legal implications. It has been used as a defense to mitigate women's responsibility for criminal acts and, on the other hand, it has undermined women's competence in some civil matters. Many treatments have been tried to mitigate the symptoms associated with PMS. None have been completely successful, however, analgesics have been used with the most success to relieve pain and discomfort in the pelvic region.

SIMONE TEN-POINT PLAN
FOR TREATING BENIGN BREAST SYMPTOMS

The Simone Ten-Point Plan outlined on page 323 has been effective for decreasing breast pain, nodularity, lumpiness, the size of many cysts, and many PMS symptoms. After adherence to the Simone Ten-Point Plan for two full menstrual cycles, 90 percent of all women will have decreased breast tenderness, decreased swelling, little or no breast pain, softer breasts, and improvement in many PMS symptoms. After approximately six months, the majority of women experience a decrease in nodularity as well. The plan is discussed at length on pages 317 through 333.

Point 1. Nutrition.

- Maintain an ideal weight. Decrease the number of daily calories if you are overweight.
- Eat a low-fat, low-cholesterol diet: fish, poultry without the skin. If you must consume dairy products, then only skim products, not whole, 1 percent, or 2 percent. No red meat, lunch meats, or oils.
- Consume both *soluble* and *insoluble* fiber (25 to 30 grams per day). Fruits, vegetables, cereals have mainly *insoluble* fibers. Pectins, gums, and mucilages have *soluble* fibers that can decrease cholesterol, triglycerides, sugars, and carcinogens.
- Supplement your diet with certain nutrients in the proper doses, form, and combination. These supplements should include: Antioxidants (beta-carotene, vitamins E and C, selenium, cysteine, flavonoids, copper, zinc), the B vitamins, calcium and calcium-enhancing agents, and others. (See Chapter 5 for additional information.)

- Eliminate caffeine.
- Eliminate salt, food additives, and smoked, barbecued, or pickled foods.

Point 2. Tobacco

Do not smoke, chew, or snuff tobacco, or inhale other people's smoke.

Point 3. Alcohol and Caffeine

Avoid all alcohol, or have one drink or less per week. Limit caffeine.

Point 4. Radiation

Have X-rays only when needed. Use #15 sunscreen, wear sunglasses. Avoid electromagnetic fields from home appliances, office equipment, and outside electric fields.

Point 5. Environmental Exposure

Keep air, water, and workplace clean by using filters.

Point 6. Sexual-Social Factors, Hormones, Drugs

Avoid promiscuity, hormones, and any unnecessary drugs.

Point 7. Learn the Seven Early Warning Signs.

- Lump in breast
- Change in wart/mole
- Nonhealing sore
- Change in bowel/bladder habits
- Persistent cough/hoarseness
- Unusual bleeding
- Indigestion/trouble swallowing

Point 8. Take Risk Factor Assessment Test

To determine your risk for disease and immune system dysfunction, take the Risk Factor Assessment Test (Chapter 3).

Point 9. Exercise and Relax Regularly.

Point 10. Have an Executive Physical Exam Yearly.

(See page 330.) Early diagnosis is important. Prevention is the key to wellness.

If you adhere to this Ten-Point Plan and still have not had significant relief from your breast pain or have not had improvement in other symptoms, then the various nutrients can be modified by an experienced clinician to attain a clinical response.

TAMOXIFEN TRIAL TO PREVENT BREAST CANCER

On April 29, 1992, the United States National Cancer Institute announced the beginning of the Breast Cancer Prevention Trial that would *last for only five years* and involve 16,000 women deemed to be at increased risk for developing breast cancer. The objective is to determine whether tamoxifen can significantly reduce the incidence of breast cancer in these high-risk individuals. Any woman over the age of 60 is eligible automatically. Women between the ages of 35 and 59 are eligible only if they have the following six risk factors:

1. Previous diagnosis of lobular carcinoma *in situ.*
2. First-degree relatives (mother, daughters, sisters) who have breast cancer.
3. Early age at menarche (first occurrence of menstruation).
4. Late age at delivery of first child.
5. No pregnancies.
6. History of having had several breast biopsies.

However, the majority of women to be entered in the study are older than 60. These women over 60 are calculated to have a 10 percent chance of developing cancer during their remaining lifetime and only a 1.7 percent risk during the five-year trial period.[15,16] A woman over the age of 35 is eligible for this protocol if her risk for developing breast cancer over the following five years is calculated to be 1.7 percent or more. This particular woman would lower her risk to 1.2 percent from 1.7 if the National Cancer Institute's prediction of a 30 percent reduction in breast cancer rates is accurate. Does that look like a significant reduction to you?

This tamoxifen prevention trial is based on the fact that eight randomized controlled trials involving breast cancer patients who took tamoxifen daily demonstrated a one-third reduced incidence of a cancer developing in the uninvolved breast.[17] But this finding may have absolutely nothing to do with women who are healthy and do not have breast cancer. Since both breasts of a breast cancer patient are exposed to identical influences, there is no reason to think that the opposite uninvolved breast of a woman with breast cancer is a healthy control. Also, premenopausal women with breast cancer rarely benefit from tamoxifen because, generally, their tumors are devoid of estrogen-progesterone receptors and the drug has not been shown to help in the prevention mode.

The people who support this trial offer another rationale for using tamoxifen in such a prevention trial. Tamoxifen was alleged to protect against osteoporosis. However, in two retrospective series[18,19] and in three prospective investigations[20,21,22] tamoxifen had no protective effect on bone density at all.

The trial's supporters also cite the alleged cardiovascular benefit of tamoxifen in older women. However, tamoxifen has been reported to decrease,[23] maintain,[24] or increase[25] high-density lipoprotein cholesterol, HDL. Tamoxifen has not had a consistent effect on total cholesterol; some studies show decrease, some studies show no change. Some reports show that tamoxifen has actually increased total cholesterol and triglyceride concentrations.[26] There have been other points of view extolling the virtues of this tamoxifen prevention trial, but the arguments do little to compensate for the well-known toxicities of tamoxifen.[27,28,29]

The principal architect of the tamoxifen prevention trial explained the rationale for use of this otherwise toxic agent. He said, ". . . the breast cancers that are diagnosed today did not begin to develop yesterday. A number of women who have what appeared to be normal breasts without detectable cancers already have the biological changes that will cause the disease. For any of these early changes an intervention such as tamoxifen may be able to halt the development or progression of breast cancer."[30]

Tamoxifen has been around for over twenty years to treat patients who have advanced breast cancer. It is the most widely prescribed cancer drug in the world. Tamoxifen used with cancer patients has been shown to be extremely helpful in cancer care. However, it is a drug used in patients who already have cancer, and it has side effects and risks, including hot flushes, vaginal discharge on a daily basis for some women, blood clots, endometrial cancer, and liver cancer.

As toxic drugs go, tamoxifen is one of the least toxic drugs. But when you have a cancer, you accept risks of drugs because you are trying to kill the cancer that can otherwise kill you. *Chemotherapy* of invasive cancer deliberately attempts to kill cancer cells—in a short period of time ranging from days to weeks. *Chemoprevention* with tamoxifen, however, is supposed to block the original initiation of the carcinogenic process. But there is a very long latency period from the initiation of a cancer cell to an outright detectable invasive cancer in humans. Many studies show that it takes at least fifteen years or more for the cancer to become obvious and detectable after the original initiation of the carcinogenic process. Hence, it would make a lot more sense to modify an entire lifestyle over a lifetime to prevent breast cancer or any other cancer.[31]

As we have said before, if a woman does have a disease like breast cancer, then treatment with a drug like tamoxifen justifies the risks associated with it. However, one can simply not justify these risks in healthy women. We must continue to identify women at high risk by using the self-assessment test in Chapter 3 combined with any available breast tissue biopsy reports to make an overall breast cancer risk assessment. We can then intervene by using the Ten-Point Plan to change the entire lifestyle so as to make it optimally healthy. One must decrease fat, increase certain vegetables like cruciferous vegetables, eliminate smoking and alcohol consumption, use certain antioxidants and other nutrients,[32] exercise more frequently, reduce stress by way of stress modification programs, and thereby change your risks for developing a breast cancer before it ever starts. We don't have the quick fix that most Americans want, a single pill like tamoxifen to get rid of all their ills.

The tamoxifen trial was halted for about a year due to improprieties. It has been reinstituted and will fail for all the reasons enumerated in the above paragraphs. Furthermore, only a five-year period of time will be investigated, and the trial does not encourage people to change their lifestyles. We will probably see all the side effects of tamoxifen in these healthy women.

If you have an illness, then take medicine for it. If you don't have an illness but are at high risk for it, change your lifestyle. It is your responsibility to keep yourself healthy. No single pill is a green light for you to continue eating the wrong foods, smoking, drinking, etc.

3
An Overview
of Risk Factors

Numerous risk factors are associated with cancer. Many of them are also risk factors for cardiovascular disease. Learn about the risks, modify them, and your risk for both illnesses will be greatly reduced.

DIET AND NUTRITIONAL RISK FACTORS

There is a strong correlation between diet and/or nutritional deficiencies and many cancers (see Table 3.1). The National Academy of Sciences and others estimate that nutritional factors account for 60 percent of cancer cases in women and 40 percent in men.[1-3] Cancers of the breast, colon, rectum, uterus, prostate, and kidney are closely associated with consumption of total fat and protein, particularly meat and animal fat. Other cancers that are directly correlated with dietary factors are cancers of the stomach, small intestine, mouth, pharynx, esophagus, pancreas, liver, ovary, endometrium, thyroid, and bladder.[4-9] Aflatoxin, a fungus product that is found on certain edible plants (especially peanuts), is related to human liver cancer.[10,11]

At one time, excessive consumption of coffee had been correlated with cancer of the pancreas,[12] but considerable doubt has been cast upon this correlation.[13,14] Obesity is also an independent risk factor for cancer, especially breast cancer. Cancers and their relationship to diet and nutritional factors are discussed in depth in chapters 7 through 10.

Table 3.1   Cancer Risk Factors

Risk Factor	Associated Human Cancer
Nutritional factors	
High-fat, low-fiber diet	**Breast**, colon, rectum, prostate, stomach, mouth, pharynx, esophagus, pancreas, liver, ovary, endometrium, thyroid, kidney, bladder
Iodine deficiency	Thyroid, **breast**
Aflatoxin (fungus product)	Liver
Obesity	**Breast**, endometrium, colon
Tobacco use	
Smoking, chewing, snuffing	Lung, larynx, mouth, pharynx, head and neck, esophagus, pancreas, bladder, kidney, **breast**
Involuntary inhalation	Lung, cervix, **breast**, oral
Alcohol consumption	Mouth, pharynx, esophagus, gastrointestine, pancreas, liver, head and neck, larynx, bladder, **breast**
Age greater than 55	Many organ sites
Immune system malfunction	Lymphoma, carcinoma
High blood pressure	**Breast**, colon
Environment	Leukemia, lung, skin, other sites
Sedentary lifestyle	**Breast**, colon, other sites
Stress	Implicated in multiple sites
Hormonal factors	
Late/never pregnant	**Breast**
Fibrocystic breast disease	**Breast**
DES (diethylstilbestrol)	**Breast**, vagina, cervix, endometrium, testicle
Conjugated estrogens	**Breast**, liver
Androgens (17-methyl position)	Liver
Undescended testicles (especially after age 6)	Testicle
Sexual-social behavior	
Female promiscuity	Uterine cervix
Poor male hygiene	Penis
Male homosexuality (promiscuity, amyl nitrite)	Kaposi's sarcoma, anus, tongue
Radiation	
X-rays, etc. (ionizing)	Skin, **breast**, myelogenous leukemia, thyroid, bone
Sunlight (UV), excessive, in fair-skinned people who burn easily	Skin
Pesticides	Lung, prostate, liver, skin, others
Occupational	
Petroleum, tar, soot industries	Lung, skin, scrotum
Boot and shoe manufacture and repair	Nasal sinus
Furniture and cabinetmaking industry	Nasal sinus
Rubber industry	Lung, bladder, leukemia, stomach
Chemists	Brain, lymphoma, leukemia, pancreas
Foundry workers	Lung
Painters	Leukemia
Printing workers	Lung, mouth, pharynx
Textile workers	Nasal sinus

CHEMICAL RISK FACTORS

Chemical and environmental factors, including diet and lifestyle, may be responsible for causing 80 to 90 percent of all cancers. Theoretically, then, most cancers could be prevented if the factors that cause them were first identified and then controlled or eliminated. Throughout their lives, people are exposed to many chemicals and some drugs in small amounts and in many combinations unique to their culture and environment. Many chemicals and drugs are now known to cause human cancer, and many more are suspected carcinogens.[15] For a full discussion, please refer to my book *Cancer and Nutrition: A Ten-Point Plan to Reduce Your Risk of Getting Cancer* (Avery Publishing Group, 1992).

Due to differences in their genetic make-up, individuals exposed to a carcinogen (a chemical substance that causes cancer) will not all have the same probability of getting cancer. Certain proteins from the liver, called enzymes, can break down or activate the carcinogen at different speeds in different people to either render it harmless or promote it to cause cancer. These enzymes destroy or activate carcinogens to varying degrees according to inherited tendencies. Some foods can induce certain enzymes to destroy certain carcinogens. The most potent food sources to induce these enzymes are vegetables of the *Brassicaceae* family, which includes Brussels sprouts, cabbage, and broccoli.[16]

ENVIRONMENTAL RISK FACTORS

Environmental factors are just as important. For example, Japanese men and women who leave Japan and settle in Hawaii or the continental United States have a lower risk of stomach cancer than those who remain in Japan. Stomach cancer in the United States has been steadily decreasing with the advent of refrigeration and the consequent removal of carcinogenic chemicals as food preservatives. Also, the Japanese generally have lower rates of breast and colon cancer, but when they immigrate to the United States, after only twenty years, they have the same rate of colon cancer as Americans. After only two generations, they have the same rate of breast cancer.

Those living in cities encounter many sources of pollution. More people in cities than in rural areas smoke cigarettes. Air pollution is a risk factor for cancer, especially lung cancer. Carcinogens derived from car emissions, industrial activity, burning of solid wastes and fuels remain in the air from four to forty days and thereby travel long distances.[17] Asbestos, a potent carcinogen, can also be found airborne in cities.

Our drinking water contains a number of carcinogens, including asbestos, arsenic, metals, and synthetic organic compounds.[18,19] Asbestos and nitrates are associated with gastrointestinal cancers; arsenic is associated with skin cancer; and synthetic organic chemicals are associated with cancers of the gastrointestinal tract and urinary bladder.

With many carcinogens, the time between exposure to the carcinogen and actual development of cancer may be quite long. Hence, a cancer initiated by trace amounts of either airborne or waterborne carcinogens years before the cancer appears may be attributed to an unrelated or unknown cause at the time of diagnosis.

We are able to detect many carcinogens in our environment, but many others exist in low concentrations. These environmental carcinogens may themselves cause cancer in certain individuals, or they may interact with other risk factors to initiate, or promote, cancers. Therefore, our imperfect environment, a risk factor for cancer, must be modified. If we avoid introducing harmful substances into the environment, it will remain clean.

RADIATION RISK FACTORS

Human studies show that the more radiation to which a person is exposed, the higher is the risk of developing cancer, especially if the radiation exposure is to bone marrow, where the blood cells are made. Women who received many chest X-rays to follow the progress of treatment for tuberculosis had an increased incidence of breast cancer with as little as 17 cGy total dose. A cGy, or centiGray, is a defined amount of energy absorbed by a certain amount of body tissue. One chest X-ray using modern equipment delivers about 0.14 cGy. Riding in an airplane at 35,000 feet for six hours exposes a person to 0.01 cGy. Other radiation risk factors for breast cancer will be discussed.

People who received radiation to shrink enlarged tonsils or to treat acne have a higher risk of developing cancer of the thyroid and parathyroid glands located in the neck. Survivors of the bombings of Hiroshima and Nagasaki have had an increased incidence of leukemia, lymphoma, Hodgkin's disease, multiple myeloma, and other cancers. People who used to paint radium on wrist-watch dials have a high incidence of osteogenic sarcoma, a bone cancer. Chronic exposure of fair-skinned, easily sunburned people to sunlight (ultraviolet light) will lead to a higher rate of skin cancer.

There has been mounting concern that people who work in or live near nuclear power plants have a higher risk of developing cancer. In the United Kingdom, a higher incidence of childhood leukemia has been reported in children living near several nuclear facilities, most notably a fuel reprocessing plant located at Sellafield in northwest

England.[20] The results of another study involving over 8,000 men who worked in the Oak Ridge National Laboratory in Tennessee between 1943 and 1972 show that these men had a higher risk of developing cancers, especially leukemia.[21] Another study shows no such increase in cancer incidence.[22]

Workers in many industries are chronically exposed to low-dose radiation and, hence, may be at risk for heart disease and cancer. We may, therefore, have to reexamine standards for acceptable radiation levels in industry.

OCCUPATIONAL RISK FACTORS

About 10 percent of all cancers are related to exposure to carcinogens on the job. The relationship between a person's job and cancer was noted in the eighteenth century when it was observed that the incidence of cancer of the scrotum was very high in chimney sweeps. Many associations between exposure to carcinogens at work and cancer have been made since then. The boot and shoe manufacture and repair industry and the furniture and cabinetmaking industry were shown to be risk factors for cancer of the nasal sinuses.[23]

Preliminary studies indicate that butchers and slaughterhouse workers are at risk for lung cancer and cancer of other parts of the respiratory system as well as some leukemias.[24,25] However, these findings need to be confirmed and controlled for those persons who also smoke before this industry can be labeled as a definite risk factor for cancer. Other occupations and their associated human cancers are listed in Table 3.1.

AGE AS A RISK FACTOR

Breast cancer is related to age. Between ages 30 and 40, there is a steep rise in the number of breast cancer cases, then there is a plateau between 40 and 55, and then another steep rise thereafter (see Figure 3.1). The incidence of breast cancer in the elderly is more than double that for younger women.

The older you get, the higher is your risk of developing any cancer. The Biometry Section of the National Cancer Institute has presented studies which show that with every five-year increase of age there is a doubling in the incidence of cancer.[26]

As you get older, your risk of getting cancer increases not only because of your age but also due to the amount of time you have been exposed to external risk factors. The elderly often suffer from nutritional deficiencies, and they have an increased number of infections, autoimmune diseases, and infantile disease patterns, as well as cancer. Werner's syndrome, which prematurely ages very young chil-

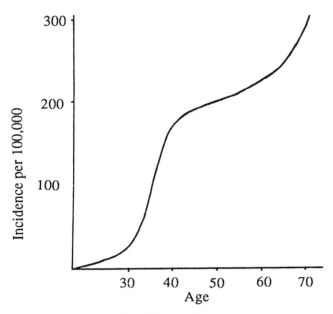

Figure 3.1 Age-related incidence of breast cancer.

dren so that they die in early adolescence, is characterized by an impaired immune system. These facts suggest that the immune system in the elderly is working inefficiently, partly due to poor nutrition.[27] Because the gastrointestinal tract absorbs nutrients less efficiently with age, the elderly need more nutrients in their diets.

Table 3.2 lists the approximate number of people aged 65 or more for each decade beginning with 1980. By 2030, the number of Americans in this age bracket will more than double the number in this group today.

GENETIC RISK FACTORS

Cancer is usually characterized by abnormal genetic chromosome material in the affected cancer cell. A cancer cell does not have the proper amount or type of genes, or, more specifically, DNA (deoxyribonucleic acid). People with certain inherited diseases are more prone to getting cancer. There are over 200 genetic conditions that have an increased incidence of cancer,[28] including mongolism or trisomy 21 syndrome, the immunodeficiency syndromes, Gardner's syndrome, and many more. *These genetic abnormalities, although important for the physician to recognize, account for only a small fraction of all human cancers.*

Table 3.2 Number of Persons Aged 65+ in the United States

Year	Millions
1980	25.7
1989	31.0
2000	34.5
2010	39.4
2020	52.1
2030	65.6

Source: American Geriatric Society. 1991. *JAMA* 265(23):3092.

ATHEROSCLEROSIS AND CANCER

Atherosclerosis and its many complications are the most common cause of death in the United States. Atherosclerosis, commonly called "hardening of the arteries," is a disease that narrows the inside diameter of the artery. This narrowing restricts the blood flow beyond the narrowed portion; therefore, less oxygen can be delivered to those tissues by the red blood cells. Death of tissues occurs when they receive little or no oxygen. The less oxygen, the more dead tissue. Pain is a symptom of either very low oxygen supply to tissues or outright death of tissues. This is why a person having a "heart attack" has pain: some tissues are dying and others are not receiving enough oxygen.

What does atherosclerosis have to do with breast cancer? Well, cancer may be responsible for the development of heart and vessel disease in a way, and, conversely, high blood pressure (a form of blood vessel disease) may lead to the development of cancer under certain circumstances.

The first step in the formation of a narrowed artery is the manufacture of cells (endothelial cells) that line the inside of the artery. Then cholesterol gets deposited in these cells after they have increased in number. The increased cells together with cholesterol is called a plaque. There is good evidence that these cells come from a single cell, that is, they are cloned from one common cell. Cloning is a form of cancer.[29] This situation can be produced in chickens by feeding them carcinogens (benzo(a)pyrene and dimethylbenzanthracene), chemical substances that produce cancer. These particular carcinogens cause an increase in the number and rate of formation of plaques without altering the blood level of cholesterol. In humans, these types of carcinogens (hydrocarbons) are carried by certain proteins (low-density lipoproteins) that also carry cholesterol. More curiously, an enzyme called aryl hydrocarbon hydroxylase, present in cells of the inner walls of arteries, can activate hydrocarbon carcinogens to start proliferating the lining cells.[30] Therefore, if we eat food contaminated with these hydrocarbons or are otherwise exposed to them so that they get into our bloodstream, atherosclerosis may begin to develop. Of course this is just one of many factors involved in the development of atherosclerosis.

R.W. Pero and colleagues have shown a relationship between high blood pressure and cancer.[31] The study shows that the higher the blood pressure and the older the person, the more alterations of DNA that occur in cells. The more abnormal the DNA content of a cell, the more often it will lose control and develop into a cancer. There is some evidence that people with high blood pressure have an increased risk of developing breast cancer,[32] colon cancer, lung cancer, and other cancers.[33]

HORMONAL RISK FACTORS

Hormones influence a cell's growth and development, so if there is an excess or deficit of hormones in the body, cells will not function properly and may grow abnormally or aberrantly and become cancer cells.

Women who have never been pregnant have a higher risk of developing breast cancer than women who do have children; women who become pregnant before age 20 have a reduced risk. Women whose mothers or other close relatives have breast cancer have three times the normal risk of getting breast cancer. Women who do not menstruate during their lifetime have a three to four times higher risk of developing breast cancer after the age of 55. A lower risk of breast cancer is seen in women whose ovaries cease to function or are removed surgically before age 35.

There has been considerable controversy over whether oral contraceptives can cause breast and liver cancer. Many studies seem to indicate that hormones used in birth control pills are a risk factor for breast or liver cancer.[34,35] Estrogens in these oral contraceptives can cause benign liver growths, which can bleed extensively and cause problems related to bleeding.

Daughters of women who received DES (diethylstilbestrol) therapy during pregnancy have developed cancer of the cervix and vagina.[36] Sons of women who took DES have a higher risk of developing cancer of the testicles because DES causes urinary tract abnormalities including undescended testicles, which, if not corrected surgically before age 6, can develop into cancer of the testicles.[37] Furthermore, women exposed to these same synthetic estrogens in adult life have a higher risk of developing cancer of the cells that line the inside of the uterus (endometrial cancer). Male hormones can predispose to both benign and malignant liver tumors.

Benign lumpy breast disease, a disease that affects 50 percent or more of all women sometime during their lives, probably represents a hormone imbalance. If a woman has had the disease over many years, she is at an increased risk of developing breast cancer. We have shown that benign lumpy breast disease has responded to certain nutrients and dietary modification.

SEXUAL-SOCIAL RISK FACTORS

Cancer of the cervix is associated with having sexual intercourse at an early age and with having multiple male sex partners. The earlier the age of the female when she first has sexual intercourse and the greater the number of male partners she has, the higher is her risk of getting cancer of the cervix. Sexual intercourse with uncircumcised male partners may also contribute to a woman's risk of developing cervical cancer.

Cancer of the penis is a very rare disease in the United States. There is almost universal agreement that one primary risk factor is responsible for this cancer—poor hygiene, especially in the uncircumcised male. Secretion and different organisms retained under the foreskin produce irritation and infection, which are thought to predispose to cancer's cellular changes.

There is an epidemic outbreak of Kaposi's sarcoma in sexually active male homosexuals. Kaposi's sarcoma is a cancer of the skin, mucous membranes, and lymph nodes. Those affected have an acquired immunodeficiency syndrome (AIDS). In addition to Kaposi's sarcoma, male homosexuality is a risk factor for two other cancers: cancer of the anus and cancer of the tongue.

Sexually active male homosexuals in good health can have a normal or abnormal immune system. Many with an abnormal immune system appear quite healthy. Some with a malfunctioning immune system have Kaposi's sarcoma and/or fatal or life-threatening infections caused by *Pneumocystis carinii*.

The immune impairment from AIDS seen in sexually active male homosexuals, intravenous drug users, prostitutes, and heterosexuals is now clearly related to infection by the HIV virus. Other risk factors leading to human susceptibility to HIV include amyl nitrite, a drug used as a sexual stimulant. Amyl nitrite produces a profound impairment of the immune system, especially the T lymphocytes. Also, immunological abnormalities are seen more often in homosexuals who have many sexual partners than in those who have only one partner.

INFECTIOUS DISEASES AS RISK FACTORS

In 1994, the International Agency for Research on Cancer (IARC) included certain infectious diseases as carcinogenic risks to humans.[38-41] Hepatitis B virus and hepatitis C virus can cause liver cancer. T cell leukemia and T cell lymphoma are caused directly by viruses. Papillomavirus can cause cervix cancer. *Helicobacter pylori*, a bacterium, can cause stomach cancer. Certain worms and flukes also cause human cancer. *Schistosoma* worms cause bladder cancer. And flukes, like *Opisthorchis*, cause liver cancer and cancer of the gall bladder.

RISK FACTOR ASSESSMENT

My Cancer Risk Factor Assessment test found on page 42 has been designed to assess your own risk factors based upon diet, weight, age, lifestyle, and other variables covered in this chapter. Take the test to evaluate your risk. We define risk for potentially developing cancer based upon the following letter combination totals:

High Risk
{
2 or more A's + any number of B's or C's
or
1 A + 4 or more B's + any number of C's
}

Moderate Risk
{
1A + 3 or fewer B's + any number of C's
or
4 or more B's + any number of C's
or
2 or 3 B's + 2 or more C's
}

Low risk
{
No A's
or
No B's or no C's
or
1 B + 2 or fewer C's
or
2 or fewer C's
}

A person in a high-risk category will not necessarily develop cancer. The high-risk category indicates only that a person in it is more at risk than a person in another category.

Following are a few examples of persons with various risk factors, their relative degrees of risk for developing cancer, and what they should do to modify those risks, thereby reducing their chance of developing cancer (and/or cardiovascular disease). After each risk factor, the score is indicated in parentheses.

Consider Linda, a 56-year-old (C) New Jersey (B) housewife (0). She is 5 feet 5 inches tall, weighs 160 pounds (B), eats red meat daily, eats several eggs per week, drinks milk daily, consumes very little fiber-containing foods, and does not eat a balanced diet (A). She also smokes two packs of cigarettes a day, and has done so for over fifteen years (A). Linda drinks socially (0) and has never had cancer (0), but her mother had breast cancer (B). She started having sexual intercourse at age 20 (0), first got pregnant at age 24 (0), has a history of lumpy breast disease (C), never had any radiation (0), and is relatively easygoing (0).

Linda's total score is two A's, three B's, and two C's. She is in the high-risk group. What can she do to modify her risk factors? She directly controls the most serious ones. I would advise her to terminate cigarette smoking abruptly and completely. Then I would suggest that she permanently modify her diet in order to reduce two other serious risk factors: her high-animal-fat, high-cholesterol, low-fiber diet, and her overweight problem. This would serve also to counter any weight gain that may occur when she stops smoking. Linda has no control over her age, the state in which she has lived, or her history of fibrocystic breast disease; but these are minor risk factors. By modifying the risk factors that she directly controls, she will, over the course of time, lessen her overall risk category and reduce her risk of developing cancer or cardiovascular disease.

The second example is Dave, a 24-year-old sexually active male homosexual who has many male partners and uses a drug called amyl nitrite (C). He smoked two packs of cigarettes a day for eleven years but quit one year ago (A). Up until a few months ago, he ate red meat daily, ate cheese daily, ate very few fiber-containing foods, and took no vitamins (A). His weight is normal (0), and he has never had cancer (0) nor have any of his family members (0). Until Dave was 21 years old, he lived in Alaska (0), but he has since lived in New York City.

Dave's total score is two A's, zero B's and one C. He is in the high-risk group, but by continuing not to smoke and by modifying his diet, he can dramatically lessen his overall risk.

Next is Nancy, a 27-year-old woman who smoked two packs of cigarettes a day until she quit eight years ago (B). She eats a well-balanced diet consisting of red meat five times a week, low-fat dairy products, and an average intake of fiber (B), and she is twenty pounds overweight (C). As a lifelong resident of Vermont (C), Nancy has been working in the furniture industry for the past seven years (B). She is taking birth control pills (B) and has been doing so for the past ten years. She is fair-skinned, sunburns easily, and enjoys sunbathing and using a suntanning booth year-round (B).

SELF-TEST

What is your risk of developing cancer? Take the following Cancer Risk Factor Assessment Test to determine your risk according to your diet, weight, age, lifestyle, and other factors discussed in this chapter. After you assess which factors pose a risk, you can begin to modify them according to my recommendations. Then take the test again to see if your overall risk has been reduced.

The test consists of a list of cancer risk factors, several statements associated with each risk factor, and a specified score associated with each statement. Choose the statement that most nearly applies to you and put a check mark in the blank. After going through the questionnaire, add up your scores. The zero scores won't count in the total.

Cancer Risk Factor Assessment Test

Risk Factor	Score

1. Nutrition

- If during 50% or more of your life two or more of the following apply to you:
  (1) one serving of red meat daily (including luncheon meat);
  (2) 6 eggs per week;
  (3) butter, milk, or cheese daily;
  (4) little or no fiber foods (3 gm or less daily);
  (5) frequent barbecued meats;
  (6) below-average intake of vitamins and minerals.　　Score A ___
- If during 50% or more of your life two or more of the following apply to you:
  (1) red meat 4–5 times per week (including luncheon meat);
  (2) 3–5 eggs per week;
  (3) margarine, low-fat dairy products, some cheese;
  (4) 4–15 gm of fiber daily;
  (5) average intake of vitamins and minerals.　　Score B ___
- If during 50% or more of your life two or more of the following apply to you:
  (1) red meat and 1 egg once a week or none at all;
  (2) poultry or fish daily or very frequently;
  (3) margarine, skim milk, and skim milk products;
  (4) 15–20 gm of fiber daily;
  (5) above-average intake of vitamins and minerals.　　Score 0 ___

2. Weight

Ideal weight for men is 110 lbs plus 5 lbs per inch over 5 ft. For women, ideal weight is 100 lbs plus 5 lbs per inch over 5 ft.

- If you are 25 lbs overweight.　　Score B ___
- If your are 10–24 lbs over.　　Score C ___
- If you are less than 10 lbs over.　　Score 0 ___

3. Tobacco

- Smoke 2 packs or more per day for 10 years or more.　　Score A ___
- Smoke 1–2 packs for 10 years or more, or quit smoking less than a year ago.　　Score A ___

- Smoke less than 1 pack for 10 years or more or smoke pipe or cigar.   Score B ___
- Smoked 1–2 packs per day, a pipe, or a cigar but stopped 7–14 years ago.   Score B ___
- Chew or snuff tobacco.   Score B ___
- Inhaled others' smoke for 1 or more hours/day up to age 25.   Score B ___
- Inhaled others' smoke for 1 or more hours/day from age 25 on.   Score C___
- Never smoked, quit smoking 15 years ago, or never inhaled others' smoke.   Score 0 ___

4. Alcohol

- If you drink 4 oz. or more of whiskey daily or equivalent alcohol content in other beverages.   Score B ___
- If you drink 2–4 drinks per week.   Score B___
- If you drink less than that indicated above.   Score 0 ___
- If you drink 4 oz. or more of whiskey daily or the equivalent alcohol content in other beverages and also:
  Smoke less than 1 pack per day, or chew or snuff tobacco   Score B ___
  Smoke 1–2 packs per day, pipe, or cigar.   Score A ___
  Smoke 2 or more packs per day.   Score A ___
- If you do not drink at all.   Score 0 ___

5. Hormonal

- If you started menstruating between ages 8 and 12.   Score C ___
- If you stopped menstruating at age 50 or older.   Score C ___
- If you never had menses at all.   Score C ___
- If your mother took DES (diethylstilbestrol) or if you took DES in your life or if you took estrogens postmenopausally.   Score C ___
- If you took oral contraceptives for 4 years or more before age 25, or 10 or more during your lifetime.   Score B ___
- If you had miscarriage or abortion in first trimester of first pregnancy.   Score C ___
- If you were first pregnant late in life (>35), or never at all, or had lumpy breast syndrome (Chapter 3).   Score C ___
- If your bra cup size is D or greater.   Score C ___
- If you don't routinely practice breast self-examination.   Score C ___

6. Breast Biopsy Report (Chapter 2, Table 2.1)

- If your biopsy report showed fibroadenoma, or papilloma, or sclerosing adenosis (well developed), or large cyst (and have first-degree relative [mother and grandmother] with breast cancer).   Score C ___
- If your biopsy report showed hyperplasia with atypia.   Score B ___
- If your biopsy report showed comedo or non-comedo carcinoma *in situ*.   Score A ___

7. Radiation Exposure
- If you received multiple X-rays or radiation treatments, or if you were exposed to radioactive isotopes used for diagnostic workups or radioactive weapons.   Score C ___
- If you are fair-skinned and sunburn easily.   Score B ___
- If neither applies.   Score 0 ___

8. Occupation
- If you are a radiologist, chemist, painter, uranium or hematite miner, luminous-dial painter, or a worker in the following industries: leather, foundry, printing, rubber, petroleum, furniture or cabinet, textile, nuclear, slaughterhouse, or plutonium. (The longer your exposure, the greater your risk.)   Score B ___
- Never was one of the above workers.   Score 0 ___

9. Chemicals
- If you have worked directly with one of the following chemicals: aniline, acrylonitrile, 4-aminobiphenyl, arsenic, asbestos, auramine manufacturing, benzene, benzidine, beryllium, cadmium, carbon tetrachloride, chlormethyl ether, chloroprene, chromate, isopropyl alcohol (acid process), nickel, mustard gas, or vinyl chloride. (The longer your exposure, the higher your risk.)   Score A ___
- If you have worked indirectly with one of the above chemicals.   Score C ___
- Never worked with one of the above.   Score 0 ___

10. Breast Implants
- If you have silicone breast implant(s).   Score C ___
- If not.   Score 0 ___

11. Sexual-social history
- If you are a female who started having sexual intercourse before age 16 and has had many male partners, particularly uncircumcised.   Score C ___
- If you are a sexually active male homosexual who has had many male partners and/or uses amyl nitrite.   Score C ___
- If neither applies.   Score 0 ___

12. Immunity, drugs, and hormones
- If your physician said you have a severe deficiency in your immune system, or you have received an organ transplant.   Score A ___
- If you've taken one or more of the following for a prolonged period of time: chlorambucil, cyclophosphamide, melphalan, or high-dose steroids (anticancer drugs).   Score A ___
- If you have taken one or more of the following for a prolonged period of time: phenacetin, thiotepa, or 17 methyl-substituted androgens.   Score B ___
- If none of the above apply.   Score 0 ___

13. **Geography**
   - Based on Figure 1.1 in Chapter 1, if during most of your life you lived in one of the states with the most cancer deaths.   Score B ___
   - If during most of your life you lived in a state that has a moderate number of cancer deaths.   Score C ___
   - If during most of your life you lived in a state with the least number of cancer deaths.   Score 0 ___
14. **Age**
   - If your age is 70 or more.   Score B ___
   - If your age is 55 to 69.   Score C ___
   - If your age is 55 or under.   Score 0 ___
15. **Personal history**
   - If you had cancer.   Score B ___
   - If you never had cancer.   Score 0 ___
16. **Family history**
   - If one or more close family members (parents, grand-parents) had cancer.   Score B ___
   - No family history of cancer.   Score 0 ___
17. **Exercise**
   - If you exercise very little or not at all.   Score C ___
   - If you exercise 3 or more times a week and get your heart rate 50% higher than normal for at least 20 min.   Score 0 ___
18. **Stress**
   - If you are frustrated waiting in line, easily angered, and unable to control stress.   Score C ___
   - If you are comfortable when waiting, easygoing, and able to control stress.   Score 0 ___

TOTAL SCORE: ___ A's; ___ B's; and ___ C's.

To evaluate your score, see page 40.

On the surface of things it looks as though Nancy's overall risk is not so bad, but when you examine the whole picture, you find she is in the moderate-risk category. Her total score is five B's and two C's. However, she is on the right track. She should do the following to modify her risk factors and thereby reduce her overall risk: continue not to smoke, lose twenty pounds, modify her nutritional status, seek another means of birth control, use sun screens when sunbathing, and avoid suntanning booths.

The last example is Bob, a 50-year-old (0) male chemist (B) who is twenty-five pounds overweight (B) and a meat-and-potatoes man all the way (A). He has smoked two packs of cigarettes a day for the past thirty years (A), drinks four ounces of whiskey every day (A), has lived in Illinois most of his life (B), and is easily angered (C). His father died of lung cancer (B).

You know that Bob is in the high-risk category: three A's, four B's, and one C. As you can see, he does have risk factors that he can directly control. He should do the following: stop smoking, drastically modify his diet and lose weight, consume alcohol in moderation, and learn how to relax. All these modifications will greatly reduce his overall risk.

What can *you* do to reduce *your* risk for cancer? You have now identified the problem areas that need modification. Simple preventive measures can be taken to help you reduce your chances of developing cancer or cardiovascular disease. This book will show you how you can make relatively minor adjustments in your lifestyle to lessen your risk. In the following chapters, I will review nutritional risk factors and other risk factors that can lead to the development of breast cancer. I will also tell you how the risk factors can be modified. Maintaining a good weight, eating a healthful diet (one that is low in animal fat, low in cholesterol, and high in fiber), choosing not to smoke or drink alcoholic beverages, avoiding or limiting exposure to the sun—all of these are just a few of the ways you can protect yourself from cancer. You must strive to maintain good health. Good health is no accident.

PART TWO

The Body's Defenses

4
Nutrition, Immunity, and Cancer

Nutrition affects immunity[1,2] and also affects the development of cancer[3,4] either directly or indirectly via the immune system. The immune system is a complex interaction of blood cells, proteins, and processes that protects you from infections, foreign substances, and cancer cells that spontaneously develop in the body.

White blood cells and antibodies are two major armies of the immune system. These armies arise separately but are related and dependent upon each other for their development and maturity. The lymphocyte, a specific type of white blood cell, is the main cell involved in cellular immunity. Lymphocytes make up only a small portion of the blood, comprising only about 15 to 45 percent of all white cells. The lymphocyte population is divided into two large groups, based on particular markings on the outer surface membrane of the cell.

T lymphocytes, or T cells, are one group of lymphocytes. They are derived from or are under the influence of the *t*hymus, which is an organ in the neck and front part of the chest that is functionally active in early childhood. T cells are responsible for your defense against cancer, fungi, certain bacteria (intracellular), some viruses, transplant rejections, and delayed skin reactions (tuberculosis skin test). T cells are further divided into several subpopulations: helper T cells and suppressor T cells, those which either help or hinder normal immune cellular function.

Proteins called antibodies or immunoglobulins are produced by the other major group of lymphocytes, the B lymphocytes, or B cells. B cells may have their origin in the *bone* marrow, from which they derive their designation. Antibodies are formed by the B cells in response to a foreign substance introduced into the body. White blood cells that kill, or complement proteins, when activated by an antibody, destroy a foreign-appearing cell by making holes in the foreign cell's membrane, thereby allowing water to rush in and explode the cell. In 1980, I showed how a white blood cell kills a foreign cancerlike cell. Figure 4.1 shows a white blood cell (center) killing several cancerlike cells. Notice that the white blood cell extends feetlike processes that aid in killing the targets.[5]

Phagocytes are another group of white blood cells that reside in the blood and body tissues and are part of your defenses against foreign invaders. These also act as policemen to recognize and dispose of abnormal cancer cells and other foreign substances. Phagocytes can perform this task alone or can recruit antibodies and complement proteins to aid in the disposal.

IMMUNOLOGY AND CANCER

The immune system is extremely intricate and finely tuned. If any one aspect of the system malfunctions because of poor nutrition, or if it is destroyed, you may become susceptible to cancer and foreign microbial invaders. The white blood cell army and the antibody army must be functioning perfectly to destroy any cancer cell or foreign invader and prevent either one from gaining a foothold in your body.

The major histocompatibility complex is part of your genetic makeup and is another component of the immune system, acting as a commander of the white blood cell and antibody armies. This complex allows the immune system to recognize the parts of your body so that it does not destroy them as it would destroy foreign substances. At the same time, it can recognize a substance or tissue (histo-) that does not belong to its body and subsequently take the necessary steps to destroy it.

In 1970, F.M. Burnet introduced the concept of immunosurveillance, which states that killer cells of the immune system watch, or keep a surveillance on, all cells in the body and immediately destroy any cells that start to have a malignant or cancerous potential.[6] There is a lot of evidence to support this concept. The most clear-cut and convincing evidence comes from observations of patients with suppressed immune systems caused by drugs or radiation or an inherited disorder. Patients with inherited immunodeficiencies, whose immune systems do not function normally from birth, or patients whose immune systems ac-

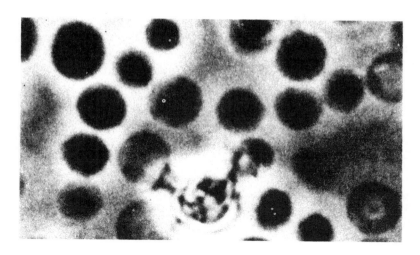

Figure 4.1 White blood cell (center) killing several cancerlike cells. Notice that the white blood cell extends feetlike processes which aid in killing the targets.

quire a malfunction later in life have one hundred times more deaths due to cancer than the expected cancer death rate in the normal population.[7,8] Kidney transplant patients, who receive drugs to suppress the immune system's ability to reject the new kidney, also have a higher rate of cancer than expected.[9,10] The cancers most frequently seen in these cases are the lymphomas and epithelial cancers; however, all other types of cancers have been reported.

The immune system is relatively immature in infancy, and then runs down and does not function well in old age. These two times of life have the highest incidence of lymphocytic leukemia. Other immune-deficiency states that can lead to cancer are seen with malaria, acute viral infections, and malnutrition.

NUTRITION AND THE IMMUNE SYSTEM

Nutritional deficiencies decrease a person's capacity to resist infection and its consequences, and decrease the capability of the immune system.[11] In old age, there is a decrease in skin hypersensitivity reactions,[12-14] a decreased number of T cells,[15,16] and impairment of some phagocytic functions. Surveys of the population have discovered nutritional deficiencies in senior citizens that also lead to impairment of the immune system.[17] It is possible that the gradual impairment of the immune system associated with aging may, in fact, be due to one or more nutrient deficiencies. Poor nutrition adversely affects all components of the immune system, including T cell function, other cellular-related killing, the ability of B cells to make antibodies, the functioning of the complement proteins, and phagocytic function. When several of these functions or processes are impaired, the ability of the entire immune system to keep a watchful eye for cancer cells, abnormal cells, or foreign substances and to dispose of them is also markedly impaired. Table 4.1 summarizes the factors that affect the functioning of the immune system.

Protein deficiency affects all the organs in the body. The number of digestive enzymes produced is reduced, and absorption of nutrients is impaired. With severe chronic protein deficiency, the heart muscle atrophies. The immune system is also severely affected. In diets that are only moderately deficient in protein, phagocytes and T cells are reduced in number,[18] and their ability to kill cancer and other abnormal cells is impaired.[19] The amount of antibody is slightly reduced as is the speed with which it attaches to an "enemy."[20] The complement proteins also have impaired function in this state. Hence, a person who is not consuming the proper amount of protein will have a malfunctioning immune system that will not be able to deal effectively with cancer cells or infection.

The immune system is affected by both hypoglycemia (low blood sugar) and hyperglycemia, as in diabetes mellitus. Phagocytic function in humans is impaired if the blood sugar level is very low.[21] Much more research has been done concerning the function of the immune system in diabetes. The number of T and B cells is normal in diabetes, but their functions are impaired: phagocytic function as well as cellular killing.[22,23] The degree of impairment correlates very well with the fasting blood sugar level and then improves when the sugar level becomes normal.

Lipids have a significant effect on the functioning of the immune system. Cholesterol oleate and ethyl palmitate inhibit antibody production.[24] The ability of the T cell to function is impaired if you eat a high-fat diet.[25] In a number of experiments, another saturated fat, methyl palmitate, was found to markedly impair phagocytosis for at least seventy-two hours after a single injection.[26]

The Epstein-Barr virus may manifest itself as entirely different diseases in different people as a result of varying degrees of impairment of the immune system. The extent to which the immune system is weakened or damaged is partly determined by the nutritional status of the individual prior to infection. Epstein-Barr virus is implicated in a relatively benign disease, infectious mononucleosis; a slow-growing cancer, nasopharyngeal cancer; and a rapidly growing, usually fatal cancer, Burkitt's lymphoma; as well as other diseases. Why does one person's immune system permit infectious mononucleosis

Table 4.1 Factors That Influence the Immune System

Enhance	Suppress
Nutrition	Nutrition
Low-fat, high fiber diet	High-fat food
Antioxidants	High sugar level
Beta-carotene, vitamins E & C,	Obesity
selenium, cysteine, flavonoids,	Soy and corn oil
copper, zinc	Tobacco smoke
B vitamins, pantothenic acid	Alcohol
Calcium	Radiation
Exercise	Heavy metals: lead, cadmium,
Stress modified, loving	mercury
Clean air and pure water	Certain drugs
	Environmental pollutants
	Ozone depletion[27,28,29,30]
	Stress
	Sedentary lifestyle
	Exhaustive exercise[31,32]

to develop and another person's immune system permit a fatal cancer to develop? The answer is very complex and not well defined at all, but nutritional status is a factor.

Your *nutritional status* is determined by how well your diet and supplementation program is meeting your nutritional needs. The better your nutritional status, the better your immune system, and the better off you will be.

5
Antioxidants and Other Cancer-Fighting Nutrients

Living cells contain proteins, nucleic acids, carbohydrates, lipids, and certain organic substances that function in very small amounts, called vitamins. Vitamins are essential to life and play a crucial role as helper enzymes in important chemical functions of the body. They are also needed for normal prenatal development. Vitamins are of great interest because of their interplay among all organ systems of the body, especially the immune system. If there are deficiencies of vitamins, a variety of diseases may occur, and the immune system will not function properly.

Vitamins interact with each other, and some can be stored for long periods of time, while others have to be supplied on a daily basis. We now know that certain drugs and hormones can produce a gradual vitamin deficiency by interfering with the ways in which vitamins are broken down for use in the body.

It is more difficult to identify a person who is only marginally deficient in vitamins than someone who is obviously deficient. Whereas a person who is grossly deficient in vitamins demonstrates many physical problems and complains about specific symptoms related to the deficiencies, a person with only marginal deficiencies demonstrates no such signs or symptoms and does not appear to be ill. RDAs (Recommended Dietary Allowances) were designed by the National Academy of Sciences for healthy people, and the values recommended may not be adequate for persons developing undetected marginal deficiencies.

Do you consider your diet to be well balanced? Do you think it is meeting your nutritional needs? Although you may believe it is fulfilling your requirements, you will most likely find that your diet is deficient in at least one nutrient. Consider the following sections.

MARGINAL DEFICIENCIES

Marginal deficiencies of micronutrients produce no frank symptoms of deficiency diseases; however, they do affect your mental acuity, your ability to cope with stress, and your body's ability to resist disease and infection and to recover from surgery. Proper wound healing requires adequate amounts of vitamins C, A, D, and K, the B-complex vitamins, and the minerals zinc, iron, and copper.[19]

Marginal deficiency is defined as a state of gradual vitamin depletion in which there is evidence of personal lack of well-being associated with impairment of certain biochemical reactions.[1,2] There are several lines of evidence that a large number of people suffer from marginal deficiencies: biochemically measured data[3–12] and data from dietary assessment studies.[13–18] Almost 50 percent of all people examined and surveyed, whether rich or poor, educated or not, had at least one, and usually two or three marginal nutrient deficiencies. With the recent discovery of a viral etiology for two human cancers (T-cell leukemia and T-cell lymphoma) and AIDS, marginal deficiencies take on an added significance.

LIFESTYLE AND EATING PATTERNS

Lifestyle and eating patterns can lead to nutrient deficiencies. Homemakers are now in the work force,[20] which leads to an increased demand for convenience foods and fast-foods. Eating patterns have also changed. About 25 percent of Americans skip breakfast,[21] 25 percent skip lunch,[22,23] almost 50 percent snack,[24] and most eat one meal a day away from home.[25]

In the federally sponsored HANES II study, people were asked to choose a food that they liked and considered "balanced." For a "balanced" vegetable, the majority chose French fries over broccoli; for meat/legume, hot dogs over split peas; and for grain, white bread over whole wheat. In the same study, favorite foods included coffee, doughnuts, soft drinks, and hamburgers. The percentage of calories in the American diet derived from fat is 42; from sugar, 24.

To eat well, you really have to take the time and have the knowledge to plan proper meals. When caloric intakes fall below 1,600 calories, there is no guarantee that all nutritional guidelines can be met.[26] And below 1,800 per day, which about 50 percent of the population consumes, trained nutritionists have trouble designing meals to provide the minimum RDA.[27] According to the 1985 Nationwide Food Consumption Survey, significant percentages of the population were consuming less than 70 percent of the RDA for the nutrients listed in Table 5.1.[28] These data demonstrate that today's eating patterns and preferences do not afford people a "well-balanced diet."

Outright vitamin deficiencies occur in two groups of people. In the first group, an individual is unable to buy the right kinds of food either because of the expense or because he is not knowledgeable about the proper foods. It is estimated that 25 percent of United States households do not have nutritionally balanced diets because people do not know what foods to buy or because vitamins and minerals are lost through cooking. The second group consists of people whose nutrient deficiency occurs as the result of a specific disease or a drug or other treatment therapy.

The results of a study on the incidence of low blood levels of vitamins in a randomly selected group of hospitalized patients are listed in Table 5.2.[29] Sixty-one percent of the total group of 120 patients were eating what is considered to be a normal American diet!

Americans continue to eat foods that are sprayed with chemicals, refined, processed, frozen, canned, stored, and trucked around the country. Many of our meats contain the hormones and chemicals that have been fed to animals. All of these foods have been depleted of nutrients to varying degrees. Some methods of cooking can totally destroy nutrients or decrease their concentration as well, and some nutrients are not stable in heat or boiling water. As a result, Americans do not or cannot eat a healthful balanced diet.

Table 5.1   America's Poor Nutrient Intake

Nutrient	Percentage of Individuals Deficient*
Vitamin B6	51%
Calcium	42%
Magnesium	39%
Iron	32%
Vitamin A	31%
Vitamin C	26%
Thiamine	17%
Vitamin B12	15%
Riboflavin	12%

* Deficiency = Intake less than 70% of RDA.

Table 5.2 Vitamin Deficiencies in Hospitalized Patients

Vitamin	Percentage of Individuals Deficient
Folic acid	45%
Thiamine (B2)	31%
Nicotinic acid	29%
Pyridoxine (B6)	27%
Pantothenic acid	15%
Vitamin A	13%
Vitamin E	12%
Riboflavin (B2)	12%
Vitamin C	12%
Vitamin B12	10%
Biotin	1%
Multiple Vitamin Deficiencies	
Two deficiencies	38%
Three deficiencies	14%
Four deficiencies	6%
Five deficiencies	10%

The average American consumes about 60 pounds of sugar each year and four to five times the amount of salt necessary, favors carbonated drinks to others when not consuming 2.6 gallons of alcoholic beverages each year (if of drinking age), and usually gets about one-third of his total calories from sources of little or no nutrient value.

In short, it is very difficult to find an individual who consistently, on a daily basis, eats a "well-balanced diet"—that is, one containing foods that are freshly prepared, varied, and nutritionally adequate.

GROUPS AT RISK FOR NUTRIENT DEFICIENCIES

There are several segments of our population that may not be "healthy" and that may be considered to be "at risk" for inadequate nutrient intake. The RDAs do not take into account the special needs of these people. The greater requirements of the groups listed in Table 5.3 need to be recognized and addressed.

STUDIES OF ANTIOXIDANTS' EFFECTS ON CANCER

Antioxidants protect normal cells and other tissues by fighting or neutralizing free radicals (see Chapter 7) and the oxidative reaction that is caused by free radicals. Antioxidant nutrients include beta-carotene, vitamin C, vitamin E, selenium, copper, zinc, bioflavonoids, and cysteine. There is a growing body of evidence that suggests

Table 5.3   United States Candidates for Nutrient Supplementation

Risk Group	Million	Nutrient Deficiencies
Alcohol Drinkers (3+ drinks/week)	90	Beta-carotene, vitamins A, B6, D, folate, thiamine[30-44]
People With Allergies/ Food Intolerance	80	Any or all
Cigarette Smokers	50	Beta-carotene, vitamins C, E, B6, folate[45-53]
Dieters	45	Any or all[54-58]
Hospitalized Patients	36	Any or all
People With Infectious Diseases	5	Any or all
Osteoporosis Patients	34	Calcium, vitamin D, others
People With Chronic Diseases	31	Any or all[59-66]
Elderly Patients	25	Folate, vitamins C and D[67-77]
Surgical Patients	23.5	Any or all
Oral Contraceptive Users	18	Beta-carotene, folate, vitamin B6[94-99]
Teenagers	17	Vitamin A, folate[78-81]
Stressed People	*	B vitamins, any or all
Athletes/Exercisers	*	B vitamins, or any
Consumers of High-Fat Foods	*	Any
Diabetics	11	Vitamins C, D, B6, magnesium[82,83]
Pregnant Women	7	All[84,85]
Strict Vegetarians	1	Vitamins B12 and D
Low Income People	*	Vitamin C, thiamine, riboflavin, niacin, iron, vitamin A[92, 93]
Premature Infants/Toddlers	*	Vitamins A, C, E, iron[86-91]
Children With Low IQs	*	Any and all[100-111]
Psychiatric Patients	*	Any and all[112]

*Unknown millions.

antioxidants keep us free of disease by protecting our tissues from the ravages of free radicals.

In a prospective study, over 11,600 residents between the ages of 65 and 84 in a California retirement community completed a diet questionnaire and answered questions on the use of vitamin supplements.[113] During 8 years of follow-up, 1,335 of these people were diagnosed as having cancer. The women who had higher dietary intakes of vitamin C, vegetables and fruits or fruits alone, showed a lower risk for developing cancer at all sites and specifically colon cancer. Supplements of beta-carotene and vitamin A as well as vitamin C and E were associated with a lower risk of getting lung cancer. Vitamins A and C were also shown to be protective against colon cancer. In men, however, there was no protective effect of dietary factors; however, bladder cancer risk was reduced in those who took vitamin C supplements. Although this is an interesting study, this like all other dietary assessment studies has a problem with patient recall.

In another study conducted by the National Cancer Institute, vitamin E supplementation had a protective effect against oral cancer cases. Supplements containing vitamin C and D protected against esophageal cancer in smokers. Vitamin E together with vegetable consumption protected against oral cancer cases, and vitamin C combined with vegetable and fruit consumption protected against esophageal cancer cases.[114]

Linxian, China Study

In north central China in the county of Linxian, which is in the Henan Province, are people who have the world's highest rates of esophageal cancer and a high rate of not only esophageal cancer but also stomach cancer. The people of Linxian also have a very high rate of marginal nutritional deficiencies. In Linxian, esophageal cancer deaths are one hundred times higher than the rate for Caucasian Americans and ten times higher than the rate for China in general. Since poor nutrition is linked to these two cancers and since marginal deficiencies are very common in the people of Linxian, an intervention trial was conducted.

Researchers from the Cancer Institute of the Chinese Academy of Medical Sciences teamed up with researchers at the United States National Cancer Institute and studied almost 30,000 adults, randomizing them over a five-year period into four different groups. This study is one of the most important studies because it purposely divided the population and randomized them to receive the antioxidants as we have discussed or other vitamins and minerals in the other three groups. Group one received 5,000 IU of vitamin A per day as well as 22.5 mg of zinc per day. Group two received 3.2 mg of riboflavin and 40 mg of niacin per day. Group three received 120 mg of vitamin C and 30 micrograms of molybdenum. And the last group received 15 mg of beta-carotene, 60 IU of vitamin E, and 50 micrograms of selenium (yeast) on a daily basis. The group of people who took the antioxidants containing beta-carotene, vitamin E, and selenium on a daily basis did the best statistically. They had a 9 percent reduction in all deaths, a 13 percent reduction in all cancer deaths, and finally a 21 percent reduction in stomach cancer deaths. This group also had a lower rate of deaths from strokes than did the other groups.

The curious thing is that it took a couple of years before any effect was seen for mortality rates for cancer. This was a progressive benefit strongly suggestive of a causal relationship and was seen only for the group of antioxidants including beta-carotene, vitamin E, and selenium and none of the other nutritional nutrients given in the study. The doses used in the study are relatively low; I recommend much higher doses. Five years is a very short time; imagine what the results would be in a population taking these antioxidant nutrients as well as other nutrients in higher doses, and over a lifetime.

In another study undertaken in China, similar results were found. High cancer death rates were seen in people who had low plasma levels of beta-carotene, vitamin C, and selenium. In this study, vitamin C appeared to confer the most protection. Selenium showed strong protection against cancers of the stomach and esophagus while beta-carotene was found to have the most protective effect, especially for stomach cancer, independent of vitamin A. In this study, one hundred randomly selected adult residents of sixty-five different counties of China were involved.[115]

To summarize:

- First large-scale intervention trial in a prospective randomized fashion demonstrated that three antioxidant nutrients together—beta-carotene, vitamin E, and selenium—significantly reduced total mortality (9 percent) especially from all cancers (13 percent) and particularly stomach cancer (21 percent).[116,117]
- These antioxidant nutrients also prevented the risk of cancer in humans.
- These antioxidant nutrients substantially reduced the prevalence of cataracts in the oldest patients (aged 65–74 years).
- Antioxidant nutrients of beta-carotene, vitamin E, and selenium also reduced the mortality from stroke in this study.

Finland Study

Between the years 1966 and 1972, over 4,500 men in Finland were examined and extensive histories of their dietary and smoking habits were taken.[118] Their dietary intakes of beta-carotene, vitamin E, vitamin C, and selenium and other retinoids including vitamin A were calculated based on their dietary history. For the next twenty years, these men were followed, examined, and monitored. Lung cancer developed in 117 of them.

The nonsmokers who had low intakes of carotenes, vitamin E, and vitamin C had high risk of developing lung cancer. Those who had the least intake of these antioxidant nutrients were twice as likely to develop lung cancer. Although no protective effects of these antioxidant nutrients were seen in the smoking population, the researchers point out that these antioxidants in the foods in Finland are generally low, and probably too low to protect against lung cancer in heavy smokers. The amount of selenium in the food of Finland also is quite low and subsequently showed no effect in these men. Hence, the antioxidant nutrients together are protective against lung cancer in nonsmokers in this particular study.

Switzerland Study

Serum levels of vitamins A, C, and E as well as beta-carotene were measured in almost 3,000 men between the years 1973 and 1985 in Basel, Switzerland.[119] At the end of the study, 204 men had died of cancer, including 68 with lung cancer, 20 with stomach cancer, and 17 with colon cancer.

Swiss men who had low levels of beta-carotene and vitamin C had a higher risk of dying from cancer. Lung and stomach cancer were more commonly seen among men who had low carotene levels, and more stomach cancers occurred in men who had low vitamin C levels. Men who had low levels of both vitamin A and beta-carotene had an increased risk of all types of cancers. The results of this study are quite meaningful because the levels of the nutrients in the blood were assayed the same day that the blood was obtained rather than freezing the blood for months or years as with most studies.

The conclusion is that there is an increased risk of death from cancer in men who have low serum levels of antioxidant nutrients. Beta-carotene, and vitamin C, and probably even vitamin A afford protection.

Hawaiian Study[120]

University of Hawaii investigators studied 230 men and 102 women with lung cancer and 597 men and 268 women with no obvious cancer.[120] The diet history was obtained and the various carotenoids were determined by assessing the amounts in the foods eaten.

There are many carotenoids found in vegetables and fruits. The one most discussed is beta-carotene. However, there are several others including alpha-carotene, lutein, zeaxanthin, lycopene, and beta-cryptoxanthin. Table 5.4 indicates the carotenoid and its source.

Beta-carotene, alpha-carotene, and lutein all conferred protection

Table 5.4 Various Carotenoids in Foods

Carotenoids	Food
Alpha-carotene	Carrots
Beta-carotene	Carrots, cantaloupe, broccoli
Beta-cryptoxanthin	Oranges, orange juice, tangerines
Lycopene	Tomatoes, tomato products
Leutein, Zeaxanthin	Collard, mustard, turnip greens, spinach, broccoli

against lung cancer. Lycopene and beta-cryptoxanthin showed no such protective effects. It was found that beta-carotene conferred the most protection.

Endometrial Cancer Study

Endometrial cancer occurs mainly in older women who are obese. High-fat food increases the risk for this tumor, and antioxidants help protect against it.[121] Patients from Japan and Finland were studied. These countries have very different intakes of dietary fat, Japan's being much lower than Finland's. Japanese and Finnish patients who had endometrial cancer and Japanese and Finnish women who did not have endometrial cancer but were simply undergoing routine hysterectomy for other reasons all had tissue samples evaluated for antioxidants. The activity of the antioxidant enzymes superoxide dismutase was found to be significantly lower in patients who had cancer of the endometrium compared to patients undergoing hysterectomy without cancer. Another important antioxidant enzyme called glutathione S-transferase was also found to be much lower in the cancer tissue compared to the normal tissue. Hence, tissue from endometrial cancer has impaired enzymatic antioxidants and, therefore, this defense system is not operational.

Cervical Cancer Studies

Many studies have shown that low blood levels of carotenoids are linked to increased risk of cervical cancer. In one instance, the level of beta-carotene was measured in cervical cells and blood samples in 105 women in New York City. Patients who had cervical cancer or cervical dysplasia had significantly lower levels of beta-carotene than women who had normal cervices.[122]

Breast Cancer Study

The Nurses Health Study published in 1992 involved 89,494 women.

Dietary intake of vitamins C, E, and A was assessed over a five-year period. A low intake of vitamin A was shown to increase the risk for developing breast cancer.[123] These women's ability to recall their diets was found to be very inaccurate. This may be one major reason why there was no recorded protective effect of vitamins C or E in this study. However, in the same group of women, vitamin E supplementation did, in fact, show protection against developing cardiovascular disease.[124]

Small Cell Lung Cancer Study

In addition to receiving conventional therapy for small cell lung cancer, eighteen patients also received antioxidant vitamins, trace elements, and fatty acids. It was found that antioxidant treatment combined with chemotherapy and radiation therapy prolongs the survival time of patients with small cell lung cancer compared to most published combination treatment regimens. The patients receiving the antioxidants were able to tolerate chemotherapy and radiation therapy better. And when antioxidant treatment was started earlier, survival was longer.[125]

Oral And Pharyngeal Cancer Study

In a population-based case control study, patients were asked about the use of vitamin and mineral supplements. People who used supplements containing individual nutrients like vitamin A, B complex, vitamin C, vitamin E were found to be at much lower risk for oral and pharyngeal cancer after controlling for the effects of tobacco, alcohol, and other risk factors for these cancers. And it was found that vitamin E had the most protective effect in combination with the others.[126]

Another study showed people with high levels of carotenoids including beta-carotene, alpha-carotene, cryptoxanthin, leutin, and lyocopine—but particularly beta-carotene—had a much lower rate of getting oral cancer than the control population. High blood levels of vitamin E and beta-carotene together provided the most protection against getting oral cancer.[127]

STUDIES OF PRE-CANCEROUS CONDITIONS

Linxian, China, Esophageal Dysplasia Study[128]

Esophageal dysplasia is a precursor to developing esophageal cancer. Over 3,300 patients in Linxian, China, with signs of esophageal dysplasia were studied by the same team of researchers from China and the United States as was described in the Linxian trial for cancer (see

**Table 5.5 Multivitamin/Mineral Supplementation
in the Dysplasia Trial[129]**

Beta-carotene (15 mg)	Calcium (324 mg)
Vitamin A (10,000 IU)	Phosphorus (250 mg)
Vitamin E (60 IU)	Iodine (300 ug)
Vitamin C (180 mg)	Iron (54 mg)
Folic acid (800 ug)	Magnesium (200 mg)
Thiamin (5 mg)	Copper (6 mg)
Riboflavin (5.2 mg)	Manganese (15 mg)
Niacinamide (40 mg)	Potassium (15.4 mg)
Vitamin B6 (6 mg)	Chloride (14 mg)
Vitamin B12 (18 ug)	Chromium (30 ug)
Vitamin D (800 IU)	Molybdenum (30 ug)
Biotin (90 ug)	Selenium (50 ug)
Pantothenic Acid (20 mg)	Zinc (45 mg)

page 59). This also was an intervention study. One group received a placebo and the other group received a multiple vitamin-mineral supplement, as listed in Table 5.5, daily for six years. The supplement contained doses of vitamins and minerals that were generally two to three times higher than the U.S. Recommended Dietary Allowance.

The group that took the supplement on a daily basis for six years had an 8 percent lower mortality rate from esophageal and upper stomach cancers. It had an overall 7 percent lower mortality rate than the other group and 4 percent lower rate of death from cancer in any site.

The duration of the trial was very short, six years. And the doses of the nutrients were far too low as compared to other trials that used 30 to 90 mg doses of beta-carotene.[130,131] Also, the dose of vitamin E was extremely low at 60 IU compared to a study that used 800 IU a day and demonstrated that patients with precancerous oral lesions responded extremely well.[132,133] The limitations of this study aside, it was found that patients who did take the supplement had a 38 percent lower risk of dying from stroke than those who took the placebo. This is similar to the findings seen in the general population of the Linxian people who had taken the combined antioxidants of beta-carotene, vitamin E, and selenium together.

Colorectal Adenomas

The abnormal growth of the mucosal lining of the colon and rectum that results in a polyp or adenoma dramatically increases the risk of a cancer. Most cancers of the large bowel are thought to arise from adenomas. Twenty patients with colorectal adenomas[134] were given vitamins A, C, and E for six months after complete polypectomy, and

Antioxidants and Disease

Recent research indicates that a host of illnesses may be caused by the action of free radicals (see Table 7.1 on page 95). It is, therefore, crucial that we be aware of the protection offered by antioxidants.

Antioxidants prevent cell damage that may lead to **cancer** *(see pages 94–96). In addition, many studies show that multiple antioxidants combined or by themselves in supplemental form (not from food intake) can confer protection against the development of* **cardiovascular disease**. *In these studies, tens of thousands of people have been investigated, measuring serum levels of antioxidants including vitamin E, vitamin C, carotene, selenium. All studies show the same findings: protection against cardiovascular disease and protection of low density lipo-protein[135–137] which is the LDL cholesterol or, as I term it, "lousy cholesterol."[138–158] It has even been shown that antioxidants are depleted during aortic coronary artery surgery, which results from the oxidative stress of clamping the aorta.[159] Antioxidants, especially vitamin C, have been shown to lower blood pressure,[161] and antioxidants, especially vitamin E, can protect against angina.[162]*

Many studies show that free radicals play a major role in the development of **cataracts** *and that antioxidant nutrients can counteract this problem. A substantial reduction in the risk of developing nuclear cataracts was another major finding of the Linxian, Chinese, intervention trial using antioxidant and nutrient supplementation. The antioxidants produced 44 percent reduction and the combination of riboflavin with niacin produced a 36 percent reduction. And although riboflavin is not an antioxidant nutrient, it is vital for optimum functioning of the body's antioxidant defenses including certain enzymes that are antioxidants. Similar findings were noted in both the cancer and esophageal dysplasia study in Linxian.[163] Other studies, including the Nurses Health Study,[164] five other United States studies,[165–169] another major study from Canada,[170] and a large study from Finland[171] all show similar findings: A high intake of antioxidants exerts a protective effect against the development of cataract formation. And people with low levels of these antioxidants like beta-carotene, vitamin E, vitamin C, and selenium have a high risk for developing cataracts. It was found that smokers have a twofold risk for developing cataracts.*

Macular degeneration, which causes blindness as a result of the degeneration of the retina, is commonly seen in elderly people. Almost 30 percent of the United States population over the age of 65 has some degree of macular degeneration. Evidence shows that free radicals cause this problem.

In patients who had the neovascular form of the degeneration, i.e., new blood vessel formation that destroys the retina (also known as "wet"), low levels of vitamin C, E, selenium, and five carotenoids were implicated in very high risk of disease progression. Results of studies involving 1,332 patients and from animal and other laboratory studies, cross-sectional studies, and case-control studies, as well as one small randomized clinical trial—a total of sixteen studies—all suggest that multiple antioxidants beta-carotene, vitamin E, and vitamin C are beneficial for macular degeneration.[174]

The first clue that antioxidants were involved in **neurological abnormalities** came from children with fat malabsorption syndrome who consequently could not absorb vitamin E. These children exhibit balance and gait disorders and may lose the ability to walk. When given enough vitamin E, all their abnormal neurological functions disappear. Patients with the following disorders have also had improvement upon use of antioxidant nutrients:

Tardive Dyskinesia[175-177]   Parkinson's Disease[181-183]
Epilepsy[178]   Lou Gehrig's Disease[184]
Alzheimer's Disease[179-180]

Patients who have **arthritis** and **inflammatory joint disease** from it have a very low level of vitamin E in the joint synovial fluid. It is suggested that vitamin E and/or other antioxidants may in fact protect the tissues of the joints from the damaging effects of free radicals associated with arthritis.[185]

Many studies are being done on the role of antioxidants in disease. If you or someone you care about is at risk for any of the conditions mentioned here, you should certainly refer to the studies cited.

twenty-one patients with adenomas received placebo. From each patient, six biopsy specimens were taken from apparently normal rectal mucosa before treatment and three and six months after treatment. These specimens were then sent to a laboratory for analysis of cell proliferation (growth of cells). Patients who received the antioxidants and vitamin A had decreased proliferation of cells in the specimens, which means that while on the nutrients they are less likely to develop future adenomas compared to the other group.

INDIVIDUAL ANTIOXIDANTS

Many nutrients have been identified as antioxidants. You should be aware of the beneficial effects, recommended doses, and possibility of toxicity of:

Beta-carotene

- Moderate intake leads to low incidence of cancer, heart disease.
- Greatly enhances immune system.[186]
- Most powerful antioxidant of free radicals and singlet oxygen.
- Toxicity: None in any amount.[187]
- Simone recommended dose: 20–30 mg/day.

Vitamin E

There is a very narrow but equal space between polyunsaturated fat molecules. One vitamin E molecule just fits snugly between them. This location and closeness to the polyunsaturated fats is extremely important. Vitamin E competes with the polyunsaturated fat for free radicals that are formed when polyunsaturated fats react with oxygen. This means that if there are more vitamin E molecules than polyunsaturated fat molecules, the radicals will be taken out of the system and neutralized by vitamin E. The more polyunsaturated fats you eat, the more vitamin E you will require. On the other hand, if the number of vitamin E molecules is low, then the radicals that are formed will not be neutralized and will proceed to cause membrane damage. Vitamin E also destroys hydroperoxides and, therefore, prevents more radical formation.

- Potent antioxidant, scavenger of damaging free radicals that produce cancer.
- Inhibits cancer.[188]
- As an antioxidant, it protects you from the cancer-inducing effects of smog.[189]
- It protects the body against the oxidation of polyunsaturated fatty acids.
- 85 percent of women with fibrocystic disease who took 600 IU of vitamin E daily for eight weeks experienced relief of the pain

associated with their disease, and some of these women had demonstrable regression of disease.[190] The women whose disease did not respond had lower vitamin E levels when checked, suggesting poor vitamin E absorption.

- Vitamin E reduces LDL levels (lipids involved in atherosclerosis) and increases HDL levels (lipids that protect against atherosclerosis).
- Supplementing with 600–1,200 IU of vitamin E daily may help prevent diabetic complications.[191]
- Toxicity: There is no case on record of vitamin E toxicity nor any indication of vitamin E toxicity. A daily intake of 800 IU of vitamin E per 2.2 pounds of body weight for five months has not been toxic. This amounts to 56,000 IU (56,000 milligrams) for an average man weighing 140 pounds, or about 5,600 times the RDA. A good dose of vitamin E seems to be 400 to 600 IU (400 to 600 milligrams) daily.

As ridiculous as it may sound, some people, including some physicians, *believe* that vitamin E causes cancer. They reason that since the molecule of vitamin E looks similar to estrogen, it can cause breast cancer. This is absolutely absurd! There are hundreds of molecules in the body that are formed from the same basic cholesterol ring structure. The body is able to discriminate one molecule from another even if there is only a slight difference between their structures. For instance, what differentiates men from women is a mere methyl group, CH3, on a cholesterol-steroid chemical compound. Obviously, Mother Nature has this under control.

Vitamin E is safe and has never been shown to cause cancer or changes in the DNA or RNA, nor has it ever been shown to cause changes in fetal development—even at very high doses of 3,200 IU.[192–194]

- Simone recommended dose: 400–1600 IU/day.

Vitamin C

Vitamin C is a major factor in controlling and potentiating multiple aspects of human resistance to many diseases including cancer. Curiously, we are one of the few animals that do not manufacture their own vitamin C.

- Potent antioxidant.
- Probably protects against breast cancer.
- Prevents the formation of nitrosamines (a potent carcinogen) from nitrites and amines, both in the test tube and in the body.[195]
- Vitamin C in foods like lettuce is partly responsible for the decreased incidence of human gastric cancer in the United States.[196]
- Vitamin C protects the body against human bladder cancer[197,198] and

destroys a very potent bladder carcinogen called N-methyl-N-nitrosoguanidine.[199] People who take high doses of vitamin C excrete most of it in the urine, where nitrosamines are also excreted. This high amount of vitamin C accumulating in the bladder neutralizes nitrosamines that would otherwise cause bladder cancer.

- Vitamin C protects the body against most carcinogenic hydrocarbons.
- Protects body's overall antioxidant defenses; marginal deficiency of vitamin C leads to decreases in all antioxidants.[200]
- Large amounts of vitamin C needed to produce sufficient collagen (the protein that forms connective tissue) to protect the body from cancer by forming a wall (encapsulating) around the cancer.[201]
- Vitamin C molecules may inhibit the spread of cancer by neutralizing an enzyme (hyaluronidase) made by cancer cells that would otherwise help the cancer to metastasize.[202]
- Smoking decreases the amount of vitamin C in lung tissue and blood.
- Vitamin C can reverse the carcinogenic effect of ultraviolet light.
- Vitamin C has a protective role in viral illnesses.
- Vitamin C greatly affects the immune system: the phagocytes require vitamin C for proper function; and a deficiency in vitamin C causes a decrease in T cells, the defensive killing cells of the immune system.[203]
- Toxicity: Doses of 3 to 30 grams of vitamin C in more than 1,000 patients since 1953 has not caused one miscarriage, kidney-stone formation, or any other serious side effect.[204] Klenner has given patients 10 grams of vitamin C daily for over thirty years without any serious toxic side effects.[205]
- Simone recommended dose: 350–6,000 mg/day or more, depending upon circumstances.

Bioflavonoids

- An antioxidant.
- Helps function of vitamin C.
- Toxicity: None reported.
- Simone recommended dose: 10–20 mg/day.

Selenium

- Selenium together with glutathione peroxidase is an antioxidant. Reacts with toxic metals (mercury, cadmium, arsenic) to form biologically inert compounds.

- The higher the selenium content of the retina, the better the vision.
- The higher the blood-selenium content, the lower the cancer incidence.[206,207]
- Selenium suppresses the development of skin tumors in animals.[208]
- Low serum levels linked to breast cancer.
- Rats depleted of selenium and fed a diet high in polyunsaturated fats developed breast cancer.[209] The antioxidant property of selenium protects your body against cancer especially if your diet is high in polyunsaturated fats.
- Deficiency corresponds to high incidence of heart attacks.[210,211]
- Toxicity: Occurs after prolonged ingestion of 2,400 to 3,000 micrograms of selenium per day.[212] Appproximately 500 micrograms of selenium per day is safely tolerated by people in Japan.[213] *Organic* selenium, as found in certain yeasts, is better than inorganic selenium for supplementation because it has less systemic toxicity at high concentrations, it resists chemical changes, and it is stable during food processing.
- Simone recommended dose: 200–300 mcg/day.

Zinc

- An antioxidant.
- Intimately involved in immune function and the development of cancer.
- Zinc deficiency decreases the number of T cells and suppressor T cells,[214,215] which could potentially lead to the development of cancer.
- Zinc deficiency is seen in patients with several different types of cancers.
- Zinc excess and zinc deficiency have both been shown to inhibit tumor growth in animals. Whereas zinc deficiency stimulates anticancer inflammatory cells, zinc-supplemented animals have augmented T cell anticancer activity.
- Toxicity: 80–150 mg/day or more.
- Simone recommended dose: 15–20 mg/day.

Copper

- An antioxidant.
- Enhances the immune system.
- Incidence of cardiovascular disease is increased with low levels of copper.
- Elevated cholesterol, elevated glucose levels, and heart-related

abnormalities are seen in people who have a marginal deficiency of copper.
- Toxicity: 10 mg/day for prolonged periods.
- Simone recommended dose: 3–5 mg/day.

Cysteine (an amino acid)

- An antioxidant.
- Protects against the cardiac toxicity of adriamycin.
- Enhances immune system.
- Toxicity: None.
- Simone recommended dose: 20–500 mg/day.

OTHER NUTRIENTS

Antioxidants are not the only nutrients that provide protection against cancer. Don't forget to include the following in your diet:

Vitamin A

- The growth of human breast-cancer cells and other types of cancer cell is decreased by vitamin A.[216]
- Clinical trials using vitamin A treatment for patients with skin, cervix, or lung cancer show very promising results.[217] Another study shows that vitamin A protects both smokers and nonsmokers from lung cancer.[218]
- Deficiency results in decreased production of antibodies.[219]
- Deficiency causes a decrease in T cells, which consequently renders the person vulnerable to cancer cells.
- Deficiency enhances the binding of a certain carcinogen (benzo(a)pyrene) to respiratory cells' DNA in our lungs,[220] which in turn can transform the normal lung cell into a cancer cell.
- Retinoic acid, a form of vitamin A, regenerates auditory hair cells, vital for hearing.[221]
- Toxicity: Daily doses of 100,000 IU (30 milligrams of retinol) have been given to adults for many months without serious side effects.[222] Children who ingest 50,000 to 500,000 IU (15 to 150 milligrams of retinol) per day do exhibit toxicity.[223] Researchers have extensively reviewed the safety of vitamin A.[224]
- Simone recommended dose: 5,000–7,500 IU/day.

Vitamin D

- Low levels linked to breast cancer.
- Vitamin D enhances the immune system.[225]

- It aids in cell growth and maturation.
- It inhibits the oncogene c-myc.[226]
- It inhibits cancer-cell growth.[227]
- Vitamin D decreases the risk of colon cancer.[228]
- Toxicity: A daily dose of 100,000 to 150,000 IU of vitamin D (250 to 375 micrograms of cholecalciferol) for many months can be tolerated by a healthy adult.[229]
- Simone recommended dose: 400–600 IU/day.

Vitamin K

- Vitamin K enhances the immune system.
- Toxicity: Not toxic in large doses.
- No supplement is needed.

The B vitamins, described below with recommended doses, all enhance the immune system.

Thiamine (B1)

- Immunological depression with thiamine deficiency.[230]
- Thiamine is required for the proper function of the heart.
- A deficiency of thiamine and folate leads to specific DNA changes that have been correlated with cancer.[231,232]
- Toxicity: None recorded.
- Simone recommended dose: 10–15 mg/day.

Riboflavin (B2)

- Deficiency results in a derease in lymphocytes and an increased susceptibility to certain infections.[233] With T cells decreased, a person can also be more susceptible to cancer development.
- Toxicity: None.
- Simone recommended dose: 10–15 mg/day.

Niacin

- It reduces cholesterol and triglyceride levels and has been shown to be beneficial to cardiac patients. The Coronary Drug Project Study showed a decrease in mortality of 11 percent in cardiac patients given niacin.[234]
- Toxicity: Those using niacin should take only the immediate-release form. The timed-release form can damage your liver. Do not exceed 1,500 milligrams of niacin per day. Take it with food to decrease the red flush to skin. Niacin may aggravate diabetes, gout, and stomach problems.

- Simone recommended dose: 40–80 mg/day for usual uses, 1000–1500 mg/day to lower cholesterol.

Pantothenic Acid

- It is required in almost all energy-producing reactions.
- It helps to regulate the blood-sugar level.
- Toxicity: None.
- Simone recommended dose: 20–30 mg/day.

Pyridoxine (B6)

- Deficiency inhibits the formation of antibodies, decreases the number of T cells, and decreases the ability of the immune system to reject foreign tissues like transplants[235] and to destroy cancer cells.[236]
- Toxicity: Damages nerve tissue at 500 mg or more for months.
- Simone recommended dose: 10–15 mg/day.

Vitamin B12

- Enhances immune system.
- Toxicity: None.
- Simone recommended dose: 18–30 mcg/day.

Folic Acid

- Enhances immune system.
- Toxicity: None.
- Simone recommended dose: 400–800 mcg/day.

Biotin

- Its deficiency results in depression, anemia, sleepiness, muscle pain, hair loss, and increased cholesterol levels.
- Enhances immune system.
- Toxicity: None.
- Simone recommended dose: 150–250 mcg/day.

Calcium

The average daily intake of calcium for an American is 450–500 milligrams, an amount well below even the US RDA of 1,000 milligrams per day for those under age 50 and 1,500 milligrams per day for those over 50.

Low calcium levels are linked to:

- Breast cancer. Current levels of calcium are far below US RDA particularly in young women, probably because of concerns about weight gain from dairy products. During puberty and adolescence, calcium and vitamin D inhibit breast carcinogenesis from a high-fat diet.[237]
- Osteoporosis.
- Hypertension.[238]
- Colon cancer.[239,240]
- Alzheimer's disease.[241]
- Asthma flares.
- Some male infertility problems.

In addition,

- Calcium supplementation reduces kidney stone risk.[242]
- Postmenopausal women should take calcium supplements because even at that age bone loss can be reduced.[243,244]
- Calcium should be taken with several other nutrients that aid calcium absorption and metabolism. Some of these nutrients, like vitamin D and vitamin C, should be taken only with food, and the others, like magnesium, boron, silicon, threonine, and lysine, should be taken with calcium at night.[245]
- Simone recommended dose: 1000 mg/day for age <50; otherwise, 1500 mg/day.

Magnesium

- Decreased magnesium will result in lower levels of calcium and potassium.
- The proper magnesium concentration is needed to maintain proper heart function.
- Decreases mortality after heart attack.[246,247]
- Simone recommended dose: 280 mg/day for age <50; otherwise, 420 mg/day.

Iron

- Women require more iron than men; however, iron should not be taken unless there is a real need, i.e. an anemia related to iron deficiency.
- Iron complexes can initiate the production of free radicals[248] and excess stores of iron increase the risk of cancer in men and in women.[249]
- Excess iron is linked to high risk of breast cancer and colon cancer.[250]

- Toxicity: Acute effects occur above 75 mg daily for adults.
- Simone recommended dose: Take only if you have iron deficiency anemia, and then only in therapeutic doses for a thirty-day period with a physician's supervision. Avoid any routine supplementation.

Dietary Fiber

During the past several decades, the consumption of dietary fiber has decreased in many industrialized countries, and, concomitantly, the consumption of dietary fat has increased. Dietary fiber includes indigestible carbohydrates and carbohydratelike components of food such as cellulose, lignin, hemicellulose, pentosan, gum, and pectin. These substances provide bulk in the diet. The major categories of foods that provide dietary fiber include vegetables, fruits, and whole-grain cereals. Americans typically consume three to five grams of fiber per day compared to the twenty-five to thirty grams consumed by rural Africans every day.

- Fiber is important for protection against cancer. High dietary fiber protects against colon/rectal cancer, breast cancer, heart disease, diverticular disease, obesity, and diabetes.[251-255]
- A low incidence of cancer is seen in people who consume large amounts of carotene-rich foods and cruciferous vegetables like cabbage, broccoli, cauliflower, and Brussels sprouts.[256-262]
- Fiber's protective action is probably due to its binding of bile acids, cholesterol, lipids, poisons, and carcinogens.
- Fiber increases the weight and amount of stool, which, in effect, dilutes carcinogens.
- Fiber decreases the gastrointestinal transit time so that the carcinogens are excreted more quickly.[263-268]
- Finally, fiber keeps the intestinal flora healthy so that they do not die and excrete fecapentaenes.
- Simone recommended dose: 25–35 grams/day.

NATURAL PROTECTORS IN FOODS

For a number of years, researchers, prompted by epidemiological evidence in the United States and abroad, have been studying the foods that can enhance your health. See Table 5.6, Natural Food Protectors. A study done by T. Hirayama showed that for those who smoked and also ate green and yellow vegetables every day, there was a slight beneficial effect not seen in a similar group of smokers who did not consume vegetables daily. This is only one study and

Table 5.6   Natural Food Protectors

Protector	Food	Protective Action
Carotene	Carrots, sweet potatoes, yams, pumpkins, squash, kale, broccoli, cantaloupe	Neutralizes free radicals and singlet oxygen radicals; enhances immune system; reverses pre-cancer conditions. High intake associated with low cancer rate.
Indoles	Cabbage family: cabbage, broccoli, cauliflower, mustard greens, etc.	Destroys estrogen, which is known to initiate new cancers, especially breast cancer.
Isoflavones	Legumes: beans, peas, peanuts	Inhibits estrogen receptor; destroys cancer gene enzymes; inhibits estrogen.
Lignans	Flaxseed, walnuts, fatty fish	Inhibits estrogen action; inhibits prostaglandins, hormones that cause cancer spread.
Polyacetylene	Parsley	Inhibits prostaglandins; destroys benzopyrene, a potent carcinogen.
Protease Inhibitors	Soybeans	Destroys enzymes that can cause cancer to spread.
Quinones	Rosemary	Inhibits carcinogens or cocarcinogens.
Sterols	Cucumbers	Decreases cholesterol.
Sulfur	Garlic	Inhibits carcinogens, inhibits cancer spread, decreases cholesterol.
Terpenes	Citrus Fruit	Increases enzymes that break down carcinogens; decreases cholesterol.
Triterpenoids	Licorice	Inhibits estrogens, prostaglandins; slows down rapidly dividing cells, like cancer cells.

should not be taken to mean that a smoker is "safe" from lung cancer if he eats vegetables every day. The research is still in progress and none of the findings are conclusive. Remember, too, that any substance can be toxic when taken in excess.

Carotene

Over thirty studies have shown that people who consume foods with high amounts of carotene have a low risk for developing cancer. Fourteen ongoing prospective randomized studies sponsored by the National Cancer Institute are currently looking at the anticancer potential of carotene in high-risk patients.

Carotene has also been shown to be the most potent antioxidant; it neutralizes free radicals and also single oxygen radicals. In addition, it has been shown to be one of the more important enhancers of the human immune system and can also reverse precancer conditions.

Eat carrots! Carrots contain carotene, one of the most efficient scavengers of singlet high-energy oxygen. When you eat carotene, it also localizes to the skin cells and partially protects them from light damage. Eating carrots or ingesting carotene in quantities large enough to color the skin slightly orange is well tolerated by the body. Vitamin E works similarly to stop high-energy oxygen (singlet oxygen) damage.

Indoles

Indoles, found in the cabbage family, can destroy or otherwise inactivate estrogen. Estrogen is known to initiate new cancers, especially breast cancer.

Isoflavones

Isoflavones, predominantly found in legumes, have been shown to inhibit or block estrogen receptors, thereby preventing the cell's normal cellular function. Isoflavones also inhibit estrogens from being effective in the first place, and have been shown to destroy certain cancer gene enzymes that can propagate and transform a normal cell into a cancer cell. This is one of the more exciting areas of cancer prevention.

Lignans

Lignans are predominantly found in flaxseed, walnuts, and fatty fish. Each of these is an excellent source of omega-3 fatty acids, which are known to inhibit the production of prostaglandins, hormonesthat modulate cell metabolism. Numerous studies have shown that omega-3 fatty acids can be used to reduce cholesterol, hypertension, heart disease, and the risk for developing breast cancer, rheumatoid arthritis, and multiple sclerosis. Lignans have also been shown to inhibit the action of estrogens on cells that are responsive to estrogen.

Phenylalanine and Tyrosine

Investigators at Washington State University found that cancer did not spread in animals if they were kept on a stringent diet that eliminated two amino acids, phenylalanine and tyrosine. Although these animal experiments have been repeated many times, human studies of this nature have not been done. The foods that have a high content of phenylalanine and tyrosine are those that are high in fats or high in protein: meats, eggs, and dairy products. Avoid or limit these, and increase consumption of fruits, vegetables, and carbohydrates.

Polyacetylene

Polyacetylene, mainly found in parsley, inhibits the action of prostaglandins and destroys a potent carcinogen called benzopyrene.

Protease Inhibitors

Protease inhibitors, mainly found in soybeans, have been shown to inhibit the development of colon cancer, lung cancer, mouth cancer, liver cancer, and esophageal cancers in animals. Protease inhibitors do this by inhibiting the action of the enzymes chymotrypsin and trypsin, as well as by preventing the conversion of normal cells to malignant cells in the early stages of carcinogenesis, but not in the late stages. These protease inhibitors have been shown to cause an irreversible suppressive effect on the process of carcinogenesis. They can also inhibit oncogene expression.

Quinones

Quinones are mainly found in rosemary. These chemical agents have been shown to inhibit carcinogens and cocarcinogens, chemicals that help carcinogens work more effectively to cause cancer.

Sterols

Sterols are mainly found in cucumbers, especially the skin of cucumbers. Sterols have been shown to decrease cholesterol; by lowering the cholesterol, you lower most of the fat content that is associated with multiple cancers, including colon and rectal cancer, breast cancer, prostate cancer, and cancer of the uterus (endometrial cancer).

Sulfur

Sulfur is found in large amounts in garlic. The National Cancer Institute, the United States Department of Agriculture, and Loma Linda University are currently studying garlic as an immune system enhancer, a cancer preventive agent, a blood clot inhibitor, and an agent to lower high blood pressure. Sulfur compounds from garlic inhibit carcinogens and inhibit the enzymes that allow cancers to spread. Garlic has been used in Japan as a painkiller.

Terpenes

Terpenes are mainly found in citrus fruits. The National Cancer Institute is sponsoring studies to investigate the use of vitamin C and citrus fruits to treat certain viruses, to lower blood cholesterol, to reduce arterial plaque, and to prevent certain forms of cancer. Terpenes also have been shown to increase enzymes known to break down carcinogens.

Triterpenoids

Triterpenoids are found in licorice. The National Cancer Institute is studying the potential of licorice to fight cancer, protect the liver, and slow cell mutation. Triterpenoids inhibit estrogens and prostaglandins, and slow down rapidly dividing cells like cancer cells to prevent them from having daughter cells.

LOWERING YOUR RISK OF CANCER

Cancer patients have vitamin deficiencies.[269] Because they do not eat, they become malnourished. I am advocating simple common sense: An apparently healthy person should take steps to avoid or eliminate risk factors that can potentially cause cancer and atherosclerosis. This includes eating the right foods and taking the right amount of those vitamins and minerals shown to have anticancer and antioxidant effects, and shown to be needed for the immune system to function well. By eliminating all known risk factors of cancer and atherosclerosis and practicing good nutrition supplemented with vitamins and minerals, your overall risk of developing cancer or atherosclerosis will be kept to a minimum.

As reported by the *Medical Tribune* on June 30, 1982, Richard S.

Table 5.7 Supplementation Program

Nutrient	Adult Amount	Adult % U.S. RDA*	Child (Age 1–4) Amount	Child (Age 1–4) %U.S. RDA
Beta-carotene	30 mg	***	1 mg	***
Vitamin A (palmitate)	5,000 IU	1,000	834 IU	33
Vitamin D (ergocalciferol)	400 IU	100	400 IU	100
Vitamin E (dl-tocopherol)	400 IU	1,333	15 IU	150
Vitamin C (ascorbic acid)	350 mg	580	60 mg	150
Folic acid	400 mcg	100	200 mcg	100
Vitamin B1 (thiamine)	10 mg	667	1.1 mg	157
Vitamin B2 (riboflavin)	10 mg	588	1.2 mg	150
Niacinamide	40 mg	200	9 mg	100
Vitamin B6 (pyridoxine)	10 mg	500	1.12 mg	100
Vitamin B12 (cyanobalamin)	18 mcg	300	4.5 mcg	150
Biotin	150 mcg	50	25 mcg	20
Pantothenic acid (d-calcium pantothenate)	20 mg	200	5 mg	100
Iodine	150 mcg	100	70 mcg	100
Copper (cupric oxide)	3 mg	150	1.25 mg	125
Zinc (zinc gluconate)	15 mg	100	10mg	125
Potassium	30 mg	#	2 mg	#
Selenium (organic)	200 mcg	**	20 mcg	**
Chromium (organic)	125 mcg	**	20 mcg	**
Manganese (gluconate)	2.5 mg	**	1 mg	**
Molybdenum	50 mcg	**	25 mcg	**
Inositol	10 mg	#	0	N/A
Para aminobenzoic acid	10 mg	#	0	N/A
Bioflavonoids	10 mg	#	10 mcg	#
Choline (choline bitartrate)	10 mg	#	5 mg	#
L-Cysteine	20 mg	#	0	N/A
L-Arginine	5 mg	#	0	N/A
Histidine	N/A	N/A	10 mg	**
Leucine	N/A	N/A	10 mg	**
Isoleucine	N/A	N/A	10 mg	**
Lysine	N/A	N/A	10 mg	**
Threonine	N/A	N/A	10 mg	**

*Percentage U.S. Recommended Dietary Allowance (U.S. RDA) for adults and children 4 or more years.
**Established as adequate and safe by the National Research Council, National Academy of Sciences; no U.S. RDA has been established.
***Can be converted to vitamin A according to body needs; 1 mg of beta-carotene = 1,666 IU of vitamin A.
No nutritional requirement established.
N/A=Not applicable

Table 5.8　Calcium Formula

Nutrient	Dosage	U.S. RDA*
Calcium (calcium carbonate)	500 mg	50
Magnesium (magnesium oxide)	140 mg	36
Silicon	2 mg	#
Potassium bicarbonate	100 mg	#
Boron	2 mg	#
L-Threonine	2 mg	#
L-Lysine	2 mg	#

* Percentage U.S. Recommended Dietary Allowance (U.S. RDA) for adults and children 4 or more years.
# No U.S. RDA established.

Schweiker, then Secretary of Health and Human Services, said that he and the Reagan Administration endorsed the research focus on cancer prophylaxis and the protective potential of vitamins and trace minerals in both normal and high-risk populations. "This new strategy holds promise for reducing the incidence of cancer more successfully than an attempt to remove from the environment all substances which may initiate the cancer process—an approach which is not always possible or practical."

I recommend taking the combination of vitamins and minerals in Table 5.7 as supplementation. These nutrients can be taken daily unless otherwise specified by your physician. Pregnant or lactating women should not follow this program unless it has been approved by their physician. The formula for young children is also shown.

I also recommend taking as a food supplement the Calcium Formula shown in Table 5.8. This formula should be taken at bedtime, never with food.

As you can see, what you eat plays an important role in your risk of developing cancer. Because you can modify your diet, *you can reduce your cancer risk.*

6
Nutritional and Lifestyle Modification in Oncology Care

By the year 2000, cancer will emerge as the number one cause of death in the United States. The successes in the treatment of cancer plateaued in the 1970s, and no real advances have been made since then. However, chemotherapy and radiation therapy continue to have a role in cancer treatment but produce morbidity. Nutritional modification, including the use of certain nutrients, and proper lifestyle can dramatically decrease the morbidity and side effects of chemotherapy and radiation therapy, and normal tissue can be better preserved. There have even been some reports that nutritional and lifestyle modification actually increases survival. Innumerable studies show that nutrients used with chemotherapy and radiation therapy can enhance tumor killing and preserve normal tissue.

VITAMINS AND MINERALS IN CHEMOTHERAPY AND RADIATION THERAPY

Do vitamins or minerals interfere with chemotherapy and/or radiation therapy? This is a question I am asked frequently by patients because their oncologists, ignorant of the subject, advise the patients not to take supplements during treatment. Many studies have been done to address this. The early studies were performed at the National Cancer Institute using an antioxidant called N-acetyl cysteine, which has a protective effect on the heart, with patients receiving a chemotherapeutic drug called adriamycin, which is toxic to the heart. The heart was protected and there was no interference with the tumor-killing performance of adriamycin. Another antioxidant called ICRF-187 offered significant protection against cardiac toxicity caused by adriamycin without affecting the antitumor effect.[1-4] Many cellular studies[5-8] and animal studies[9-13] demonstrate that vitamins A, E, and C, as well as beta-carotene and selenium, all protect against the toxicity of adriamycin and, at the same time, actually enhance its cancer-killing effects.

Vitamins and minerals have also been studied with other chemotherapies and radiation. Studies using beta-carotene and other retinoids, vitamin C, or vitamin K show that normal tissue tolerance was improved in animals undergoing both chemotherapy and radiotherapy and that tumors regressed.[14-20] Vitamin E produced similar findings: There was no interference with the killing of tumors by either radiation or chemotherapy in animals given concomitant vitamin E.[21-23] Animals given both beta-carotene and vitamin A with radiation and chemotherapy had more tumor killing than with chemotherapy and radiation alone, normal tissues were more protected, and there was a longer period of time without tumor recurrence.[24,25] Selenium and cysteine also heighten tumor killing by chemotherapy and radiation, and at the same time protect normal tissue.[26,27]

All cellular studies using vitamins (C, A, K, E, D, beta-carotene, B6, B12), minerals (selenium), and cysteine concomitantly with chemotherapy and radiation show the same effect: increased tumor killing and increased protection of the normal tissues.[28-37]

In human studies, vitamin E reduced the toxicity without affecting the cancer-killing performance of 13-cis-retinoic acid, used in the treatment of patients with head and neck, skin, and lung cancers.[38] At 1,600 IU of vitamin E per day, hair loss in patients receiving chemotherapy was reduced from the expected 30–90 percent.[39] Treating 190 head and neck cancer patients with vitamin A, 5FU, and radiation resulted in more-than-expected tumor killing while preserving normal tissue.[40] And vitamin A combined with chemotherapy for postmenopausal patients with metastatic breast cancers significantly increased the complete response rate.[41] In thirteen patients with different cancers receiving different chemotherapies, vitamin K decreased tumor resistance.[42] Vitamin B6 at 300 milligrams per day decreased radiation therapy toxicity.[43] In twenty patients receiving chemotherapy with vitamins A, C, and E, there was a greater response rate.[44] Glutathione, part of the selenium complex, protected 150 women with ovarian cancer against cisplatin toxicity with no loss of anticancer effects as shown in double-blind studies at nine British oncology centers. In fact, more women treated with glutathione had an objective response (73 percent vs. 62 percent) and completed more cycles of cisplatin (58 percent vs. 39 percent)[45] than those who were not so treated. And studies show that WR-2721, an antioxidant, protects against the harmful side effects of chemotherapy and radiation without the loss of antitumor activity.[46]

An increase in survival for cancer patients, which is uncommon with any treatment, has been shown using antioxidants combined with chemotherapy or radiation. In fact, eleven patients who were given beta-carotene and canthaxanthin while undergoing surgery, chemotherapy, and radiation lived longer with an increase in disease-free intervals.[47] And antioxidant treatment with chemotherapy and radiation prolonged survival for patients with small cell lung cancer compared with patients who did not receive antioxidants.[48,49]

The effects of one chemotherapeutic agent, methotrexate, can be reversed with folinic acid, which is an analog of the vitamin folic acid. Folic acid itself does not reverse methotrexate's effects. In order to reverse the effects of methotrexate, folinic acid has to be given in extremely high doses. It cannot be obtained over the counter; it must be prescribed.

Studies of supplements all show that vitamins and minerals do not interfere with the antitumor effects of chemotherapy or radiation therapy. In fact, on the contrary, some vitamins and minerals used in conjunction with chemotherapy and/or radiation therapy have been shown to protect normal tissue and potentiate the destruction of cancer cells. In my own preliminary studies, I have found a decrease in side effects from chemotherapy and/or radiation therapy in breast cancer patients who followed my Ten-Point Plan, which, among other things, advocates the consumption of certain vitamins and minerals.[50]

BREAST CANCER TREATMENT USING
ADJUNCTIVE THERAPEUTIC LEVELS OF NUTRIENTS

Using Quality of Life Scales, fifty patients with early staged breast cancer evaluated treatment side effects of radiation and/or chemotherapy while taking therapeutic doses of nutrients.[50] Quality of Life Scales, which are a series of qualities of life, are an acceptable way of evaluating any treatment or side effect not by the physician, but rather by the patient. The patient decides whether the treatment is beneficial or not in terms of side effects incurred. These scales have been successfully used to evaluate treatments for cardiovascular disease, cancer, and other chronic illnesses.[51-60]

The scoring system for the Quality of Life Scales is simple. The patient decides if the nutrients used during the radiation and/or chemotherapy treatments has improved, worsened, or has made no change in her life during the treatment period. The qualities of life tested were: physical symptoms, performance, general well being, cognitive abilities, sexual dysfunction, and life satisfaction.

Fifty consecutive patients with early staged infiltrating ductal adenocarcinoma of the breast were treated with lumpectomy (re-excisional lumpectomy if indicated), axillary node dissection, and radiation therapy. Depending upon the nodal status, chemotherapy was used. In Group I, twenty-five women with T1 or T2, N0, M0 were treated with primary radiation therapy, receiving 4500 cGy to the whole breast, and a total dose of 6000 cGy to the tumor bed. In Group II, twenty-five patients with T1 or T2, N1, M0 were treated with primary radiation therapy to the same doses as with Group I and also received modified CMF chemotherapy consisting of cytoxan and 5-FU (methotrexate was omitted until radiation was completed). A total of six cycles of this modified regimen was given.

Each patient was instructed to follow the aspects of the Simone Ten-Point Plan pertinent as an adjunct to treatment. (A general-use version of the plan appears on page 317.) These points are:

POINT 1. NUTRITION.

- Maintain an ideal weight—lose even 5 or 7 pounds if needed.
- Low-fat (about 20 percent of calories), high-fiber (25 gm) diet.
- Micronutrients (as outlined at the end of Chapter 5) taken 30 minutes before each therapeutic modality:

Beta-carotene 30 mg, vitamin A 5000 IU, vitamin D 400 IU, vitamin E 400 IU, vitamin C 350 mg, folic acid 400 mcg, vitamin B1 10 mg, vitamin B2 10 mg, niacinamide 40 mg, vitamin B6 10 mg, vitamin B12 18 mcg, biotin 150 mcg, pantothenic acid 20 mg, iodine 150 mcg, copper 3 mg, zinc 15 mg, potassium 30 mg, selenium (organic) 200 mcg, chromium (organic) 125 mcg, manganese 2.5 mg, molybdenum 50 mcg, inositol 10 mg, and L-cysteine 20 mg.

In addition, the women took the following at bedtime: calcium carbonate 1000 mg, magnesium 280 mg, boron 2 mg, L-lysine 2 mg, L-threonine 2 mg, and silicon 2 mg.

- Eliminate salt, food additives, and caffeine.

POINT 2. TOBACCO. Do not smoke, chew, snuff, or inhale other's smoke.

POINT 3. ALCOHOL. Avoid all alcohol.

POINT 4. RADIATION. Avoid unnecessary X-rays; sunscreens to be used. Avoid electromagnetic fields.

POINT 5. ENVIRONMENT. Keep air, water, and work place clean.

POINT 6. HORMONES, DRUGS. Avoid all estrogens and unnecessary drugs.

POINT 7. KNOW THE SEVEN WARNING SIGNS OF CANCER.

POINT 8. TAKE SELF-TEST (see page 42) to identify organs at risk.

POINT 9. EXERCISE AND RELAX REGULARLY.

POINT 10. HAVE EXECUTIVE PHYSICAL ANNUALLY and its pertinent components.

The majority of the nutrients ingested were free radical scavengers (antioxidants) in high doses, combined with the B vitamins, and other important minerals. The rationale for this combination has been previously outlined. Radiation and many chemotherapeutic agents exert their killing effects and morbidity by generating free radicals.

Table 6.1 presents the responses of the fifty patients. Patients generally indicated improvement, a few indicated no change, and none indicated worsening. Multiple *in vitro*, and animal and human studies have addressed this question. Vitamins and minerals do not interfere with the tumor-killing effects of radiation and chemotherapy, and they actually enhance tumor kill while at the same time protect normal cells. In summary, this study demonstrates that patients who followed the Ten-Point Plan and used certain vitamins and minerals had few side effects from chemotherapy and radiation therapy.

THE HOFFER-PAULING STUDY

Researchers Hoffer and Pauling asked whether therapeutic nutrition helped cancer patients.[61] All 129 cancer patients in their study were to follow a low-fat diet supplemented with therapeutic doses of vitamins C, E, A, niacin, and a multiple vitamin/mineral supplement, in addition to following the advice and treatment of traditional oncology care. Those who did not follow nutritional modification (31 patients) lived an average of less than 6 months. The other 98 patients fell into three categories: Females with breast, ovarian, cervix, and uterus (32 patients) cancer had an average life span of over 10 years; patients who had leukemia, lung, liver, and pancreas cancer (47 patients) had an average life span of over 6 years; and patients with end-stage terminal cancer (19 patients) lived an average of 10 months.

Other studies show similar findings: Patients who undergo conventional oncology therapy and modify lifestyle, which includes diet

Table 6.1 Patient Responses to Qualities of Life

Life Quality	GROUP I*			GROUP II*		
	Improve	No Change	Worsen	Improve	No Change	Worsen
Physical symptoms	25			24	1	
Skin reaction						
Fatigue						
Mouth sores						
Nausea/vomiting						
Dizziness, vertigo						
Lightheadedness						
Muscle cramps						
Performance	23	2		23	2	
General well-being	25			25		
Cognitive abilities	25			22	3	
Sexual dysfunction	25			15	10	
Life satisfaction	25			25		

*Group I patients had radiation only; Group II had radiation and chemotherapy.

and nutrient supplementation, generally live longer.[62-66] It has also been found that patients who undergo chemotherapy, in fact, have lower serum levels of vitamins and minerals, which return to near baseline levels thereafter.[67]

JAPANESE EXPERIENCE

The older generation of Japanese women rarely get breast cancer, but when these women do, they live longer than American women stage for stage[68-73] because of only two reasons: (1) they are less obese, and (2) eat a low-fat, high-fiber diet with vitamins and minerals. This is not necessarily true for younger Japanese women who have now adopted a more Western culture and diet.[74]

Obese breast cancer patients have a greater chance of early recurrence and a shorter life span compared to nonobese patients.[75-79] And breast cancer patients who have a high-fat intake and a high serum cholesterol also have a shorter life span than patients with normal or low-fat intake and low serum cholesterol.[80] Fat can initiate and also promote a cancer, especially a dietary cancer like breast cancer. If cholesterol intake is dramatically limited, cancer cell growth is severely inhibited.[81]

NATIONAL CANCER INSTITUTE "EFFORT"

Armed with this information, NCI attempted a research protocol in the mid-80s to see if a low-fat diet would increase the life span of breast cancer patients. However, in January 1988, after only a brief time and an expenditure of about $90 million, the Board of Scientific

Counselors of NCI's Division of Cancer Prevention and Control decided to end the proposed 10-year study because: (1) physicians did not "believe" that there was a relationship between breast cancer and fat or other nutritional factors and, subsequently, did not refer patients to the study; and (2) once a woman was enrolled in the protocol, she subsequently "failed out" because she did not want to give up pizza, ice cream, and other high-fat foods. In 1991, NCI decided to try, in the near future, another low-fat cancer study in women aged 45 and 69.

CONCLUSION

My own experience, as already discussed, supports the above studies. It behoves cancer patients to modify their lifestyles, which includes modifying nutritional factors and taking important vitamins and minerals in doses outlined in Chapter 5, especially if they receive chemotherapy and/or radiation.

PART THREE

The Risks

7
Free Radicals

Free radicals are made in our bodies all the time and, if not destroyed, can lead to the development of cancer and other diseases. Free radicals cause oxidation to occur: rusty metal, rancid butter, the greenish hue on outdoor copper statues. Antioxidants, like beta-carotene, vitamins C and E, selenium, and others, can neutralize the harmful free radicals and thereby prevent disease and protect us.

By definition, free radicals are chemical substances that contain an odd number of electrons. Every atom has a nucleus and a certain number of electrons that orbit around the nucleus. This setup is very much like our solar system, with the sun in the middle and all the planets orbiting around the sun. The nucleus has a positive charge, and the electrons have a negative charge. The negative charges of electrons balance out the positive charge of the nucleus to give an overall charge of zero. Hence, the energy of a single atom is very stable at zero.

When high energy in any form (from light and radiation to smog, tobacco, alcohol, polyunsaturated fats, etc.) hits an atom, an electron is kicked out of orbit. All of the energy that forced the electron out of orbit is transferred directly to the electron, making it highly energetic and unstable. Because it is so unstable, this electron quickly seeks *another* atom to reside in. This excited high-energy electron transfers very high energy to the new atom, which then becomes extremely unstable because of the newly acquired high energy. The process is depicted in Figure 7.1. (An analogy to this state is a nine-month-old

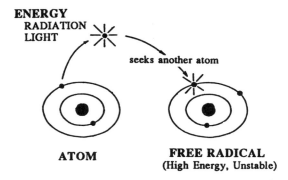

ENERGY
RADIATION
LIGHT

seeks another atom

ATOM

FREE RADICAL
(High Energy, Unstable)

Figure 7.1 Free radical formation. When high energy from any source hits an atom, it knocks an electron out of orbit. This high-energy electron goes into another atom, making it extremely unstable.

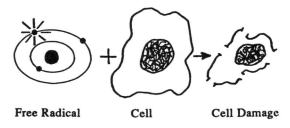

Free Radical   Cell   Cell Damage

Figure 7.2 Cell damage by free radicals. Free radicals can destroy the layer of fat in the cell membrane.

child who has a great deal of energy but is extremely unstable if left unattended.) This excited high-energy atom with its extra electron is called a free radical.

A free radical is unstable and must get rid of all the extra energy for the atom to become stable once again; hence the radical transfers its energy to nearby substances. (All these reactions take place within a fraction of a second.) When free radicals are made in the body, the high energy is transferred to body tissues, particularly to the polyunsaturated fats found in the cell membranes. The more polyunsaturated fats you eat, the more of them will be absorbed by the cell membranes and the higher the risk will be for membrane disruption by free radicals as seen in Figure 7.2. If not counteracted, this process can lead to the development of cancer in the tissue affected by the radical.

FORMATION OF RADICALS

The following produce free radicals and can lead to the development of cancer:

Oxygen. Can be activated or split with high energy into very potent damaging radicals (superoxide) or a high-energy, unstable nonradical called singlet oxygen. Singlet oxygen has extremely high energy and is very unstable, and thus is very destructive to normal body tissues and cells.[1]

Polyunsaturated Fats. React with oxygen or enzymes to release their energy and thereby form a free radical. This free radical reacts with another polyunsaturated fat to produce a lot of hydroperoxide.[2,3] The more unsaturated the fat is, the more hydroperoxides are made. And hydroperoxides produce more radicals, damage cell membranes, and can lead to the development of cancer.

Metals. Accumulate in the body and can also initiate free radical formation by activating oxygen. Iron is one example.

Radiation. Produces free radicals and electrons that react to yield many different kinds of free radicals. At high levels of radiation, hydroperoxides are produced in addition to all the other free radicals.[4]

Sunlight (Photolysis). Produces free radicals in skin cells, which can damage the skin[5] and lead to skin cancer. Chronic sun exposure in Caucasians directly damages the uppermost skin cells and results in wrinkling, the formation of tiny networks of blood vessels, and the appearance of discrete small raised bumps on the skin called actinic keratosis (which are precancerous). And ultraviolet light adversely affects the immune system.

Skin cancer is the most common of all human cancers. There are three main types: basal cell cancer, squamous cell cancer, and melanoma. Squamous cell cancer is directly caused by sun exposure, and about 66 percent of all basal cell skin cancers occur in areas of the body exposed to sunlight. The influence of sunlight on the development of melanoma, a very deadly cancer, is not conclusively established, but a number of surveys do suggest that sunlight does cause the development of melanomas.

Smog. Causes more tissue damage than does background radiation.[6] Ozone reacts with almost every type of molecule in the body to form free radicals, which then damage cells. Ozone in normal amounts in the air can even form radicals with polyunsaturated fatty acids.[7] Other components of smog, peroxyacetyl nitrate and nitrogen dioxide, can form radicals. The components of smog, tobacco smoke, and other air pollutants can form radicals, especially in the lungs.

Protect Yourself
From Harmful Effects of Sunlight

What defenses do we have against the harmful and cancer-pro-ducing effects of sunlight? There are many common-sense pre-ventive measures that we can take to lessen our risk for skin cancer. First of all, before sunbathing, use one of the several commercially available sunscreens on areas of your body that will be exposed. Don't stay out in the sun for a prolonged period of time at one sitting. If you work out-of-doors, wear protective clothing to minimize the chronic prolonged exposure to sunlight. Don't seek a suntan from a suntanning booth, because the rays it usually emits are more damaging on the whole.

Alcohol and Chloride-Containing Compounds. Certain chloride-containing compounds (vinyl chloride, chloroprene, carbon tetra-chloride) react with some enzymes (specifically microsomal mixed function oxidase system) in the liver to produce free radicals.[8,9] These radicals can then locally damage liver cells and potentiate liver cancer or other deadly liver diseases.

FREE RADICALS AND DISEASE

It has become quite clear that free radicals play an important role in the development of many human diseases. The free radical connection to human diseases is so exciting that two new medical journals have been created to deal solely with this subject. It is now thought that once free radicals are made, they are the primary cause of certain human diseases involving many organs. This theory is supported by a multitude of data.[10–12] Table 7.1 lists medical conditions associated with free radical formation.

Free radicals cause damage to the nucleus of the cell and subsequently to the DNA. When certain segments of the DNA are affected, a malignant change occurs, altering the genetic code and leading to cancer.[13,14] Substances called antioxidants (see Chapter 5) can protect against agents that cause cancer.[15–17] Antioxidants work against oxidation (the process in which oxygen reacts with another chemical) and thereby prevent the harmful effects of oxygen on tissue via free radical formation. These protective substances occur naturally in the body, and various nutritional supplements also act as antioxidants (see page 67).

Table 7.1 Conditions Associated With Free Radicals

- Heart and cardiovascular disease
  Alcohol heart condition (Alcoholic cardiomyopathy)
  Selenium heart condition (Keshan disease)
  Atherosclerosis
  Adriamycin toxicity
  Heart attack

- Cancers: all types

- Lung disease
  Emphysema
  Pneumoconiosis
  Respiratory distress syndrome
  Bleomycin toxicity
  Air pollutant toxicity

- Alcohol-related diseases
  Cirrhosis

- Immune-system-related diseases
  Glomerulonephritis (kidney disease)
  Vasculitis (inflammation of blood vessels)
  Autoimmune diseases: lupus, Sjögren's, etc.
  Rheumatoid arthritis

- Eye diseases
  Cataracts
  Retinal damage

- Central nervous system diseases
  Senile dementia
  Parkinson's disease
  Hypertensive stroke
  Encephalomyelitis
  Aluminum overload
  Worsening of traumatic injury
  Ataxia-telangiectasia syndrome

- Iron overload

- Radiation injury

- Kidney diseases

- Gastrointestinal diseases
  Free-fatty-acid-induced pancreatitis
  Nonsteroidal anti-inflammatory drug (NSAID) lesions
  Liver injury from toxins
  Carbon tetrachloride injury

- Skin diseases
  Solar radiation damage
  Thermal injury
  Contact dermatitis
  Dye reactions

- Aging

- Red blood cell diseases
  Falconi's anemia
  Sickle cell anemia
  Favism
  Malaria
  Protoporphyrin photo-oxidation

The preponderance of evidence suggests that free radicals damage the cells that line the inside of all blood vessels.[18] Due to this initial injury, fats and fibrin (blood-clotting protein) and other elements of the blood ultimately form clots and block the arteries.[19] It has also been shown that once a person sustains a heart attack, the injury that occurs within the first twelve to twenty-four hours is secondary to free radical damage.[20,21] Therefore, antioxidants (also called free radical scavengers because they neutralize the free radicals) may have an important role not only in the prevention of cardiovascular disease but also at the time of an ongoing heart attack.

OUR BODY'S DEFENSES AGAINST RADICALS

We know that all life requires oxygen, but sometimes oxygen can produce radicals and high-energy (singlet) oxygen. Because of this, most animals have developed many lines of defense against free radical formation to preserve their very existence and to lessen the chance of abnormal cell (cancer) development.

Mechanisms that prevent or decrease the occurrence of radicals and the formation of hydroperoxide thereby decrease the amount of cell membrane damage. The most obvious mechanism is the *protective protein coat* that lines the surface of the cell membrane. This protective coat prevents oxygen from reacting directly with lipids in the membrane, a reaction which would produce many free radicals.

A second defensive mechanism involves the *protective enzymes* that float around in all cell membranes. These enzymes also act as antioxidants, preventing radical formation and prevent radical damage to the cell membrane. They include *superoxide dismutase,*[22] *catalase,*[23] and *selenium-containing glutathione peroxidase.*[24]

Vitamin E is also an antioxidant and is the third mechanism that inhibits formation of free radicals, thereby preventing their destructive damage. Vitamin E and selenium also protect vitamin A because vitamin A is a polyunsaturated compound. Lipid antioxidants prevent cancer.[25] The process of aging is also most probably related to hydroperoxide action on lipids. Aging is thought to be due to the process of oxidation.

Free radicals are unstable chemical substances with high energy. Normal enzymes can produce free radicals, which can form more radicals and singlet oxygen (very-high-energy oxygen). Oxygen reacting with lipids to free its stored energy may also produce hydroperoxides. All of these will cause tissue damage and may lead to the development of cancer. As will be seen in Part III, the body does have defenses to protect itself against these, including the protective protein coat of the cell membrane, protective enzymes (catalase, superoxide dismutase, and selenium-containing glutathione peroxidase), and vitamin E. There are other vitamins as well as minerals that can protect us against the effects of free radicals. These are discussed at length in Chapter 5.

8
Nutritional Factors

It is now widely accepted that an estimated 60 percent of all women's cancers and 40 percent of all men's cancers are related to nutritional factors alone.[1-3] Overall, it has been estimated that 75–90 percent of all cancers are related to lifestyle: nutritional factors, smoking, alcohol consumption, occupational factors, chemicals, environmental factors, etc. All the major agencies in the United States—the National Academy of Sciences, the National Cancer Institute, and the American Cancer Society—have supported the contention that nutritional factors are linked to certain cancers.

Nutritional factors are most closely associated with the following cancers, listed in order of their prevalence in the United States: lung, gastrointestinal cancers, breast cancer, prostate cancer, and endometrial cancer. With each year, the number of new cancers continues to rise; with the great majority of these being diet-related cancers, you can readily understand the enormous impact that proper nutrition can have in lowering the overall incidence of cancer in the United States and the world.

NUTRITIONAL EVOLUTION

The human race has existed for about two million years, and our prehuman ancestors existed for at least four million years. Today, we are confronted with diet-related health problems that were previously of minor importance or totally nonexistent. Dietary habits adopted by Western society over the past hundred years have greatly contributed to the development of coronary heart disease, hypertension, diabetes, and cancer. These illnesses have dominated the past ninety-year history of humanity and are virtually unknown among the few surviving hunter-gatherer populations, like the Bantu tribesmen in Africa, whose way of life and eating habits today resemble those of people before agricultural development. Members of primitive cultures today who survive to the age of sixty or more are relatively free of these illnesses unlike their Western "civilized" counterparts.[4,5]

With the development of agriculture over 10,000 years ago, we began eating less meat and more vegetables. With less protein in our diets, our height declined by six inches. After the Industrial Revolution, the pendulum started to swing back, and we started to increase the protein content of our diets. Height increased and we are now nearly the same height as were the first biologically modern people. But our diet is still very different from theirs: We are affluently malnourished.

Investigating the wild game in areas of the world where people are still quite primitive today, we find that these wild animals have less fat than domesticated ones because they are more active and have a less steady food supply. Also, domesticated animals are fed high concentrations of fat to produce tender meat. Wild game has fewer calories and more protein per unit of weight. Even modern vegetable foods have more fat than noncommercially grown vegetables and fruits. Table 8.1 lists the various nutrients consumed by primitive people compared with those eaten by Americans today.[6]

Table 8.1 Diet Comparison of Primitive and Modern Person

Nutrient	Primitive Person	Modern American	My Recommendations
Percentage of Total Calories			
Protein	34%	12%	10%
Carbohydrate	45%	46%	70%
Fats	21%	42%	20%
Daily Consumption			
Cholesterol	591.0 mg	600 mg	250 mg
Fiber	45.7 g	19 g	30–45 g
Sodium	690.0 mg	5,000 mg	1,000 mg
Calcium	1,580.0 mg	740 mg	1,500 mg
Vitamin C	392.3 mg	88 mg	400 mg

Given a primitive person's wide variety of collected plant foods, and assuming that his vitamin C intake is representative of his overall vitamin intake from foods, the diet of primitive people contained substantially greater amounts of vitamins than ours does. The vitamin and mineral content continues to decrease in our food supply because of: pesticides, processing techniques like refrigeration and freezing, thawing, transporting around the country, etc. The protein content of primitive people's food was approximately two to five times that of ours. The early human diet contained much less fat than ours, and the fat that it did contain was of a very different mix from ours. Its cholesterol content was about the same, but its total fat was much less than ours. In addition, primitive people consumed many more essential fatty acids than we do today. Since chronic diseases have been with us for only a few decades, and the incidence of cancer is spiraling ever upward, we should perhaps model our modern diet after that of our ancestors.

We have created a food supply very different from that of our ancestors with the development of food technology and the chemicals used for its growth and production. This "advancement" is costly to the human race.

EPIDEMIOLOGICAL PATTERNS

Large epidemiological studies demonstrate that a high-risk diet for cancer as well as cardiovascular diseases is one that has high-fat, high-cholesterol, low-fiber, salt-cured, pickled, charred, smoked, or burned foods, and a low consumption of vitamins and minerals. Human breast cancer is associated with a high-fat diet, particularly animal fat.

Consumption of five food items has been associated with breast cancer: fried potatoes, hard fat (butter and margarine) for frying, all fried foods, some dairy products, and white bread. All these foods, except white bread, are excellent sources of dietary fat. About forty years ago, Dr. A. Tannenbaum showed that dietary fat significantly favored the development and growth of both spontaneous and induced breast cancer in animals.[7] Since then, a high-fat, low-fiber diet has been associated with human breast cancer, colon cancer, prostate cancer, cancer of the endometrium, and coronary artery disease, suggesting that similar modifications of the diet would be beneficial in decreasing the risk of developing all these major diseases. Over the past half century, Americans have been consuming more fat, more cholesterol, more animal protein, more refined sugar, and less fiber. Likewise, an ever-increasing incidence of cancer has been seen for the same period in the United States.

Epidemiological studies are very important to assess cancer trends. They show that there is a sixfold variation in breast cancer incidence in different parts of the world. High-risk countries such as the United States are characterized by high standards of living with diets rich in cholesterol and animal fat. In high-risk countries, there is a constant increase in the rate of breast cancer development with age, but in low-risk countries the rate decreases after menopause.

The Bantu people of rural Africa have an extremely low incidence of cancer compared to people in industrialized nations. They have a low-fat, very high-fiber diet. Except for Japan and Finland, the more industrialized a country is, the higher is the rate of "diet-sensitive" tumors, that is, colon/rectal cancer, breast cancer, endometrial cancer, and prostate cancer. People in industrialized countries usually eat a diet higher in fat than do people in nonindustrialized countries. The people in western Europe and in English-speaking countries have the highest colon cancer incidence rates, while the peoples of Asia, Africa, and South America (except Uruguay and Argentina, where the rates are similar to those of North America) have the lowest colon cancer incidence rates.

If a person emigrates from a country with a low incidence rate of colon cancer to a country with a high rate, such as the United States, the higher colon cancer rate shows up within the first generation. Japanese immigrants to the United States have the same colon cancer rate after only twenty years of consuming the American diet and have the same incidence of breast cancer after only two generations. Only 20 percent of the daily caloric intake in Japan is derived from fat compared to 40 percent in America.

About half of the Seventh-Day Adventists in the United States follow a vegetarian diet, and most do not eat pork. Their breast cancer mortality is one-half to two-thirds the breast cancer mortality seen in the United States population in general. Seventh-Day Adventists and Mormons also have a substantially lower incidence of colon cancer than the general population in the United States as well.[9–11] Both of these groups consume dietary fiber in great amounts and little or no beef or animal fat.

American-born Jews of European descent are at high risk for developing colon and rectal cancer. A twenty-year prospective study conducted in Israel has recently shown that a diet high in fiber, with foods of high vitamin C content, and with polyunsaturated fats, substantially reduces the number of colon and rectal cancer cases in that group.[8]

People in Finland have a high fat intake, with the majority of their fat calories derived from dairy products rather than beef. The incidence of heart attacks is quite high in that country; however, the incidence of colon cancer is very low. The latter statistic may seem surprising, but it is probably due, in part, to the large amount of fiber the Finnish get from rye. Hard evidence to explain this seeming discrepancy was unavailable until the recent discovery of fecapentaene. Fecapentaenes are found in the stools of people on fiber-depleted diets who have a high incidence of colon cancer. This chemical, produced by bacteria in the large bowel and then released by them when they die, is not present in fiber-eating populations who are free from colon cancer.[12,13] Fecapentaene is a very potent mutagen, as potent as one of the most potent carcinogens that we know, benzopyrene. When fiber is added to the diet, the bacteria stay healthy: they don't die and they don't release the fecapentaene.

Breast cancer and its association with fat intake is among the most widely and well studied of all cancers and risks. People who migrate from low to high risk countries start increasing their fat consumption and thereby increasing their risk for developing breast cancer.[14] For example, the diet in Japan began changing in the 1950s. The Japanese began to eat more fat and consume more calories and, as a result, they actually grew in stature. With the changing diet, especially among the younger women, the rates of breast cancer, colon cancer, and prostate cancer began to climb.[15] When Japanese immigrated to California and adopted United States eating habits, their breast cancer and colon cancer rates rose. The same phenomenon is seen when women move from Southern Italy where the breast cancer rates are generally low to Australia where they are high. When the women adopt the high-fat Australian diet, the breast cancer rates begin to rise. Dietary changes may have an impact on hormonal changes especially in young women when the breast tissue is forming, and this might affect breast cancer risk over a lifetime. There is probably a benefit of changing dietary factors even when you are older as well.[16] All other migration studies show a relationship between changing diet and increased cancer risk.

In another group of epidemiological studies, newly diagnosed breast cancer patients are asked what foods they had eaten. Of the sixteen well controlled studies like this, eleven show a positive association between the intake of fat and the occurrence of breast cancer.[17-26] All these human studies have been backed up and supported by innumerable studies showing the same association in animals: A high-fat diet is linked to a high risk for developing breast cancer. So there is good evidence from animal studies, international migration studies, and time trend studies all supporting the fact that high fat, low fiber is linked to breast cancer and other cancers.

In 1992, results of the Nurses Health Study, which involved 89,494 women,[27] were published. The authors wrongly concluded that there is no relationship between fat intake and the risk of breast cancer. There are a number of flaws in this study, now reviewed by many scientist-physicians, which led to the improper conclusion. First of all, the questionnaire was sent through the mail, which can lead to self-reporting errors. Most people tend to underestimate their consumption of fat and/or other unhealthy foods particularly when they have heard in the media for the last ten years that a high-fat diet is not healthy. Secondly, this study involved only eight years, most cancers take decades to develop. Thirdly, the study targeted mainly middle-aged women and totally ignored diet earlier in life, a time which is extremely critical in breast cancer development. And further, the great majority of women consumed 32 percent of their total calories from fat, a number that is not that low at all. And, in fact, another group of investigators showed that the women involved in the Nurses Health Study demonstrated both recall and selection bias when describing their dietary habits and the percentage of calories from fat is actually higher than 32.[28] Yet another study shows similar faulty recall by patients.[29] In countries like Japan where breast cancer rates are comparatively low, Japanese women consume 20 percent of their calories in fat. And the author of the Nurses Health Study freely admits that low-fat diets, 20 percent or less fat calories, probably do have a beneficial effect on lowering the risk of breast cancer and dietary tumors.[30] Other studies that are similar to the Nurses Health Study all show that fat consumption is related to an increased risk of developing breast cancer.[31-38]

Another study shows that breast cancer mortality significantly correlates with an intestinal enzyme called lactase.[39] Lactase is responsible for the digestion of the milk sugar lactose. The enzyme is present in all mammals at birth and then starts to decrease after weaning, so that the adult human usually is incapable of digesting milk and many milk products. Exceptions to this pattern include populations of northwestern European origin (including the United States, Australia, and Canada) and scattered groups in other areas of the world in whom the enzyme is still present in varying amounts. These people historically consume a large number of dairy products compared to other populations. Asians, Africans, and Mexicans, on the other hand, rarely have the enzyme lactase after childhood, and breast cancer mortality is only a small fraction of that seen in peoples who originate from northwestern Europe. This study confirmed the findings of other investigations showing that breast cancer mortality is closely associated with the consumption of animal fat, milk, butter, and total calories.

Milk may be related to cancer in several ways. Milk consumption may contribute to the production of carcinogenic estrogens and other carcinogens by changing the type of bacteria in the intestine (more anaerobes) or by increasing the amount of cholesterol and bile acids available for the production of estrogens and other carcinogens. Also, it is known that mouse milk harbors a certain virus that can cause breast cancer in mice. When mouse milk is fed to baby mice, the cancer-producing virus is passed along and causes breast cancer. Milk from cows with leukemia harbors a cancer-producing virus that is infectious for several species. It is altogether possible, but not proven, that a cancer-producing virus in cow's milk may be passed along to humans who consume milk. Virus particles that can cause cancer have been found in human milk. In addition, a person is exposed to other contaminants in milk. For example, DES (diethylstilbestrol) is used as a growth promoter for cattle. The amount of DES in milk is very small and probably cannot cause human breast cancer. However, there is no information concerning chronic low-level exposure to DES and its effect on cancer development. Additional contaminants that may inadvertently be included in milk are pesticides, industrial contaminants, and heavy metals.

A high-animal-fat diet can favor the development of breast cancer for many reasons. First, the typical high-fat American diet produces large amounts of sterol chemicals and bile acids in the intestine. Bacteria that normally live in our intestines can alter the sterol chemicals and bile acids produced by a high-fat diet to produce certain carcinogenic estrogens and other carcinogens affecting the breast.[40-42] This fact is supported by a great amount of research that has been reviewed by S.H. Brammer and colleagues.[43]

Second, large amounts of fatty tissue in the breasts may lead to greater amounts of estrogens in these tissues locally, which can be carcinogenic. An increased incidence of breast cancer is seen in heavier women who tend to have larger breasts and subsequently more fatty tissue in them.

Third, it has been shown that dietary polyunsaturated fats enhance cancer development. They do so more than saturated fats, presumably by increasing the hormone called prolactin.[44] A woman who eats a high-fat diet, especially one high in unsaturated fats, has a very high blood prolactin level.[45] High prolactin levels are also found in women who have their first pregnancies late in life; this may account for such women's high risk of developing breast cancer.

Polyunsaturated fats not only increase prolactin levels but can also be easily attacked by chemical-free radicals. As we discussed in Chapter 7, this is another mechanism by which polyunsaturated fats can lead to the development of cancer. Furthermore, polyunsaturated fatty acids in the serum may inhibit the normal function of the immune system and thus favor cancer development. And finally, the more polyunsaturated fats there are in cell membranes, the more susceptible the cell is to carcinogenic agents.

Substances in breast fluid may also have an influence on the development of breast cancer. Breast fluid secretion occurs in most women, but in varying amounts. For example, Oriental women have much less breast fluid secretion than white women, and they also have a lower incidence of breast cancer. Breast fluid bathes the ductal cells of the breast gland. Many of the breast cancers originate in the ductal cells of the gland, so the fluid that bathes the cells may have an effect on the development of cancer. A study involving 252 Finnish women revealed that about one-third of them had very high prolactin levels in their breast fluid compared to the amount in their blood. However, this study by P. Hill has not yet been extended for a long enough period of time to determine whether this group will eventually develop breast cancer. The prolactin content of breast fluid from Oriental women has not yet been determined, so no conclusion can be made concerning breast fluid prolactin level and its effect on the development of breast cancer.

A chemical substance derived from cholesterol called cholesterol epoxide has been found in human breast fluid.[46] The higher the blood cholesterol level, the higher the cholesterol epoxide level in breast fluid. Cholesterol epoxide is carcinogenic in animals. Its carcinogenic potential in humans is very real. Hence, this is another reason to keep your blood cholesterol level low—so that your breast fluid level of cholesterol epoxide is also low and lessens the potential risk of cancer development.

Nicotine and its close relative cotinine have been shown to appear in breast fluid within five minutes after smoking. So far no studies have shown a conclusive relationship between smoking and the development of breast cancer. However, it is well known that there are fifteen carcinogens derived from smoking. And the fact that nicotine can be detected in breast fluid indicates that many other environmental factors may be present, a number of which may be carcinogenic. Chemicals may be held in breast fluid longer than in the blood because there are more lipids inside the breast. Therefore, known risk factors for cancer in general, such as tobacco smoking, should be eliminated altogether because carcinogens get into breast fluid, bathe breast tissue for long periods of time, and may lead to the development of cancer.

The bottom line is that high-fat diets are correlated with a higher risk of developing breast cancer and other cancers like colon, prostate, endometrium, etc. There is no rational reason to suggest or recommend any diet other than one low in fat. I recommend 20 percent or less of your calories be derived from fats.

Some women substitute soy products for red meat and dairy products thinking soy has less fat. *Not only is soy high in fat, it is also high in estrogen compounds, substances that women, especially breast cancer patients, should stay away from.*

Epidemiological Study of Dietary Factors

One of the largest epidemiological studies done of dietary and other factors in both China and the United States has been completed by Cornell University. This study was begun in 1983 and completed in 1990. A total of 6,500 Chinese participated in the study, and each contributed 367 facts about his or her eating practices and other habits.

The study found that the Chinese consume 20 percent more calories than Americans but that Americans are more obese. Chinese people eat only one-third of the amount of fat that Americans do and eat twice as much starch. Our government agencies recommend that Americans reduce calories from fat to 30 percent; however, I recommend only 15–20 percent of total calories from fat. The level of 30 percent may not be little enough to curb the risk of heart disease and cancer, as demonstrated by this Chinese study.

The Cornell University study also showed that Americans consume 33 percent more protein than the Chinese and that 70 percent of this protein comes from animal sources, compared to only 7 percent coming from animals for the Chinese. The Chinese who eat the most protein have more heart disease, cancer, and diabetes.

Diets rich in fat and high in calories and protein also promote growth and early menarche, which, as we discussed, has been associated with higher cancer rates, especially breast cancer. Chinese women rarely suffer from these cancers and start menstruating three to six years later than American women.

Osteoporosis is very uncommon in China. Unlike Americans, the Chinese do not consume dairy products; instead they get all their calcium from vegetables. They consume only half as much calcium as Americans and yet do not have osteoporosis. This indicates that calcium derived from dairy products is certainly not needed, and since dairy products contribute to the fat content of your diet, it is wise to limit or avoid their consumption.

While Chinese people are a genetically similar population, there are differences in dietary habits, environmental exposures, and disease rates in China from region to region. For instance, the cancer rate varies by a factor of several hundred from one region to another. In poor areas of China, infectious disease is the leading cause of death. In areas that are more affluent, heart disease, diabetes, and cancer are more often seen. These differences are typical and confirm what we have said: Chronic illnesses including cancer, diabetes, and heart disease are more prevalent in affluent countries than in poorer ones. These facts make this an important study, since the genetic contribution to cancer in China is minimal. Any differences in cancer rates and other chronic illnesses, like heart disease, can therefore be attributed to dietary and other environmental exposures.

As with most other studies, high cholesterol levels were shown to be predecessors of cancer, heart disease, diabetes, and other chronic diseases. The Chinese study showed that low cholesterol protects against heart disease and also cancer, especially colon cancer. What is considered to be a high cholesterol level in China is thought to be low in the United States. In other words, the range of normal cholesterol levels for the Chinese is much lower than our levels.

The Chinese diet contains three times the dietary fiber of the typical American diet. The average intake of fiber in China is 33 grams a day with a high of 77 grams in some regions. Those with the highest fiber intakes also had the least diseases as outlined on tables 8.2 and 8.3.

FATS

Dietary animal fat is found in all red meat, luncheon meats, and all dairy products, including milk, cheese, and eggs. Dietary animal fat promotes and initiates carcinogenesis.[47-67] Epidemiological studies have repeatedly shown an association between consumption of dietary fat and the occurrence of cancer at several sites, especially the breast, the prostate and colon/rectal area, the endometrium, and, to a lesser extent, the ovary. High fat consumption is related not only to the high incidence of breast cancer but also to the high mortality rates from breast cancer.[68-73] Some studies show a correlation with saturated fats, but other studies show a correlation with both saturated and unsaturated fats.[74] Low breast cancer rates are seen in peoples who consume low-fat diets, such as the Japanese, Seventh-Day Adventists, and Mormons in the United States.

Early life exposures are the important determinants of breast cancer risk for dietary fat. The studies citing changing rates of colon cancer as well as breast cancer in some Japanese immigrants to the United States suggest that the older the Japanese immigrant to the United States, the less her risk of developing breast cancer and colon cancer. However, you must remember, older Japanese women would be less apt to adopt American dietary customs.

The issue of an inverse relationship between serum cholesterol and cancer of the colon was thought to be significant at one time. However, a thorough examination of all the data revealed that the information was

Table 8.2 Comparison of Chinese and Western
Normal Blood Values

Blood Component	Chinese Range	Western Range
Cholesterol	88–165 mg/dl	155–274 mg/dl
HDL cholesterol	25–60 mg/dl	30–70 mg/dl
LDL cholesterol	41–128 mg/dl	90–205 mg/dl
Hemoglobin		
men	11–16 gm	14–17 gm
women	10–15 gm	12–15 gm

Table 8.3 Comparison of Chinese and Western Daily
Nutrient Consumption

Nutrient	Chinese Consumption	Western Consumption
Total protein	40–90 gm	39–192 gm
Plant protein	31–98 gm	27 gm
Dietary fiber	8–77 gm	3–21 gm
Starch	190–610 gm	120 gm
Vitamin C	6–429 mg	7–315 mg
Calories	1,800–3,700	1,090–3,800
Fat (percentage of calories)	5.9–25%	40%

Source: Nutrition, Environment and Health Project, Chinese Academy of Preventive Medicine—Cornell-Oxford.

inconclusive and did not point to a causal relationship between low cholesterol levels and the risk of colon cancer. In fact, the National Institutes of Health Consensus Conference stated that there was no relationship between low blood cholesterol and colon cancer.

The prognosis for patients with breast cancer differs from one country to another. A better survival rate is seen in Japanese patients than in United States patients.[75-77] The differences are thought to be related to fat consumption.[78-83] Neither the clinical extent of disease nor histology was the basis for the differences seen in survival. Disease-free survival was also greater for Japanese women than American women.[84] In a study conducted in Hawaii, the medical care given to Japanese women and Caucasian women was the same, so the differences in survival could not be attributed to differences in treatment.[85]

Several studies have indicated that increased body weight may decrease both disease-free survival and overall survival in breast cancer patients.[86-88] The lowest five-year disease-free survival in patients was noted in patients with high weights (more than 150 pounds) and high cholesterol (above median), and the highest five-year disease-free survival rate was noted in those with low weights (less than 150 pounds) and low cholesterol (below median).[89] Dietary fat and obesity clearly influence the patient's prognosis, but the mechanism by which it does is not well understood. Several theories have been posed to explain the reactions that are triggered by increased body weight and dietary fat, including abnormalities in the pattern of prolactin secretion,[90] decreased levels of gonadotropins,[91] increased conversion of androstenedione to estrone,[92] or altered sex hormone binding globulin, free androgen, and free estrogen.[93]

There are several mechanisms by which dietary animal fat promotes and initiates carcinogenesis. It increases bile acids and bile steroids. It also significantly increases the number of colonic anaerobic bacteria, which then form carcinogens from bile acids. Certain bacterial enzymes are induced by beef for its digestion. These same enzymes can change cocarcinogens into carcinogens. As was already discussed, a potent fecal mutagen called fecapentaene probably also plays an important role in the development of colon cancer.

Dietary animal fat also weakens the immune system by decreasing antibody production and impairing the function of T cells and phagocytes.[94] Cholesterol oleate and ethyl palmitate inhibit antibody production, probably because these lipids do not allow the immune system to recognize a foreign substance.[95] In addition, the structure of a fat makes it easily susceptible to attack by free radicals and increases the cell's susceptibility to carcinogens. This is more true for unsaturated fats than it is for saturated fats, because the unsaturated fats act as a natural sink for these highly unstable free-radical chemicals.

Because of the preceding data, it is worthwhile to put breast cancer patients on a low-fat, high-fiber diet to test the hypothesis. Another reason to increase dietary fiber in breast cancer patients is that it has been shown to increase the fecal excretion of estrogen and to decrease the plasma concentration of estrogen.[96] In fact, it might be wise to extend this modified diet to other diet-sensitive tumors—colon and rectal, prostate, and endometrial cancers, for example—in an attempt to increase disease-free survival as well as survival in general.

PROTEIN AND CARBOHYDRATES

High amounts of daily protein cause a high incidence of carcinogenesis in animals.[97] In many animal studies, carcinogenesis was suppressed when animals were fed levels of protein that were at the minimum or below the minimum required for optimal growth.

There has been a fair amount of epidemiological human data to support the contention that total protein intake will correlate with the incidence of and mortality from cancers of various sites.[98] This correlation has been seen for breast cancer[99–101] and colon and rectal cancer.[102,103] There has also been a weaker association between high protein intake and other cancers, specifically pancreatic cancer, prostate cancer, and endometrial cancer.

Many of the studies included the consumption of fat as well as protein. Because there are two variables, it is not possible to say with any certainty that high protein per se will be a factor in the cancers described.

The evidence linking pure sugars to the incidence of cancer is much weaker. A high dietary intake of refined sugar was one of the dietary components linked to the increased incidence of breast cancer in several studies.[104,105] To date, the evidence from both epidemiological and laboratory studies is too inconclusive to suggest any role for carbohydrates in carcinogenesis. But as we have already discussed, excessive carbohydrate ingestion contributes to obesity, which, in turn, has been implicated in carcinogenesis.

NATURALLY OCCURRING CARCINOGENS AND MUTAGENS

Some foods have naturally occurring carcinogens or mutagens. Plants have certain molecules to protect them against microorganisms and insects, and some of these are carcinogenic or mutagenic in humans.

For instance, certain human foods contain nicotine, especially plants from the family *Solanaceae* (potatoes, tomatoes, eggplant). Table 8.4 lists various vegetables assayed,[106–109] their content of nicotine, and importantly, the amount of that vegetable that must be consumed to equal the amount of nicotine absorbed over three hours by a person inhaling other people's smoke in a room with a minimal amount of tobacco smoke. Eggplant has the highest amount of nicotine compared to the other foods assayed. Although there is no cotinine (breakdown product of nicotine) in these foods, it may show up in the bloodstream of people eating these foods.

Some other foods and the carcinogens they contain are: black pepper (piperine and safrole), bruised celery (psoralen), herbal teas (pyrrolizidine, phorbol esters), mushrooms (hydrazines), and all foods containing mold (aflatoxin) or certain bacteria (nitrosamines).[110–116] A complete review of these is given by Ames.[117] Many of these are occasional contaminants, whereas others are normal components of relatively common foods, as you can see. All foods contianing mold, which produces toxic compounds called aflatoxin, are carcinogenic, as are foods containing certain bacteria (nitrosomonas).

Some foods also contain mutagens, which are chemical com-

Table 8.4   Nicotine Content in Vegetables

Vegetable	Microgram Nicotine Per Gram Vegetable	Portion of Vegetable Needed to Attain 1 Microgram Nicotine
Eggplant	0.1	10 grams
Potato	0.007	140 grams
Tomato (ripe)	0.004	244 grams
Cauliflower	0.0038	260 grams
Green Peppers	0	0
Black Tea	0	0

pounds that cause heritable changes in the genetic material of cells. Many vegetables contain mutagenic flavonoids, and mutagens are seen in charred and smoked foods. Mutagens can also be produced at lower temperatures, such as from the normal cooking of meat. Other commonly consumed items like coffee and horseradish also contain mutagens (quinones and allyl isothiocyanate, respectively).[118] The overall risk of human beings' developing cancer from mutagens is thought to be minimal.

DIETARY TRENDS FOR FAT AND CHOLESTEROL

It has been estimated that if Americans reduce their caloric fat content from 40 percent to just 30 percent, about 42,000 of the 2.3 million annual deaths in the United States could be deferred.[119] This represents about a 2 percent benefit of three to four months increase in life, mainly to those over age sixty-five.

The third National Health and Nutrition Examination Survey (NHANES III), conducted by the National Center for Health Statistics of the Center for Disease Control and Prevention (CDC), showed that there is a continuing decline in serum cholesterol levels among adults in the United States.[120] However, the federally sponsored study called Healthy People 2000 had a goal of reducing the average cholesterol level of United States adults to 200 mg/dL; this goal may or may not be attainable.[121] And if this goal is to be attained, it has been estimated that one-third of American adults will require dietary intervention.[122,123]

I don't think this goal can be attained and one-third is a *gross underestimation* because when one examines how well patients follow through and adhere to dietary advice given them, a very different picture emerges.

A large study was done to determine if dietary advice could prevent a second heart attack in people who had just suffered their first. Over 2,000 patients were divided into three groups. One group received dietary advice on how to reduce fat intake, another group received advice on how to increase fatty fish intake, and the third group received advice on how to increase cereal fiber. The group given advice on fat intake had no difference in mortality—their serum cholesterols did not change. Those advised to eat fatty fish had almost a 30 percent reduction in two-year mortality compared with those who were not advised. The third group evidenced no difference in mortality. This study indicates that even after getting advice about the proper thing to do, people rarely follow the advice. The study group simply would not reduce their red meat intake. One group did increase the fatty fish consumption and benefited from that.[124] This study indicates that unless there is a strong motivating factor, and it is hard to imagine that a person's life is not such a motivating factor, people simply will not change habits even though they are told it will benefit them medically.

And this is not one isolated study. Other studies and polls show people are no longer following sound medical advice about life-style even though they have been given this information in one form or another.[125–128] People who are aware of the health benefits of a low-fat, high-fiber diet supplemented with certain nutrients chose, instead, to eat high-fat snacks, and gained an average of two to four pounds in 1993. This "pleasure revenge," as *The New York Times* labels it, is seen most often among the affluent and well-educated people who previously led the health and fitness frenzy ten years ago. People now are giving themselves permission to be unhealthy—not worrying about weight or smoking cessation. Consider the facts:

- In a 1992 survey, 30 percent of the respondents said they were smokers, compared to 25 percent in 1991 (Princeton Survey Research, 1,250 adults polled).
- In 1992, 39 percent of diabetics said they did everything "they could to eat a healthy diet" compared to 44 percent in 1991 (American Dietetic Association, 1,000 polled).
- A major fast-food chain's lean hamburger is doing less well now compared to its new half-pounder with cheese.
- In 1993, 850,000 copies of an anti-diet book were printed, compared to 450,000 copies of an anti-heart disease book in 1992. The trend for non-self-help books is increasing.
- Massage is more popular than exercise.
- Spending on diet-product advertising was down $309 million in 1993, on non-diet, up $1.6 billion.
- People who worked out four times a week several years ago are now going to the gym only two or three times a week.

- Beef sales rose in 1993.
- Cheese sales reached an all-time high in 1993.
- Sale of high-fat superpremium ice cream rose 8 percent in 1993.

Table 8.5 Total Sales of High- and Low-Calorie Foods in 1993

High-Calorie Foods	Low-Calorie Foods
Butter ↑$362 million	Margarine ↓$116 million
Soda ↑$122 million	Diet soda ↓$41 million
Sugar ↓$4 million	Sugar substitute ↓$49 million
Ice cream ↑$45 million	Yogurt ↑$16 million
Fast food ↑$418 million	Fruit ↓$4 million
Cookies ↑$154 million	Popcorn ↓$35 million

Source: Competitive Media Reporting, January 1994

People know what is good for their health, but the trend, apparently, is for many people to indulge themselves (see Table 8.5) and do what they want, when they want. This unhealthy trend is happening at a time when the cost for health-care is rising. Who do you think is going to pay for all this indulgence? And why should people who are striving to be healthy pay for others who indulge themselves?

9
Obesity

Obesity affects about 35 percent of all Americans. Being obese carries with it a social stigma as well as a general health risk. One study calculated that there are 832 million pounds of excess fat on American men and 1,468 million pounds of excess fat on American women, for a total of 2.3 billion pounds.[1] More obesity occurs in middle-aged people and in people with low socioeconomic status. The percentage of African-American women who are obese is greater than the percentage of white women. Adopted children become obese if adoptive family members are obese.

The fat cell *size* is increased in all types of obesity. An increased *number* of fat cells is found in children and adults who were obese before the age of two. Statistics show that if a child is obese before the age of two, he will likely be obese in adulthood because he already has an increased number of fat cells. It is ideal, then, not to allow a baby to become fat; otherwise, the resulting fat cells will remain for the rest of his life. It is more difficult for an obese patient to lose weight if she was obese before age two; in other words, it is more difficult for an obese patient to lose weight if she has more fat cells than normal. Only 1 percent of obesity is caused by a disease or medical problem; 99 percent of all obesity is directly related to overeating—make no mistake about that!.

Because obese individuals tend to develop a variety of diseases, some of which are life-threatening, obese adults have a higher than normal death rate for their age group. The risk of death correlates almost directly with how much a person is overweight. Even if you are only a little overweight, you still have an increased risk of death compared to a person who is not overweight.

There have been several studies suggesting that longevity is correlated with factors that limit the adult body size. In 1935, C.M. McCay showed that feeding rats a low-protein diet yielded lean animals that lived much longer than animals fed high-protein diets.[2] Many more of these types of experiments were completed by Dr. Robert A. Good and colleagues at Memorial Sloan-Kettering Hospital in New York City.[3,4] They have had similar results: animals with lean body mass live much longer. Many human studies have now been done and show that obesity decreases longevity.[5] This finding has been corroborated. In addition, investigations by Tannenbaum,[6] Kraybill,[7] and others[8-10] have shown that animals with lean body masses have lower rates of cancer development as well as greater longevity.

Epidemiological studies also show the same correlation. In one study, when per capita total caloric intake was examined relative to cancer incidence in twenty-three countries and to cancer mortality in thirty-two countries, a significant correlation was found between total calories and each of the following: the incidence of rectal cancer in males, the incidence of leukemia in males, and the rate of mortality from breast cancer in females.[11] Another researcher found obesity to be a factor in breast cancer in the United States as well.[12] Among postmenopausal women studied in the Netherlands, heavier and taller women were found to have a higher rate of breast cancer.[13] This same correlation was seen in other studies.[14,15] Because of all these well-planned studies, the National Dairy Council issued the following statement in 1975: "Of all dietary modification studies, caloric restriction has had the most regular influence on the genesis of neoplasms in experimental animals."[16]

The American Cancer Society sponsored a study from 1959 to 1972 in which mortality from cancer and other diseases among 750,000 men and women was recorded and compared with their weights. Those who were overweight by 40 percent had a significantly higher cancer mortality rate. For men, the mortality was from cancer of the colon and rectum; for women, from cancer of the gallbladder, biliary passages, breast, cervix, endometrium, and ovary. Many other studies confirm the relationship between obesity and increased risk of cancers in various sites.

Obese postmenopausal women have a higher rate of breast cancer because they have more estrogens circulating in their bodies than those who are not obese. More estrogens are produced from the adrenal glands and fat cells.[17-20] The main site of this higher amount of estrogen production is in the fat cell, converting adrostenedione to estrone, a more carcinogenic estrogen.[21]

After the age of thirty-five, a woman accumulates more fat in the breast regardless of overall body weight. Breast fat then serves as a local source of estrone (a hormone) production. In fact, estrogen and estrone levels in breast fluid are ten to forty times the levels normally found in serum of menstruating, nonlactating women.[22,23] This alone will increase the risk for developing breast cancer.

Armed with this information, women should reduce their weight by restricting calories and fat. This should lower the production of estrogen and estrone, which in turn should decrease the risk of breast cancer. Several studies, including the Women's Health Trial, have been done to assess hormone production on a low-fat diet.[24-28] Although these studies only reviewed the effects of modifying dietary fat instead of total weight reduction (which would include calorie restriction), some conclusions can be made:

1. Reducing dietary fat from 35 percent to 23 percent resulted in a decrease of estrogen and estrone levels by 30 percent in three to six months.

2. Reducing dietary fat modestly and adding 35 grams of fiber per day resulted in a decrease of estradiol levels by about 15 percent.

Multiple studies have repeatedly shown that obesity is associated with more advanced breast cancers at the time of diagnosis, higher recurrence rates, and shorter survival times[29-34] even after allowing for other factors that do shorten survival like tumor size, lymph node involvement, etc. (see chapters 21 and 22).

When a statistical analysis of eleven studies was done, body weight and body mass (surface area) were significant risk factors for causing breast cancers that were, in fact, more advanced.[35] Originally this was explained as a result of delayed diagnosis in obese women (more difficult to find tumor, which is still, in part, true) rather than more aggressive cancer promotion from higher amounts of estrogen. But recently, it has been shown that postmenopausal women who have estrogen-receptor positive tumors have more invasive cancers than women whose receptor status is negative.[36] Among women who had breast cancers with positive estrogen receptors and positive axillary lymph nodes, about 66 percent were obese, and 33 percent were not obese. No such association with obesity and lymph nodes was demonstrated for patients with negative estrogen receptors indicating that obesity with its hormonal changes accounts for breast cancer promotion and aggressiveness.

The risk of postmenopausal breast cancer is higher in adults who gain weight, particularly in the abdomen, and this is independent of original body weight.[37-41] Postmenopausal women who have a waist size much larger than their hips, also have a higher rate of breast cancer.[42] Obese women with a large waist who lose more than 4.5 kg (10 pounds) can lower their increased risk of breast cancer by 45 percent.[43]

Obesity is a major risk factor for the development of endometrial cancer (cancer of the inner lining of the uterus) in postmenopausal women. Obese postmenopausal women produce a lot more of the female hormone called estrone, which is directly related to the number and size of the woman's fat cells. Estrone constantly stimulates the uterus, and this is believed to cause endometrial cancer. Similarly, postmenopausal women who take estrogens daily for symptoms of menopause also have a higher incidence of endometrial cancer. The mechanism is presumably the same. Most obese women have lesser symptoms of menopause than thinner women, presumably because of their increased production of estrone.

People who are obese usually consume more fats in their diet; this is a major risk factor for the development of breast cancer and colon cancer.[44] Both height and weight are positively associated with cancer in postmenopausal women. An animal study showed that if food intake was reduced (the number of calories decreased) during a "critical period" after a carcinogen was given to induce breast cancer, the development of the cancer was inhibited[45] as a result of low production of two hormones, prolactin and estrogen. Leaner animals produce less of these two hormones, which in high amounts can lead to the development of cancer.

In addition, obesity can adversely affect the body's response to infection. Obese animals have more severe infections and higher death rates from the infections.[46] Diets that are high in fat depress a person's resistance to tuberculosis, malaria, and pneumococcus (an often severe pneumonia). The incidence of pneumonia is significantly higher in obese infants than in nonobese infants.[47] Adverse effects on the immune system or poor lung ventilation due to obesity have been suggested as possible reasons for severe pneumonias in these infants. The antibody response also diminishes with obesity in women.[48]

An obese person has a two or three times higher risk of developing diabetes. Obesity interferes with the action of insulin, the hormone that normally packs sugar into the cells of the body. When insulin is interfered with, the blood-sugar level goes very high. If this person loses weight, insulin can then work properly and usually return the blood-sugar level to normal.

An obese person has an increased risk of developing cardiovascular disease. The reasons for increased heart attacks are not clear but may be related to increased blood lipids associated with obesity. Obese people tend to have higher blood cholesterol and triglycerides. If the obese person loses weight, the high blood levels of cholesterol and triglyceride return to normal.

A prospective study showed that even women who are only mildly to moderately overweight have an increase in their risk of developing coronary heart disease.[49] Obesity was found to be an independent risk factor again. Another study showed that men who are obese in the central portion of their bodies, that is, those who have a "beer belly," also have a higher risk of developing coronary artery disease independent of all other risk factors.[50] An older person who is only moderately overweight has a twofold higher risk of death.[51]

Overweight people have a higher incidence of hypertension, which itself contributes to the risk of coronary heart disease, heart attacks, and stroke.[52] The left ventricle of the heart, which is the chamber that pumps blood into the arteries, becomes thickened in mass with hypertension and other heart diseases. Obviously, this impairs heart function and is detrimental to health. It has been found, however, that when people start to lose weight, the thickness of the left ventricle becomes less.[53]

Obesity contributes to the development of gallbladder disease and also is a risk factor for major respiratory problems. Some massively obese individuals have trouble breathing because the weight of the chest is so great that the individual's chest muscles have difficulty lifting it. Being overweight also causes too much wear and tear on bone joints and leads to the early development of joint problems.

ATTAINING YOUR IDEAL WEIGHT

How much should a person weigh? There is no one answer, but here is a good rule of thumb. Men who are 5 feet tall should weigh 110 pounds. For every one inch over 5 feet, add another 5 pounds. Thus, if a man is 5 feet 11 inches tall, his ideal weight is about 165 pounds. Women who are 5 feet tall should weigh about 100 pounds. For every one inch over 5 feet, add 5 pounds. Therefore, if a woman is 5 feet 6 inches tall, her ideal weight is about 130 pounds.

Attaining your ideal weight is not always easy. Although it is crucial that you give up smoking, quitting can lead to weight gain. Those who quit often crave sweets. Unfortunately, many sweets—cookies, cakes, chocolate bars—are laden with fat, and fat consumption increases your risk of breast cancer. In addition, people who quit smoking have a much lower energy output than smokers regardless of whether they are busy at work or home or even resting.[54] It appears that nicotine is responsible for increasing the rate at which smokers burn calories. Hence, people gain weight when they stop smoking because they eat foods that are high in calories, and they burn less calories when working or resting.[55]

If you do need to lose weight, you should do it gradually. Losing one or two pounds a week is safe, and that loss will probably be maintained. Do not lose more weight than called for by the formula. Successful weight loss and maintenance of that loss will be achieved only if you totally modify your eating habits. Many people are put on high-protein liquid diets consisting of 800 calories a day and lose a great deal of weight within the first few weeks. But on a long-term basis, these pounds come right back on because the person did not learn new eating habits. Diets containing less than 800 calories per day may be dangerous if the person is not closely monitored by a physician.

Most people do lose weight on reducing diets, but they invariably gain it back along with some additional pounds. This self-inflicted fluctuation in body weight usually happens many times in a person's life. A number of studies have shown that repeated fluctuation in body weight per se has negative consequences on a person's health.[56–58] A person whose body weight fluctuates often or greatly has a much higher risk of developing coronary heart disease and dying than does a person who has a relatively stable body weight. Those aged thirty to forty-four were shown to suffer the most detrimental effects of weight fluctuation. These harmful effects of weight fluctuation were independent of degree of obesity or existing cardiovascular risk factors.

To lose weight, you must eat less and increase your physical activity. Every pound of fat you have contains about 3,500 calories. Therefore, to lose one pound, you have to burn off 3,500 calories more than you eat. You will lose a pound a week if you burn off 500 calories per day more than you consume. In other words, if you eat a diet containing 1,200 calories per day and burn off 1,700 calories per day, you will lose one pound a week.

Before you start a physical exercise program, you should be checked by a physician. An exercise program should start out gradually, with new goals set every week. Walking is very good exercise. Table 9.1 shows approximately how many calories are used up by a 150-pound person performing various activities.

If you lose weight suddenly or without a good reason, see a physician. Unexplained weight loss can be a sign of cancer or another serious medical problem.

Table 9.1 Activities and the Calories They Burn

Activities	Calories Used Per Hour	Activities	Calories Used Per Hour
Job		**Recreation (cont.)**	
Answering telephone	50	Calisthenics	500
Bathing	100	Card playing	25
Bed making	300	Cycling slowly (5 ½ mph)	300
Brushing teeth or hair	100	Cycling strenuously	
Chopping wood	400	(13 mph)	660
Dishwashing	75	Dancing, slow step	350
Dressing, undressing	50	Dancing, fast step	600
Driving automobile	120	Fishing	150
Dusting furniture	150	Football	600
Eating	50	Golfing	250
Filing (office)	200	Handball	660
Gardening	250	Hiking	400
Housework	180	Horseback riding	250
Ironing	100	Jogging	600
Mopping floors	200	Kissing vigorously	6–12
Mowing lawn	250	Lovemaking	125–300
Preparing food	100	Painting	150
Reading	25	Piano playing	75
Sawing	500	Running, fast pace	900
Sewing	50	Singing	50
Shoveling	500	Skating leisurely	400
Sitting	100	Skating rapidly	600
Sleeping	80	Skiing (10 mph)	600
Standing	140	Soccer	650
Typing	50	Swimming leisurely	
Walking upstairs		(¼ mph)	400
and down	800	Swimming rapidly	800
		Tennis, singles	450
Recreation		Tennis, doubles	350
Badminton	400	Volleyball	350
Baseball	350	Walking leisurely	
Basketball	550	(2 ½ mph)	200
Boating, rowing	400	Walking quickly (3 ¾ mph)	300
Boating, motor	150	Watching television	25
Bowling	250		

Source: Department of Agriculture, 1980, from data prepared by Dr. Robert Johnson at the University of Illinois.

Even though it is very difficult to lose weight, you must try if you are overweight because of the tremendous benefits of being at your ideal weight. Obesity has no benefits, and its risks are very great.

10
Food Additives, Contaminants, and Pesticides

Chemical food additives and food contaminants have been quite extensively studied, more so than most other chemicals that come into contact with our bodies—with good reason. Only carefully selected chemicals can prevent contamination and spoilage of food that has to be produced in great quantities, stored, and transported. Chemicals are also used for flavoring and appearance. Chemical contaminants may develop as a result of food processing procedures such as irradiation, cooking, pickling, or smoking. The trouble with the use of chemicals in food is that we are exposed to them constantly, repeatedly, and at low doses. For this reason, it is difficult to ascertain from studies whether these chemicals can cause cancer; therefore, laboratory investigations rather than large population studies must be conducted to find out whether the chemicals are potentially hazardous.

The "Delaney clause" of the Federal Food, Drug, and Cosmetic Act, written because of food additives, prohibits the addition of any known carcinogens to food. Currently there are about 3,000 intentional food additives. One is nitrite, which can be converted in the body to a potent carcinogen, nitrosamine. There are over 12,000 occasionally detected unintentional additives from packaging, food processing, and other phases of the food industry. Those in the unintentional category that are of some concern to us are vinyl chloride and diethylstilbestrol, which are used in food packaging and processing and in the foods fed to much livestock. The overall risk of human cancer from food additives is thought to be quite minimal at this time, however.

Chemical food additives are divided into several groups. *Intentional* food additives are chemicals that are purposely added to food. Some of these definitely produce cancers in animals, but others do not produce such clear results. Thiourea[1] and butter yellow[2] produce cancers in animals and are no longer used in food. A very important antioxidant presently used in foods, butylated hydroxytoluene, is reported to enhance certain animal cancers[3] but inhibit some carcinogens.[4] Red No. 2 and Red No. 40 dyes have both been banned because they are not safe according to the Food and Drug Administration.

Cyclamate has not been shown to be carcinogenic in humans, but its metabolite (chemical breakdown product) does produce testicular atrophy (shrinking) in rats. Saccharin, another highly publicized intentional food additive, does produce bladder cancer in rats when comprising 5 percent or more in the diet.[5] Epidemiological studies show that saccharin does not pose a major cancer risk to man;[6] however, it is generally agreed that additional studies are needed concerning the effects of saccharin on man before conclusive statements can be made. Xylitol, a new sweetener compound, also has been reported to give rise to bladder cancer in mice and to adrenal cancer in rats.[7]

Nitrite is a most important food additive. Nitrites are used as preservatives in meats to prevent botulism. They also add color to certain meats, especially bacon and hot dogs. Look at the label of ingredients on your package of bacon or hot dogs—nitrites are probably listed. Nitrites can react with other compounds to form potent carcinogens called nitrosamines.[8] When bacon is cooked, nitrosamines form. There is a low level of nitrites in our saliva and in some vegetables, but there is no information on whether these nitrites can be activated to form nitrosamines. Vitamin C, also found in vegetables, can inhibit the formation of nitrosamines and is usually added to meat cures. Some research has suggested that nitrite itself might be carcinogenic.[9]

A certain wine additive, diethylpyrocarbonate, interacts with alcohol to cause levels of 0.1 parts per billion of another strong carcinogen, urethan.[10] This chemical is now banned in many countries.

Unintentional food additives are those chemicals used to prepare or store the food product; small amounts of these chemicals subsequently, unintentionally, become part of the food. An example of this is trichloroethylene. Decaffeinated products were made by using trichloroethylene to extract the caffeine. Trichloroethylene was found to be a carcinogen and was removed from the market. Another example of unintentional contamination of food involves certain processes used to make the paraffin wax that lines many food containers. Carcinogens were formed during certain of these processes, and once the problem was discovered, these processes were discontinued.

Pesticides are also unintentional food additives. Some, like DDT, aldrin, and others produce liver cancer in mice and are probably carcinogenic in other species. It is important to realize that most pesticides get into our bodies and are stored in fat cells, since they are fat soluble. These pesticide-laden fat cells can then act as reservoirs to slowly, but constantly, release the pesticide into the bloodstream. Another chemical that is used in agriculture is DES (diethylstilbestrol). DES is used to fatten cattle and has been found in trace amounts in dairy products and beef. DES causes human cancer: cancer of the vagina in young women and cancer of the testicles in men whose mothers had taken DES. (Cancer of the testicles is rare, however, especially in this situation.) Keep in mind that a large amount of DES is needed to cause cancer, and only a small amount is in our food. But small amounts accumulate and do affect us.

Some food contaminants, like aflatoxin, which causes human liver cancer, are of natural origin. Aflatoxin is a product of a fungus, *Aspergillus flavus*, which grows mainly on peanut plants. Other fungal products have been implicated in human cancers, but these findings have not yet been substantiated. *Gyromita esculenta*, a common mushroom used in cooking, contains a compound called N-methyl-N-formylhydrazine, which is a most potent animal carcinogen.[11] Related chemicals in other mushroom types are now under investigation.

Certain food processing techniques, such as smoking and charcoal broiling, are known to produce carcinogens.[12] Smoked food is associated with an increased incidence of gastric cancer in the Baltic States and Iceland. The carcinogens that result from charcoal broiling appear to come from the fat that drips from the meat and is burned, forming the carcinogen, which then rises with the smoke back up into the meat.[13] If the fat drippings were eliminated, the carcinogens would probably also be eliminated.

As yet, there are no definite proven cases of human cancers directly related to food additives, but many authorities agree that additives and contaminants do account for a very small percentage of human cancers. Those chemicals implicated in animal cancers were removed from the market for the most part. However, nitrites are bothersome sources of carcinogens and should be avoided. It is altogether possible that the reduced incidence of gastric cancer in the United States is directly related to better methods of food preparation and smaller amounts of nitrites being used in foods with the advent of refrigeration. Also it seems that certain naturally occurring food components like aflatoxins do cause human cancer and should definitely be eliminated. And finally, think twice before you make a habit of eating a great many mushrooms.

PESTICIDES

Pesticides, though not commonly used before the 1940s, are now in widespread use throughout the world. I am defining pesticides as chemicals that control or kill pests or affect plant or animal life. Herbicides are, therefore, included under the general term of "pesticide." Pesticides are commonly used around your home to control pests and weeds. Their presence permeates many areas other than the home; they are used in agriculture, horticulture, public parks, and gardens, among others. Table 10.1 is a partial list of different types of pesticides and their functions.

Pesticides have made an important contribution to both food production and disease control. It is estimated that 45 percent of the world's potential food supply is lost to pests: 30 percent to weeds, pests, and diseases before harvest, and another 15 percent between harvest and use. Some estimate that at least one-third of the crops in Third World countries are lost to pests.[13]

Despite the fact that pesticides have aided in the control of malaria, schistosomiasis, and filariasis in tropical countries, there are still 150 million cases of malaria and about 250 million cases of schistosomiasis and filariasis each year in the world. There is no way of knowing and no way of calculating how many lives will be saved or improved by the use of pesticides to control diseases and increase our food production. Likewise, there is no way to calculate how many lives will be lost from pesticide use. Some dangerous pesticides that are banned or restricted in North America and Europe have been unloaded on Third World countries.

There were about 1,200 pesticide chemical compounds, combined in 30,000 different formulations and brands in the United States in 1981. The United States used about 900 million pounds of pesticides in that year. Approximately 334 million pounds of pesticides or 5–10 percent of the entire world's supply was used by California alone in 1977.[14]

Pesticides enter your body by inhalation, absorption through the skin, or ingestion. And unlike industrial chemicals, which are used in a very controlled manner, pesticides are sprayed, powdered, or dropped as pellets or granules in and around places where the general public may walk or play. In fact, pesticide residues are commonly

Table 10.1 Pesticide Class and Function

Pesticide	Function
Insecticide	Controls or kills insects.
Herbicide	Controls or kills weeds.
Fungicide	Kills fungi.
Bactericide	Kills bacteria.
Disinfectant	Destroys or inactivates harmful microorganisms.
Defoliant	Removes leaves.
Desiccant	Sometimes used to speed drying of plants.
Repellant	Repels insects, mites, ticks, dogs, cats.

found in human tissue in almost everyone in the United States, averaging six parts per million (ppm) in fatty tissue.[15] Pesticide residues have been found in breast milk and cow milk and have been found to cross the placental barrier to the human fetus.[16]

Breast Cancer and Pesticides

Because pesticides are soluble in oil or fatty tissue like that of the human breast and its milk, it is theorized that pesticides may be a contributing factor to breast cancer.[17] Incidental findings in experiments involving exposure of rats and mice to pesticides show a significant increase in breast cancer in the exposed animal group. Women are at greater risk than men when exposed to the same amount of pesticides because the Allowable Daily Intake for pesticides as determined by the federal government is calculated on the basis of a 70-kilogram man, not a 50-kilogram woman with larger breast tissue.

Politicians, who are influenced by PAC lobbyists, passed the General Agreement on Tariffs and Trade (GATT) in December 1994. The GATT rules allow for substantially higher levels of pesticide residues on U.S. import produce. Specifically, 5000 percent higher levels of DDT than current U.S. standards are permitted on imported peaches, bananas, grapes, strawberries, broccoli, and carrots. Hence, the health of American women is apparently subordinate to political pressure.

Certain pesticides, such as DDT (an insecticide), are animal carcinogens. They get into fatty tissue and are slowly released from the fat. Between 1985 and 1991, blood specimens from over 14,000 women in New York City were analyzed for content of these pesticides in the University Women's Health Study.[18–20] Women who developed breast cancer had much higher levels of these two pesticides than women who did not.[21] Since DDT is used extensively in the environment and food chain, and since it is another risk factor for the development of breast cancer, the public health implications are far-reaching.

In another study, the pesticide HCH (betahexachlorocyclohexane) was found in the breast fat of forty-four breast cancer patients and thirty-three patients with benign breast disorders. Here again, the pesticide was found more often in women with breast cancer.[22]

Three pesticides that have been shown to cause many types of cancer in animals were found to be 100 times as concentrated in Israeli milk compared to levels demonstrated in United States milk. It was estimated that their concentration was about 800 times greater in breast tissue than in the blood. The pesticides involved included: alpha-BHC, gamma-BHC (lindane), and DDT. After public pressure and court action in Israel by consumer groups, those pesticides are no longer used in Israel. Immediately after the ban, a sharp drop in pesticide levels in milk was shown. Breast cancer rates have now dropped according to epidemiological and laboratory findings.[23]

The link of pesticides to breast cancer is not direct, but the findings from these studies and others below, are enough to dictate the reduction in pesticide use from a public health standpoint.

Table 10.2 lists several different pesticides and their roles as human carcinogens.[24-27] Some are definitely associated with human cancer, some are probably associated with human cancer, and some are possibly associated with human cancer. You will recognize a number of them. Many other pesticides not included in this table, like malathion and Mirex, have been linked to cancers in animal studies. Some of them are also familiar to you because they are commonly used in household and garden settings. Currently there is no definite evidence that the pesticides causing animal cancer also cause human cancer. However, we should continue to be on the alert and await future studies that may link these pesticides to human cancer.

The human cancers associated with pesticide use include the following:

- Breast cancer.
- Leukemia.
- Multiple myeloma.
- Lymphoma.
- Soft-tissue sarcoma.
- Prostate cancer.
- Stomach cancer.
- Melanoma.
- Brain cancer.
- Liver cancer.
- Skin cancer.
- Lung cancer.
- Central nervous system tumors: gliomas.
- Cancer of esophagus.
- Ovarian cancers.

There is a correlation between these cancers and a variety of pesti-

Table 10.2   Pesticides as Human Carcinogens

Pesticide (Chemical Name)	Definite	Human Carcinogen Probable	Possible
Aldrin and dieldrin			√
Amitrole		√	
Arsenicals	√		
Benzal chloride			√
Benzotrichloride		√	
Benzoyl chloride			√
Benzyl chloride			√
Carbon tetrachloride	√		
Chlordane			√
Chlorophenols		√	
p-Dichlorobenzene		√	
2,4-Dichlorophenoxyacetic acid esters (2,4-D)			√
p,p^1-Dichlorodiphenyl trichloroethane (DDT)		√	
Ethylene dibromide		√	
Ethylene oxide		√	
Formaldehyde		√	
Heptachlor			√
Lindane (-hexachloro cyclohexane)			√
(4-chloro-2-methyl phenoxy) acetic acid			√
Methyl parathion			√
Pentachlorophenol			√
Phenoxy acids		√	
2,3,7,8-Tetrachloro dibenzo-p-dioxin		√	
2,4,5-Trichlorophenol			√
2,4,6-Trichlorophenol		√	
2,4,5-Trichlorophenoxy acetic acid			√
Vinyl chloride		√	

cides and pesticide uses. This does not mean, however, that pesticides are the direct cause of these cancers.

Other Dangers of Pesticide Use

Some cases of Parkinson's disease as well as other neurological diseases have been linked to various pesticides.[28] Hypertension, cardiovascular disease, and abnormal blood cholesterol and vitamin A levels have been linked to pesticide exposure. Pesticides are also associated with allergies, liver disease, skin diseases, and fertility problems as manifested by changes in the egg and sperm, and changes in the RNA and DNA. Regular spraying of pesticides in homes and gardens was linked with the development of acute leukemia in young children in the Los Angeles area.[29] Other cancers have also been associated with pesticides.[15,30]

Pesticides also pose an environmental hazard. They pollute the rainwater of many U.S. states when they are vaporized or when the wind blows soil particles treated with pesticides.[31]

If you were exposed to toxic amounts of pesticide, that is, if a large dose were inhaled or made contact with your skin, you would experience acute effects. These effects usually appear within minutes to hours after contact. However, the effects of low-level or prolonged pesticide exposure, particularly to those that may have carcinogenic potential, are very different. Cancer does not appear immediately after exposure to a pesticide; it may not be apparent until long after exposure has occurred. Unfortunately, by the time the medical and scientific community becomes aware that a particular pesticide causes cancer, a large number of persons can be exposed without their knowledge. For example, R-11, which is a chemical found in insect repellants, has just been shown to cause cancer in animals.

Dioxin, otherwise known as Agent Orange, and one of its associated contaminants, TCDD, was extensively used toward the end of the United States's conflict in Vietnam.[32] Hundreds of thousands of people were exposed to these agents, and Vietnam veterans and other persons raised serious allegations that Agent Orange and TCDD[33] caused malignant tumors, sterility, spontaneous abortions, birth defects, disfiguring skin diseases, and other illnesses.

Endometriosis, affecting over 5 million women in the United States, is a disease whereby tissue from the uterus travels to the abdomen, ovaries, bowels, and bladder, and causes bleeding, infertility, extreme pain, and other problems. Although specific causes of this disorder are not definite, dioxin has recently been implicated. Researchers have found that dioxin can cause endometriosis in female rhesus monkeys.

Researchers around the world are assaying for dioxin in the bloodstream of women with endometriosis. The U.S. National Institutes of Health and the U.S. Environmental Protection Agency are both investigating the link between endometriosis and this pesticide and many others in the family of pesticides to which dioxin belongs.

We do know that TCDD is very toxic and causes tumors in rats, in which it acts as a promoter of cancer.[34] It can also initiate carcinogenesis in animals.[35,36] A number of human epidemiological and toxicological studies have suggested an association between TCDD, or the chemicals it contaminates, and soft-tissue sarcoma,[37-39] Hodgkin's,[40] non-Hodgkin's lymphoma,[41-43] stomach cancer,[44,45] nasal cancer,[46] and liver cancer.[47,48] However, other studies did not show a correlation between TCDD and other cancers.[49-54] Most of these studies involved a short period of time between exposure and disease. It now appears that the longer the time from exposure to TCDD, the higher the risk for the development of cancer and the higher the incidence of cancer.[55,56]

Minimizing Pesticide Use

In this age of organic farming, the debate over pesticide use rages on. Othal Brand, who was recently appointed to the Texas Pesticide Regulatory Board, said of the termite killer Chlordane, "Sure, it's going to kill a lot of people, but they may be dying of something else anyway."[57] Farmer Clarence Hopmann of Dumas, Arkansas, decreased the use of agricultural pesticides because he developed an allergy to them. However, in order to qualify for bank loans, the bankers demanded that he use large doses of pesticides on his crops. He has resumed using them.[58]

There are several things that can and should be done to minimize the use of pesticides in our country and the world. Before the 1940s, pesticides were not used very much at all. Hence, there have always been alternatives to the artificial chemical pesticides currently in use.

Nature provides us with biological controls, that is, natural predators that can be introduced to control insects. For example, ladybugs can be used to fight off aphid predators. Beetles were used to control weeds in the western United States in the 1950s and parasites, to control the citrus fly in Barbados in the 1960s. You can minimize the number of pests by providing food and habitat for the pest's natural enemies. Certain traditional farming practices may be employed as well. Crop residues may be removed by plowing or flooding. Pest deterrents, crop rotation, proper drainage methods, and physical controls like traps or blocking of insects and/or other pests can be used. These techniques, along with biological controls, have been used successfully by many countries, including China, Nicaragua, certain areas of England, and also some parts of the United States.

While chemical pesticides certainly benefit populations by increasing food production and decreasing certain diseases, it is important to use them only when they must be used and to use the pesticides that cause the least toxicity in human beings and the least damage to the environment around us. Treat them all as hazardous and minimize their use in public areas and in and around your home. For example, since the pesticide 2,4,5-T is very hazardous, substitute the less hazardous Amcide or Krenite. Silicon and soap can be used in gardens as a nontoxic insecticide rather than the other commonly used pesticides for the garden. Wasps have been controlled by parasites in greenhouses more effectively than with chemicals. And the bacteria called *Bacillus thuringiensis* has also been shown to be a good alternative to several toxic insecticides.

What Can Be Done

The number of tons of pesticides has increased thirty-three times since 1940, and their toxicity has grown tenfold. However, crop losses to microorganisms, insects, and weeds have gone up 31–37 percent. There are a number of reasons for this. As new pesticides are developed, insects develop resistance to them. But even more importantly, the government supports prices of various crops, which encourages farmers to produce only a single crop instead of rotating crops to inhibit the pests.

By using crop rotation and biological pest control, pesticide use could be cut in half. Food prices would rise by one percent—about $1 billion a year—but the benefits would be enormous. The United States would save $4–$10 billion per year as a result of decreased damage to fish and water supplies, decreased costs of regulating pesticides, and decreased health-care costs for the 20,000 people poisoned each year from pesticides.[59]

You should learn as much as you can about any pesticides you do use. Acquiring such information is not easy but neither is maintaining good health. Acquire information and use alternatives to the current pesticides. Exposure to pesticides can be controlled. This is yet another risk factor for disease over which you have control.

11
Smoking

Smoking is one of the biggest health hazards today. The scientific evidence of the dangers of smoking is tremendous. In 1979 Joseph Califano, then Secretary of the Department of Health, Education, and Welfare, wrote: "Smoking is the largest preventable cause of death in America."

Projections by the World Conference on Smoking and Health sponsored by the World Health Organization (WHO) show that even if present consumption rates of cigarettes stay steady—and all data indicate a continued increase—the annual number of premature deaths caused by tobacco will rise from about 3 million worldwide in the 1990s to 10 million by the year 2025. Over half a billion people alive today, including 200 million currently under the age of 20, will die from tobacco-induced disease, and half of these will be in middle age.[1]

The WHO Conference said that the tobacco companies have targeted expansion in Third World countries, countries in Eastern Europe, Thailand, and other Far Eastern countries. Also targeted are women and girls, and young boys.[2]

Smoking among children has increased dramatically. Since 1968, the number of girls between the ages of 12 and 14 who smoke has increased eightfold. Six million children between the ages of 13 and

19 are regular smokers, and over 100,000 children under 13 are now regular smokers. Smoking among blacks exceeds that among whites. However, on a positive note, about 30 million Americans have become ex-smokers since massive educational warnings were issued by the federal government.

More deaths and physical suffering are related to cigarette smoking than to any other single cause: over 228,700 deaths (and rising) each year from cancer, over 325,000 deaths from cardiovascular disease, and more than 50,000 deaths from chronic lung diseases. Compare these figures with the number of people who died in the following wars (combat and noncombat fatalities): World War I (from 1917 to 1918), 116,708; World War II (from 1941 to 1946), 407,316; Korean War (from 1950 to 1953), 54,246; and Vietnam conflict (from 1964 to 1973), 58,151. (See Table 11.1.) The cigarette industry's own research over a ten-year period (1964–1974), which cost over $15 million, confirmed the fatal dangers of smoking cigarettes.[3] In a one-year period, a one-pack-a-day smoker inhales 50,000 to 70,000 puffs that contain over 2,000 chemical compounds, many of which are known carcinogens. Many tobacco product ingredients, such as flavoring additives, are kept secret even from the government.

The cost of smoking-related diseases is staggering. Health care in the United States costs over $500 billion each year. Smoking accounts for approximately one-fifth of that cost per year.[4] A great deal of this cost is paid by nonsmokers as well as smokers through ever-increasing health insurance premiums, disability payments, and other programs. It doesn't seem fair that nonsmokers have to pay one penny for self-induced smokers' diseases.

The longer a person smokes, the greater is his risk of dying. The earlier a person starts smoking, the higher is his risk of death. A person who smokes two packs a day has a death rate two times higher than a nonsmoker. Smokers who inhale have higher mortality rates than smokers who do not. Life expectancy is eight to nine years shorter for a two-pack-a-day smoker of age 30 to 35 than it is for a nonsmoker, and those who smoke cigarettes with higher contents of "tar" and nicotine have a much higher death rate. Overall, the greatest mortality is seen in the 45 to 55 age groups. Hence, death from smoking is premature death!

If a smoker stops smoking, his mortality rate decreases progressively as the number of nonsmoking years increases. Those who have stopped for fifteen years have mortality rates similar to those who never smoked, with the exception of smokers who stopped after the age of 65. Persons who smoke cigars and pipes also have an increased risk of death.

Table 11.1 U.S. Deaths: Wars Vs. Smoking

World War I	116,708
World War II	407,316
Korean War	54,246
Vietnam conflict	58,151
Smoking annually	603,700
Involuntary smoking annually	53,000

SMOKING AND BREAST CANCER

Because it was found that cigarette smoking decreases estrogen levels in body fluids, it was hypothesized by some investigators that smoking could be protective against breast cancer.[5,6] The results of their studies were not statistically significant, however. Furthermore, it is beyond me how any investigator of science or medicine could say that smoking is beneficial to any degree for any reason.

A number of case-control studies were done to refute that hypothesis.[7-12] In all, over 300,000 women were part of these studies and there was no evidence that showed smoking reduced the incidence of breast cancer in these women.

A higher incidence of breast cancer in smokers compared to nonsmokers was seen in a study that involved over 95,000 American women.[13] In other studies, no significant difference was demonstrated for developing breast cancer in smokers versus nonsmokers.[14,15]

Hence, the majority of the statistically significant data show that there is a positive relationship between smoking and breast cancer. The notion that smoking is protective has been completely discounted.

Smoking Plus Breast Radiation Therapy Leads to Lung Cancer

After about 10 years, women with breast cancer who smoked at the time they received breast radiation therapy have a high risk, about 75 percent, for developing a lung cancer on the same side as the breast that was treated.[16] The overall risk for developing lung cancer in a woman who smokes and gets radiation therapy is about thirty times that of a woman with breast cancer who doesn't smoke, and over seventy-five times for the same side lung as the treated breast. If this high-risk woman is not willing to stop smoking, then maybe she should have a mastectomy instead of radiation to decrease the future risk of a new lung cancer.

LUNG CANCER

Cigarette smoking is the major risk factor for lung cancer in both men and women. The scientific evidence for this and for other cancers related to smoking is overwhelming. The risk of developing lung cancer is increased by the amount of smoking, duration of smoking, age at which smoking starts, and content of tar and nicotine. Female lung cancer deaths are rising at an alarming rate, and have become the leading cause of cancer deaths among females. Smoking now accounts for 25 percent of all cancer deaths in women.

Evidence suggests that certain lung cancer cells come from precursor abnormal cells found in smokers.[17] These precursor cells are present for years before an overt cancer develops and can be eliminated if one stops smoking. However, there is an undetermined point of no return at which time the precursor cell develops into a cancer cell.

Smoking acts in combination with certain occupational exposures to produce lung diseases. The carcinogenic potential of smoking is greater when it works together with the occupational exposures than when it works alone. The cooperative action between these carcinogens is called synergism.

There has been much concern about marijuana and its effects on the human body. In 1982, the National Academy of Sciences released the report "Marijuana and Health," which states that there is a "strong possibility" that heavy marijuana smoking may lead to lung cancer. In fact, marijuana tar extracts have produced genetic changes in cells, and the smoke has 50 percent more carcinogenic hydrocarbons than cigarette smoke.

OTHER TOBACCO-RELATED CANCERS

Smoking cigarettes, pipes, and cigars is directly related to cancer of the larynx in men and women, and the more alcohol a smoker consumes, the higher is his risk of developing laryngeal cancer. Asbestos exposure has this same synergistic effect. Other cancers related to smoking include cancer of the mouth, esophagus, and pancreas. Here again, alcohol acts to intensify the effects of tobacco smoking. Cancer of the kidney and the urinary bladder are also directly related to smoking. Chewing tobacco or snuff dipping in nonsmokers causes a fourfold increase of oral cancers and a sixfold increase in those who were both tobacco smokers and heavy alcohol drinkers.[18] Furthermore, countries such as India, Ceylon, China, and the Soviet Union have the highest rates of death from oral cancer because the people there combine snuff and/or chewing tobacco with other ingredients such as betel nut. A chemical in the betel nut (N'nitrosonornicotine) can initiate tumors in animals. Hence, these findings should discourage the use of chewing tobacco or snuff as a substitute for smoking; you would simply be exchanging one type of cancer risk for another.

Cigarette smoking is associated with cancer of the cervix.[19] Cigarette smoking also causes dysplasia of the cervix,[20] an abnormality detected by Pap smears.

Smoking has been associated with both adenomous and hyperplastic colon polyps in women and men.[21,22] Adenomatous polyps are precursors to colon cancer.[23-25] A smoker has a 2.7 higher risk for developing an adenomatous colon polyp than a non-smoker.[26]

CARCINOGENS IN TOBACCO SMOKE

There are over 2,000 chemical compounds generated by tobacco smoke. The gas phase contains carbon monoxide, carbon dioxide, ammonia, nitrosamines, nitrogen oxides, hydrogen cyanide, sulfurs, nitriles, ketones, alcohols, and acrolein.

The "tars" contain extremely carcinogenic hydrocarbons, which include nitrosamines, benzo(a)pyrenes, anthracenes, acridines, quinolines, benzenes, naphthols, naphthalenes, cresols, and insecticides (DDT), as well as some radioactive compounds like potassium-40 and radium-226. Do you recognize any of these compounds? Some of them, already described in Chapter 3, are known to be risk factors for human cancer.

Tobacco smoke, through its many carcinogens, produces harmful free radicals, which have been shown to change the DNA. Experiments with free radical scavengers show that some of them can inhibit, to a degree, the radicals' damaging effects.[27]

OTHER SMOKING-RELATED ILLNESSES

Many serious illnesses have been directly associated with smoking:

- Cardiovascular illnesses[28-32]
- Osteoporosis, especially in women[33]
- Emphysema and other lung diseases
- Female infertility, higher risk of miscarriage or spontaneous abortion, more genetic mutations[34-37]

SMOKING AND THE IMMUNE SYSTEM

Cigarette smoking adversely affects the human immune system. It affects certain anatomical parts as well as cellular components of the immune system.

Smoking destroys the hairlike structures that line the mucosa of the respiratory tract. These hairlike structures normally beat upward synchronously to remove mucous and any microorganisms. With these hairlike cilia gone, the mucous remains in the respiratory tract and is a perfect medium for the growth of microorganisms, including bacteria and viruses.

Another finding is that smoking causes an increase in macrophages, cells of the immune system that defend the lung against invading organisms and abnormal cells. Macrophages secrete enzymes and other cellular products against the invaders, which also inadvertently causes emphysema, the breakdown of the walls of the respiratory tree.[38-40] The secretion of these enzymes and cellular products by macrophages generates free-radical chemicals, which are responsible for the breakdown of the walls. When this breakdown occurs, organisms can take hold and infect the person because the functional capacity of macrophages to kill invading microorganisms is greatly diminished. Certain micronutrients, like carotene, vitamins E and C, selenium, zinc, and copper, can neutralize free radicals and prevent the invasion of microorganisms and the breakdown of the respiratory wall.

Smoking has been shown to cause reversible changes in the immunoregulatory T cell lymphocytes.[41,42] The ratio of T4 to T8 lymphocytes is decreased in heavy smokers, as in patients with AIDS, but returns to normal six weeks after these heavy smokers stop smoking. Other studies have corroborated these findings: suppressor T cell activity is significantly enhanced by smoking.[43]

Smokers also show a significant decrease in natural killer cell activity,[44,45] which may explain the reported increase in survival of cardiac transplants in patients who resumed smoking postoperatively. Antibody levels are adversely affected by smoking as well.[46] IgA, the antibody in the mucous membranes, and one of the first lines of defense against viruses and bacteria, is decreased in smokers.[47] Other antibody classes are at lower levels also.

Studies show that smokers have lower blood levels of vitamin C and several other free radical scavengers. Nutrition in smokers is generally poorer also. Nutritional deficiencies, especially of vitamin C, compromise the immune system of the smoker. Smoking is associated with many infections, cancers, heart disease, and many other chronic illnesses. Smoking suppresses the immune system, but early data indicate that this is reversible.

INVOLUNTARY SMOKING

A nonsmoker who is exposed to tobacco smoke from other smokers has many adverse reactions and is unjustly and unnecessarily subjected to risk factors detrimental to his or her health.[48] The smoke that comes from the lighted end of a cigarette contains more hazardous chemicals than does the smoke that is inhaled by the smoker. It is almost unavoidable to inhale tobacco smoke because it is so prevalent in homes, work places, public areas, and private establishments. In a large study of nonsmokers and former smokers, 64 percent of the nonsmokers reported daily exposure. Thirty-five percent were exposed to second-hand smoke at least ten hours per week. Under experimental conditions, nonsmokers in England inhaled smoke equivalent to one cigarette per day, and up to two cigarettes a day in Japan.

The controversy over passive smoking began to heat up in 1983, and on March 19, 1984, R.J. Reynolds Tobacco Company paid for a one-third-page advertisement in the *Wall Street Journal* entitled "Smoking in Public: Let's Separate Fact From Fiction." The company asserted, "But, in fact, there is little evidence—and certainly nothing which proves scientifically that cigarette smoke causes disease in nonsmokers."

The Surgeon General's report in 1986 was a landmark, asserting for the first time that involuntary inhalation of cigarette smoke by nonsmokers causes disease, most notably lung cancer.[49,50] The report also states that the number of people injured by involuntary smoking is much larger than the number injured by other environmental agents that have already been regulated. The National Research Council of the National Academy of Sciences reported similar findings.[51]

Separating smokers from nonsmokers within the same physical space is not always successful because the smoke travels on the same floor and between floors. A movement to ban all smoking in public areas has culminated in the ban of smoking on all domestic flights in the United States since early 1990. Forty-two states have legislated smoking restrictions in various areas like public transportation, hospitals, elevators, indoor areas, cultural or recreational facilities, schools, and libraries.

Lung Cancer

The National Research Council has estimated the effect of passive smoking on nonsmokers to be significant in the development of lung cancer. Of the 12,200 annual deaths from lung cancer in the United States that are not due to smoking, between 2,500 and 8,400 of these may be attributable to passive smoking.[52] This equates to about 7.4 deaths from lung cancer among nonsmokers per hundred thousand person years. (Person years are computed by taking the age of each person and adding them together. For example, a 70 year old and a 20 year old would equate to 90 person years. If the study were of 1,000 people each of whom was 100 years old, this would equate to a hundred thousand person years [1,000 x 100 = 100,000].)

Over a dozen studies have been done to assess the relationship between passive smoking and lung cancer. There have been at least three significant prospective studies showing that nonsmokers married to smokers have a greater risk for lung cancer than do those married to nonsmokers. The lung cancers most frequently seen in these studies were squamous cell carcinoma and small cell carcinoma of the lung. A review of these studies made by the National Academy of Sciences and the Surgeon General found that the risk of developing lung cancer in a passive smoker is 1.34: one hundred times higher than the person exposed to asbestos for twenty years.[53]

A study published in 1990 shows that about 17 percent of lung cancers in nonsmokers are a result of exposure to tobacco smoke during childhood and adolescence.[54] For the first time, this study confirms that innocent children are at tremendous risk for lung cancer because they inhaled tobacco smoke in their household. Smoking during pregnancy increases by 50 percent the fetus's risk of developing cancer later in childhood. This, too, is alarming.[55]

Cervical Cancer

Studies show that cigarette smoking increases your risk of cervical cancer. Passive smoke exposure for three or more hours per day has been shown to increase almost threefold a nonsmoker's risk of developing cervical cancer. It is quite alarming that this amount of exposure increases your risk of cervical cancer by such a significant factor.[56]

Bladder Cancer

Nonsmokers have a higher risk of getting bladder cancer if they are exposed to other people's smoke at home, at work, or during transportation.[57]

STOP SMOKING

More than 95 percent of former smokers quit on their own, usually at the recommendation of their physician. A common mistake a "quitter" makes is to think it is all right to have one or two cigarettes every once in a while. If you could have done that before, you would have.

Your local chapter of the American Lung Association has courses on how to stop smoking. These sessions are inexpensive and quite comprehensive. I encourage you to participate in them.

Smokers who have existing heart disease can reduce their risk of future heart attacks and death if they quit smoking.[58] Prospective findings in a study that involved over 7,000 people who are 65 years old or older indicate that smokers who continue to smoke will have a higher rate of mortality, but those who quit will have an improved life expectancy.[59] So it's never too late to quit.

Many studies indicate that if a person quits smoking for at least ten years, his risk of developing coronary heart disease is the same as a nonsmoker of the same age. On the other hand, a person must quit smoking for fifteen years before his risk of developing cancer will equal that of a nonsmoker.

Many people say that they do not want to stop smoking because they fear gaining weight. Weight gain may occur in those who stop smoking, but it is likely to occur only in a small percentage of them.[60] It is important to guard against possible weight gain, and this can be accomplished by following the Ten-Point Plan in Chapter 26.

CURRENT PUBLIC POLICIES

Federally sponsored programs support tobacco prices, benefiting allotment holders (a unique monopoly situation) and tobacco growers. In addition, other federally sponsored programs benefit the tobacco industry. The programs and their cost to the taxpayer—both smoker and nonsmoker—are the following: tobacco inspection and grading, $6.1 million; market news service, $10.5 million; research, $7.4 million; short-term credit, $69.2 million (1979). Total cost to the taxpayer: over $157 million in 1979.

On the other hand, federal funds are spent to discourage smoking, to research the health effects of smoking, and to provide a great portion of the cost of medical care for people who are suffering from and dying of smoking-related diseases. Patients with *self-induced* smoking-related diseases and families of these patients receive Social Security benefits.

The American Medical Association's official policy since 1986 has stated that it:

1. Opposes any efforts by the government or its agencies to actively encourage, persuade, or compel any country to import tobacco products; and
2. Favors legislation that would prevent the government from actively supporting, promoting, or assisting such activities.

However, the AMA's Political Action Committee has been giving money to United States representatives who actively oppose the AMA's official policy and who are responsible for getting tobacco into foreign markets.[61]

TIME FOR NEW PUBLIC POLICIES

On the basis of the evidence citing the dangers of passive smoking, I believe it is prudent for all individuals, specifically employers and those who develop public policy, to consider tobacco smoke a threat to the health of nonsmoking adults and children alike. The data have been thoroughly reviewed,[62] and it is time now to prohibit smoking in all public areas and work places.

Not only do nonsmokers experience many harmful health effects from tobacco smoke, but they also have to pay higher health insurance premiums for diseases related to smoking (cancer, cardiovascular diseases, lung diseases, etc.). Moreover, nonsmokers subsidize the tobacco industry through their tax dollars. We should pressure our senators and congressmen to force the American government to stop subsidizing the tobacco industry.

The United States has adopted uncompromisingly restrictive measures concerning food additives, but only a verbal statement of caution is required on every package of cigarettes. The Delaney Clause legislation prohibits the sale of any product to the American people that has been shown to be carcinogenic to humans and animals, and thus applies to situations in which the human hazard may be minimal. Tobacco is a major risk factor for cancer, cardiovascular diseases, lung diseases, and other illnesses.

CONCLUSION

If you smoke, you should stop. If you have not started, don't! Seek professional help if you must, but stop smoking.

12
Alcohol and Caffeine

Industrial losses in the United States due to alcohol consumption cost about $45 billion every year. Many more billions of dollars are added to this figure when you consider that alcohol is involved in 50 percent of all traffic fatalities, 30 percent of small-aircraft accidents, and 66 percent of all violent crimes. The totals are higher still when you consider the losses due to diseases aggravated by alcohol use, and losses due to alcohol-induced poor decision-making in government, industry, education, law, the military, and medicine. About 68 percent of adult Americans abuse alcohol.

It is estimated that 100 million Americans drink alcohol, and over 28 million—1 of every 8 Americans—are children of alcoholics. Alcohol-related costs total about $117 billion every year; for abuse of other drugs, the cost is $60 billion a year. This total of $177 billion a year represents about $63 a month for every man, woman, and child in the United States.

All of society pays for substance abuse. Employers lose productivity, taxpayers pay the bill for programs and services, and consumers pay higher insurance premiums. Society pays for tobacco abuse as well.

Alcohol-related hospitalizations among elderly United States citizens are common and vary according to each state.[1] The states with the highest rates of alcohol-related hospitalizations include: Maine, New Hampshire, Massachusetts, Wisconsin, Minnesota, Montana,

Wyoming, Washington state, Oregon, Nevada, Alaska, and Hawaii. In 1989, the charges to Medicare for this preventable problem were close to $250 million. And the median charge per hospital stay was $4,515.

Excessive alcohol consumption is a risk factor for cancers of the breast, mouth, pharynx, larynx, esophagus, pancreas, liver, and head and neck. Alcohol acts synergistically with tobacco smoking in the development of other gastrointestinal cancers and urinary bladder cancer. A greater frequency of these cancers occurs in men, blacks, people on the low end of the socioeconomic scale, and older people. Alcohol is directly responsible for causing cirrhosis of the liver, which is the seventh leading cause of death in the United States. Fifty percent of alcoholics die from cardiovascular diseases and 20 percent from accidents, suicides, and homicides.

Nutrition and Alcoholism

Alcoholics have more nutritional deficiencies than all other groups of people. Alcohol is a source of calories, and alcoholics consume this rather than foods with much better nutritional value. Alcoholics will consume about 20 percent of their total calories as alcohol.

Many vitamin deficiencies are severe in alcoholics. The most important is thiamine (vitamin B1) deficiency. A severe brain disease called Wernicke-Korsakoff syndrome can be rapidly reversed by the administration of thiamine. Folic acid and vitamin B12 deficiencies are responsible for anemias, among other things. Pyridoxine (B6) deficiency causes peripheral nerve problems. Alcoholics have a deficiency of vitamin C because of their liver disease. Because of their vitamin deficiencies, alcoholics may complain of visual problems and sometimes infertility, since their sperm production may be impaired. In addition to vitamin deficiencies, alcoholics have several mineral deficiencies including calcium, zinc, and magnesium. Since alcohol can interfere with the absorption of iron from the gut, some alcoholics develop the Plummer-Vinson syndrome, which is characterized by a cluster of symptoms including difficulty swallowing; a red, smooth tongue; and iron deficiency anemia. People with this syndrome have a high rate of cancer of the mouth.

Alcohol and Immunity

Not only does consumption of alcohol rob the body of many nutrients, it also increases complications from cirrhosis of the liver, gastrointestinal hemorrhage, trauma, cancer, and infection. The high incidence of infection among alcoholics is attributed to dulled mental function;

breakdown of the protective mucous lining of the nose, mouth, and airways; aspiration of saliva into the lungs; exposure out-of-doors; and malnutriton. The frequency and severity of infections are so pronounced among alcoholics that most physicians believe that alcohol itself directly inhibits the body's immune defense mechanisms. Clinical observations and laboratory studies support the long-held conviction that alcohol depresses the function of the immune system.

The clinical evidence linking alcohol intake and depressed immune function dates back to 1785. There is a strong correlation between the amount of alcohol consumed and the degree of immune dysfunction. Even moderate users of alcohol have very high rates of infections, especially pneumonia. Alcohol interferes with normal immune defense mechanisms (see Chapter 4 for a review).

The neutrophil leukocyte, a kind of white blood cell, is decreased in number and its function is retarded with chronic or acute ingestion of alcohol. As you may remember from Chapter 4, the function of these cells is to fight and kill invading bacteria. Alcohol consumption of this type also causes a decrease in the number of lymphocytes and impairs their function, especially the T cells and natural killer cells, which seek out and destroy viruses and cancer cells. Monocytes, too, are impaired by alcohol ingestion. Suppression of this cellular arm of immunity leads to a high rate of tuberculosis infection and viral infections. Because cellular killing is inhibited, latent viruses, like the Epstein-Barr virus, become activated and there is a high degree of susceptibility to all viruses.

Alcohol ingestion significantly interferes with the ability of the immune system to make antibodies against a new invading antigen, like a virus or bacterium. The complement protein defense system is also adversely affected by alcohol consumption.

Thus, both acute and chronic use of alcohol interferes significantly with our defense mechanisms. Chronic use of alcohol adversely affects the cellular arm of the immune system and increases the risk for tuberculosis, viral infection of all types, and cancer. Alcohol should be considered an immune suppressive drug with far-reaching effects.

ALCOHOL AND BREAST CANCER

Women who consume two to four alcoholic drinks per week, *not per day*, have a two to three times higher risk for developing breast cancer independently of other breast cancer risk factors. Twelve ounces of beer equals four ounces of wine, which equals one and a half ounces of whiskey in alcohol content. So any two or three of these a week will put you into this very high risk category. The preponderance of evidence from acceptable studies indicates this relationship, especially for younger women.[2-9]

Alcohol may actually speed up an existing cancer, especially breast cancer.[10] Animals were injected with breast cancer, which always spreads to the lungs. At the time of injection, the animals were allowed to get drunk. Those with a blood alcohol content of 0.15 percent, which represents about four to five drinks an hour, later developed more than twice the number of new lung metastases compared to the animals that did not drink alcohol. Those with a blood level of 0.25 percent had eight times more tumors in their lungs.

These same levels of alcohol are seen in humans who drink excessively in one hour. Alcohol suppresses natural killer cells of the immune system that ordinarily would destroy cancer cells in the bloodstream. Women who drink this amount are at an increased risk for developing cancer and also for developing metastatic disease.

ALCOHOL, OTHER CANCERS, AND OTHER DISEASES

Alcohol may exert its carcinogenic effects by direct topical action on the mouth, pharynx, and esophagus. The evidence that alcohol is a topical carcinogen is that mouthwash users have a high rate of oral cancer and mouthwash is rarely swallowed. Alcohol and tobacco account for 75 percent of all oral cancers in the United States. And a considerable amount of evidence shows that alcoholism, because of the nutritional deficiencies associated with it, significantly increases the risk of smoking-related cancers.

The rate of liver cancer in alcoholics who have cirrhosis is rising. In addition, there are many other complications of cirrhosis, including varicose veins in the esophagus, which can bleed; ascites (fluid in the abdomen); muscle wasting; and kidney failure. Alcohol induces an inflammation of the pancreas and other abnormalities of the pancreas, and the heart can become severely enlarged and nonfunctional with alcoholism. Moderate alcohol consumption is also an independent risk factor for the development of heart disease and stroke.[11,12]

Premature testicle and ovary shrinkage are seen in alcoholics. Peptic ulcers are also common and are often quite large. Infants born of alcoholic mothers may have a variety of problems including defects in the brain, in intellectual development and physical growth, and in the facial features. This is called the "fetal alcohol syndrome," in which alcohol acts to transform normal cells of the fetus into abnormal cells. The number of persons affected in this way is grossly underestimated.

CAFFEINE AND CANCER

Caffeine is the most popular drug in North America and in many other parts of the world. It is found in coffee, tea, cola beverages, and chocolate.

Coffee drinking may be related to cancer of the lower urinary tract, including the bladder.[13] Studies show that the risk for these cancers is independent of other factors like tobacco smoking, and these cancer rates are very high in persons who drink more than three cups of coffee a day. This risk is probably related to other compounds in coffee as well as caffeine.

It is well known that caffeine can cause damage to genetic material,[14,15] thereby potentially leading to the development of cancer by altering DNA. It also interferes with the normal repair mechanisms of DNA and other genetic material. Caffeine can act as an agent that causes mistakes in gene production which lead to malformations of a fetus.

Excessive coffee consumption by pregnant mothers can lead to lower infant birth weights.[16] Fetuses in women who consume 600 milligrams or more of caffeine per day have a higher incidence of abortion and prematurity.[17]

In a study of coffee consumption in 1,130 male college graduates for nineteen to thirty-five years after graduation, it was found that those who drank five or more cups of coffee a day had a 2.8 times higher risk of developing heart disease.[18] This study also showed coffee to be an independent risk factor for the development of heart disease.

Drinking two cups of caffeinated coffee per day over a lifetime for close to 1,000 postmenopausal women put them at a much higher risk for developing osteoporosis compared to women who do not drink caffeinated coffee.[19] This study showed statistical significance especially for regions of the hip and lumbar spine.

CONCLUSION

Although alcohol and caffeine are two important risk factors for cancer, the decision to consume them is *yours*. You can again decide about the status of your health!

13
Hormonal and Sexual-Social Factors

Hormonal factors and sexual-social behavior have become increasingly important in the development of cancer in modern times. The relaxation of sexual mores has increased promiscuity, which is a major risk factor for certain cancers. There has also been a concomitant increased use of hormones, which can lead to the development of other cancers.

As early as 1898, scientists recognized a connection between the immune system and the hormones of the body. More recently, both clinical and experimental evidence support the hypothesis that the sex hormones regulate immune function. This is based on the following observations: (1) immune response is slightly different in men and women; (2) immune response is altered by decreasing or increasing hormones; (3) immune response is altered during pregnancy when sex hormones are increased; and (4) immunological cells have specific receptors for sex hormones. Female and male sex hormones regulate the immune system, indicating an important interaction between the nervous system, endocrine system, and immune system. The immune system, in turn, can control the circulating levels of these hormones. As we see again, the immune system is very delicate and can orchestrate a great many things.[1]

Apart from their regulatory effect on the immune system, excess hormones can increase the chance of an error in normal cell division and lead to a cancerous transformation. This occurs because hormones can affect cell division rates of normal, hyperplastic, and even cancer cells. The more often these cells try to divide, the higher the risk is for them to make a mistake and hence change or transform into a cancer cell.

Female sex hormones, at certain times of life, can be protective also.[2] Between ages 11 and 19, the rates for developing certain types of cancer (epithelial types) are about 50 percent lower for females compared to males. Before age 11 or after age 19, female sex hormones do not have a protective effect. It may be that female sex hormones prevent the establishment of distant metastases in certain cancers. Mother Nature seems to be very protective of this child-bearing age group.

NATURE'S INFLUENCE

Many events and processes in a person's life increase the risk of developing breast cancer. A number of these factors are natural or biological.

Menstrual History

A woman's menstrual history is another risk factor for developing cancer. The longer the body is bathed with estrogens, the higher is a woman's risk of developing cancer. The earlier a woman starts menstruating and the later she stops, the higher is her risk for cancer, especially breast cancer. For instance, American women typically begin menstruating at around age 11 and experience menopause in their early 50s. Chinese women start menstruating at an average age of about 17 and the incidence of breast cancer per 100,000 people is less than in the United States. But 200 years ago, North American women were like the Chinese in that they too started to menstruate at about age 17.[3] Though it is difficult to specify at what age the risk increases, studies done in Norway indicate the risk for developing breast cancer increases about 4 percent for every year earlier than 17 that the first menstruation begins, and the risk increases about 4 percent for every year later that menopause begins.[4]

It is well known that a high-fat, low-fiber diet initiates an earlier menarche or time of first menstruating. High-fat food triggers the early release from the brain of a hormone called prolactin, which starts menstruation. The higher the fiber content of food per day, the later the age of menarche, no matter where in the world you live.[5] This is because a high-fiber diet generally is linked to a low-fat diet, and/or fat is reduced by the high-fiber component.

If a woman has had few or no pregnancies and many reproductive years, she has a higher risk of getting breast cancer. The older a woman is when she first becomes pregnant, the higher is her risk of developing breast cancer. A woman who delivers her first child after the age of 35 has a threefold higher risk of developing breast cancer than a woman who bears her first child before the age of 18. Women who never become pregnant and women who never menstruate have a three or four times higher risk of developing cancer, especially breast cancer. Women are less at risk for developing breast cancer, however, if they have an early menopause of if they have their ovaries removed surgically so that early menopause is induced.

Although the majority of studies have always concentrated on the time of the first full-term pregnancy and its association with risk for developing breast cancer,[6-8] a Brazilian study demonstrated that the last full-term pregnancy and the total number of pregnancies may be just as important in determining breast cancer risk.[9,10] When statistical analyses were applied to the Brazilian women, the number of total pregnancies became the single most important factor in determining risk of breast cancer and not when the woman had the first or last full-term pregnancy. Eleven other studies also demonstrate that a high number of pregnancies is independently protective against breast cancer.[10] Five or more pregnancies seems to be the number that confers protection against the risk for developing breast cancer, regardless of when they occur in a woman's life.

Termination of First Pregnancy and Breast Cancer Risk

A woman who had an abortion in the first trimester of her first pregnancy, whether it was spontaneous or induced, is two and one-half times more likely to develop breast cancer.[11-20] When conception occurs, hormonal changes influence the breast. The milk duct network grows quickly to form other networks that will ultimately produce milk. During this period of tremendous growth and development, breast cells are undergoing great change and are immature or "undifferentiated"; hence, they are more susceptible to carcinogens. But when a first full-term pregnancy is completed, hormonal changes occur that permanently alter the breast network to greatly reduce the risk of outside carcinogen influence. When a termination occurs in the first trimester, there are no protective effects, and many of the rapidly dividing cells of the breast are left in transitional states.[21,22] It is in these transitional states of high proliferation and undifferentiation that these cells can undergo transformation to cancer cells.

Prebirth Exposure to Estrogen and Breast Cancer Risk

A human fetus exposed to estrogen has another risk for breast cancer when it matures into an adult.[23] Fetal breast tissue is undifferentiated and, therefore, susceptible to transformational change especially by estrogen. The estrogen concentration *in utero* is about ten times the amount in the adult state.[24] Estrogens can initiate carcinogenesis, the process by which normal cells change into cancer cells.

An ongoing study from Harvard involves Sweden's Uppsala University Hospital's records of women who delivered daughters between 1873 and 1957 and the number of breast cancer cases that occurred between 1958 and 1986. The hypothesis is that the estrogen level during pregnancy may influence a daughter's subsequent risk of breast cancer because a female gets her largest exposure to estrogen while *in utero*, her mammary glands being undifferentiated then and very susceptible to the effects of estrogen. Symptoms related to high estrogen levels in pregnant mothers include: severe nausea, obesity, or sometimes high birthweight. A correlation will be made between these symptoms and the subsequent development of breast cancer in daughters.

The Swedish study,[25] data from the Breast Cancer Detection Demonstration Project,[26] and a review of other studies[27] demonstrate that, indeed, the high levels of estrogens *in utero* can increase the risk for breast cancer in adult life.

Breast-Feeding (Lactation) and Breast Cancer Risk

It was generally believed that breast-feeding does not confer protection against the development of breast cancer. Based on two studies[28,29] that may have been flawed statistically because menopausal status was not recorded, this fallacy persisted for decades.

However, a review published in 1985 suggests that breast-feeding can reduce the risk for breast cancer.[30] Studies since then in Western cultures showed mixed results, which are probably related to the shorter length of time a Western woman actually breast-feeds and to the relatively small number of Western women who elect to breast-feed at all. Most studies do not take into account women's ages when they breast-feed or whether these breast-feeding mothers are part-timers who also use formula when they wish. Chinese studies, on the other hand, show that over half of Chinese women breast-feed and do so for at least three years, which confers protection against breast cancer.

Most studies[31–38] demonstrate that breast-feeding protects against breast cancer in premenopausal women rather than postmenopausal women. In order to see a protective effect, a woman must breast-feed for between four to twelve months[32] and six to eight years.[35] The younger a woman is when she breast-feeds, the lower the breast cancer risk. This may be related to having an early pregnancy, which is known to confer protection.

Women who consistently use only one breast to breast-feed have a higher risk of developing breast cancer in the unsuckled breast in postmenopausal years.[39] The Tanka people who live in boats in China breast-feed with only the right breast, probably for convenience, with the opening of the clothing on the right side. However, non-Tanka Chinese women who live on land and have the same style of clothing with the opening on the right, use both breasts to breast-feed. The Tanka women who use only their right breasts have smaller and softer left breasts. Postmenopausal Tanka women have a much higher rate of left-breast cancers than non-Tanka women. This study demonstrates that it is important to breast-feed using both breasts to confer protection to each breast.

Breast-feeding may reduce the risk of breast cancer simply by interrupting ovulation and thereby reducing the overall time that estrogen bathes the body.[40,41] Anatomical changes in the breast from breast-feeding may also contribute to the protection. Animals that are breast-feeding generally resist the effects of chemical carcinogens to the breast during that period of time.

Human breast milk is rich in immune components, like antibodies, that protect the baby. Human breast milk is economical, nutritious, and uncontaminated. In undeveloped countries, use of breast milk may be the single most important factor in an infant's physical survival. In developed countries, like the United States, where commercial formulas are available without fear of contamination, and where the pace and social stigma of society may decrease the willingness to breast-feed, the infant's physical survival is less dependent on breast milk.

Human breast milk can, however, pass the human immunodeficiency virus (HIV) as well as other infectious disease agents to the infant.[42] But new evidence suggests that HIV may not be the important factor in causing AIDS. Also, an infant will have the same alcohol level as her/his mother's serum level if the mother drinks alcohol.[43] Infants taste and, hence, react differently to various foods that mothers eat.

Infants who drink the milk of mothers who have silicone breast implants may be at risk for developing autoimmune diseases with the same frequency as the mother who has the implant.[44] In almost all of the infants who fed from silicone implanted breasts, systemic sclerosis developed which included esophagus-related problems in swallowing. Bottle-fed children of mothers with silicone implants were unaffected.

Breast-feeding has multiple advantages:

- Decreases breast cancer risk if lactation continues for six to twelve months or more;
- Decreases severity of baby's gastrointestinal infections;

- Enhances maternal-infant relationship;
- Enhances woman's confidence about motherhood.

Bilateral breast-feeding is preferable to unilateral.

Breast cancer may be reduced in premenopausal women by 11 percent if they breast-feed for four to twelve months. If they breast-feed for twenty-four months or more, the incidence may be reduced by almost 25 percent.[31]

Cancer and Pregnancy

There are not many situations in medicine that arouse the anxiety of the physician and patient as much as the discovery of cancer in the pregnant woman. Cancer during pregnancy is not an infrequent occurrence. About 1 of every 1,000 pregnancies involves cancer, and about 1 of every 118 women who are found to have cancer will be pregnant at the time. The cancers most often seen in pregnant women in order of their prevalence are breast cancer, cervical cancer, ovarian cancer, lymphoma, and colorectal cancer.

Cancer and pregnancy are the only two biological conditions in which cells foreign to the mother, that is, the cancer cells and those that make up the fetus—foreign because half of the genetic make-up of the fetus is from the father—are tolerated by what appears to be a relatively normal immune system. These conditions are permitted because some aspects of the immune system are not working to peak capacity. Hormones like estrogen, progesterone, alpha fetal protein, and human chorionic gonadotropin all have an immunosuppressive effect on the mother's immune system, without which the fetus would not grow. Other changes that occur during pregnancy are depression of the cellular killers, enhancement of certain blocking antibodies, and alteration of other esoteric factors of the immune system. The hormonal mechanisms that ensure the survival of the fetus and consequently suppress the immune system are the same mechanisms that also favor the progress of a cancer. However, the important point is *pregnancy*, per se, *is probably not a risk factor for the development of cancer nor is it likely that it will cause existing cancer to spread.*[45-48] Only one study from Sweden suggests a slight and transient risk for the development of breast cancer in a woman who has just given birth.[49]

Poor results seen in the treatment of cancer in pregnant women have largely been due to late diagnosis or inadequate treatment.[50] Signs of cancer can often be mistakenly attributed to changes due to pregnancy or lactation. If you discover you have a cancer during pregnancy, treatment should be instituted without delay by delivering the fetus if it is viable. However, data suggest that treatment should not be delayed to obtain a viable fetus. Since the symptoms of the cancer are usually attributed to the pregnancy, the diagnosis is usually somewhat delayed, and generally speaking, the prognosis is slightly worse in patients who are pregnant and who have cancer, especially those who have breast cancer.

Should you become pregnant after having been diagnosed as having breast cancer? This is a very common question since breast cancer is one of the leading causes of death in women. A review of the data reveals that pregnancy is not associated with excessive risk of cancer recurrence; hence, there is little evidence for advising against subsequent pregnancy for women who want to become pregnant and are free of any recurrences at the time. However, it is still recommended that breast cancer patients do not become pregnant. Given the fact that most cancer recurrences appear within the first two years, it is prudent to advise a woman not to become pregnant until she has been free of cancer for at least two years. Should a pregnancy occur before two years have elapsed, the decision for a therapeutic abortion should be based on the patient's treatment program and other factors.

Most of the time, a physician attending a patient who has had a cancer or a patient with a newly diagnosed cancer will decide whether to recommend an abortion based on his feelings or religious beliefs. When the supporting data concerning these patients as outlined above are presented to physicians, these data fly in the smack of what has been taught, handed down, or otherwise believed. Hence, abortions are commonly recommended. The data for this section involve well over 300 references and have been reviewed in two major investigations.

Benign Breast Disease

Lumpy breast disease is influenced greatly by a number of factors: hormonal changes, dietary practices such as consumption of caffeine and foods high in fat and inadequate intake of certain vitamins and minerals, and nicotine exposure. A randomized trial involving twenty-one patients who had painful breasts premenstrually for at least five years showed these women benefited from a diet that reduced the fat content to 15 percent of their total calories and increased complex carbohydrate consumption to maintain the normal caloric intake. There was a significant reduction in the severity of the breast tenderness and swelling after six months. Physical examination also showed reduced breast swelling, tenderness, and nodularity in 60 percent of the patients.[51]

Since 1979, I have treated women with breast cancer and benign breast disorders, specifically lumpy breast disease. All the patients with lumpy breast disease followed my Ten-Point Plan as presented on pages 317 through 333, with particular attention paid to low-fat, high-fiber foods, supplementation with certain vitamins and minerals, abstinence from alcohol and smoking, and avoidance of passive smoke. Almost 90 percent of the patients had decreased breast pain premenstrually, and about half of the patients experienced a decrease in the size of their cysts. In most cases the size of the breast diminished somewhat; however, in about 10 percent of the women, the size of the breast increased slightly.

Prolactin

A number of studies indicate that high levels of prolactin, a hormone secreted by the pituitary gland in the brain, may be a risk factor for breast cancer. Normally, prolactin levels rise during pregnancy and then promote and maintain lactation for breast-feeding. Although there is wide range of normal values for prolactin in the nonpregnant state, values two to two and one-half times higher than normal have been associated with breast cancer.[52]

In a provocative study, investigators have shown that a first pregnancy causes a significant decrease in the normal secretion of prolactin. This effects long-term changes lasting twelve to thirteen years regardless of the age of the pregnant woman. Researchers have proposed that the long-term depression of prolactin after an early first pregnancy may be a protective factor against the development of breast cancer.[53]

HORMONES ADMINISTERED TO PATIENTS

Several hormonal risk factors stem from external factors (exogenous).

DES

A little more than two million women took diethylstilbestrol, commonly known as DES, to avert miscarriages in the 1940s and 1950s. Adding this figure to the number of children exposed to DES brings the total to an estimated six million. DES is associated with vaginal and cervical adenocarcinomas and dysplasia in women who were exposed to the drug as fetuses.[54,55] Women who took DES during pregnancy have a higher risk of developing breast cancer.[56-58]

In addition, sons of DES-exposed mothers have reproductive and urinary tract abnormalities. One of these is undescended testicles, which may lead to cancer of the testes if uncorrected before the age of 6.[59]

In Italy, between the years 1977 and 1979, there was an epidemic of breast enlargement in children that, when investigated, proved to be caused by the presence of DES in the meat the children ate.[60] Although it was known that cattle were being treated with hormones including DES, the potential consequences were not realized until the late 1970s. We must continue to keep abreast of the amount and type of hormones used in the animals we consume.

It is recommended by a research task force that women who were exposed to DES inform their physicians and:

1. Tell your daughter or son about your DES exposure.
2. Try to obtain the details of your DES dosage and the duration you took it.
3. Have an annual physical examination (the same type of examination all women should have if they are over twenty or sexually active). The examination should include:

   - A pelvic examination with a Pap smear.
   - A breast examination by a physician.
   - Mammography (X-ray study of the breast) *if you have no symptoms of breast cancer*; annually if you are over 50. (Do not have a mammography screening if you are younger than 35.)

4. Practice breast self-examination every month. Report anything suspicious to your doctor; however, 80 percent of all breast lumps are not cancer.
5. Report any unusual bleeding or discharge from the vagina to a physician immediately.
6. Avoid exposure to other estrogens. This includes oral contraceptives, estrogens as a "morning-after" pill, and estrogens used as replacement therapy during or after menopause.

The recommendations for a daughter of a DES-exposed mother are similar:

- If unusual bleeding or discharge occurs from the vagina at any age, see your physician immediately.
- If you have no symptoms, you should have a pelvic examination including a Pap smear at least once a year starting at age 14 or when you begin to menstruate—whichever is first.
- During the pelvic exam, the vaginal walls should be temporarily stained so the physician can see any abnormalities.
- Follow-up examinations are most important.

It is recommended that sons of DES-exposed mothers have a physician check their reproductive and urinary systems to make certain there are no abnormalities.

Oral Contraceptives

The risk of developing cancer, specifically breast cancer, with the use of oral contraceptives has been the focus of much controversy and media attention. It is a topic that evokes dramatic swings of emotion in patients, physicians, and newscasters. Scores and scores of studies have been done on the subject. A number of studies show no increased risk in cancer, including breast cancer, but the great majority of studies show an increased risk of developing breast cancer in those who use oral contraceptives.[61]

Recent studies show that early use of oral contraceptives is linked to a high incidence of breast cancer. Women who have used oral contraceptives with a high progesterone content, the so-called "safer pills," for five years prior to age 25 are four times more likely to get breast cancer than those who did not.[62] Another study of women less than 45 years old showed a correlation between risk of breast cancer and use of oral contraceptives. Women who used birth control pills for four or more years had a threefold increase in their risk for breast cancer.[63,64] The most recent study involving a large number of women has come from the UK National Case Control Study Group. The risk of breast cancer among women under age 36 was found to be increased by 74 percent by long-term use—eight years or more—of oral contraceptives. Those who took the contraceptives for four to eight years had a 43 percent greater chance of developing breast cancer. Oral contraceptive use accounted for 20 percent of all breast cancers among the women studied.[65] Two more major studies have been done that confirm this relationship: There is an increased risk of breast cancer when a person begins using oral contraceptives at an early age.[66,67] Comprehensive reviews of all previous epidemiological studies that have been reported confirm that oral contraceptives are a risk factor for breast cancer.[68,69]

Oral contraceptives have also been associated with cancer of the cervix. The incidence of cervical cancer increases from the second through eighth years of using oral contraceptives. In addition, oral contraceptive users have a higher incidence of carcinoma *in situ* and premalignant conditions like dysplasia of the cervix than do women who do not use birth control pills.[70] Oral contraceptives have also been linked to primary liver cancer.[71] In addition to its correlation with cancer risk, oral contraceptive use has been associated with lumpy breast disease, stroke, heart attack, pulmonary embolus, and other cardiovascular illnesses.

Oral contraceptive use does not increase the risk of all types of cancer. Two studies have reported that oral contraceptive use may marginally reduce the risk of getting ovarian cancer and endometrial cancer.[72,73]

The preponderance of evidence suggests that oral contraceptive use is a strong risk factor for the development of breast cancer. The earlier in life a woman uses it, the higher is her risk. Oral contraceptives also have contributed to other forms of cancer and cardiovascular illness. The *minimal* protection allegedly seen for ovarian cancer and endometrial cancer in a few studies should not entice people to use the contraceptive. The U.S. Food and Drug Administration inserts a warning in all oral contraceptive packages which states that oral contraceptive use is associated with cancer, cardiovascular disease, and other illnesses.

Progesterone as a Contraceptive

Injection of medroxyprogesterone as a contraceptive has been shown to increase the risk of developing breast cancer, cervical cancer, uterine cancer, and ovarian cancer in women.[74,75]

Estrogen Use in Menopause

Life expectancy in women today is 86. This life expectancy has increased by thirty years since the turn of the century, but the average age for the onset of menopause is 51½, which has not changed significantly. One-sixth of the United States population are postmenopausal women, and the number of women age 65 or older is expected to double by the year 2000. Estrogens are used to prevent osteoporosis, decrease cardiovascular risk,[76] and minimize the effects of menopausal symptoms, like vulvovaginal dryness, urinary frequency, urgency, incontinence, dyspareunia, and skin and hair changes associated with inadequate estrogen and relative androgen excess.

Despite the benefits of estrogen use, there is also a down side. Exogenous estrogens (estrogens taken by mouth) affect some cells' division and may make them abnormal. Normally the hormones produced by the body are in a very delicate balance. If you take additional hormones, the tissues that respond to them may become abnormal and cancerous. An extensive review of the literature indicates that estrogens taken by mouth increase the risk of cancer of the endometrium (uterus lining).[77-80] In addition to an increased risk of cancer of the endometrium, exogenous estrogens are also implicated in an increased incidence of breast cancer. Estrogens administered in large amounts have been associated with breast cancer in male transsexuals[81-83] as well as in male heart and ulcer patients.[84,85] The use of estrogens by postmenopausal women to relieve menopausal symptoms increases their risk of developing breast cancer.[86-88] Other risks seen in postmenopausal women using estrogens have been an increased risk of myocardial infarction (heart attack), stroke, gallbladder disease, porphyria, liver disease, and other cardiovascular illnesses.

Estrogen replacement therapy was thought to preserve cognitive function in older women. But in a well-designed study involving over 800 postmenopausal women, estrogen replacement did not preserve or heighten cognitive abilities.[89]

In all, there have been over sixty epidemiological studies that support the fact that postmenopausal use of estrogens increases the risk for developing breast cancer.[90-92] The longer estrogens were used, the higher the risk for breast cancer. After fifteen years of estrogen use, there is a 30 percent increase in breast cancer risk. The increased risk is the same for a woman who uses estrogens after natural menopause or menopause caused by ovarian ablation from surgery or radiation.

Some clinicians thought to add progesterone to estrogen in postmenopausal replacement in an attempt to decrease the risk. Hormones, in general, increase mitotic activity of cells, that is, make them turn over more quickly. Estrogens alone can induce quite a bit of cell division, but when progesterone is added to the mix, much more cell division is induced.[93]

A study done in Sweden involving over 23,000 women aged 35 or more who had both estrogen and progesterone showed that the women had a higher risk for developing breast cancer. In fact, progesterone did not protect against the harmful effects of estrogen and actually increased the breast cancer risk over and above the risk associated with estrogen.[94]

Estrogen Replacement for Patients With Prior Breast Cancer

Although there are no hard data, estrogen replacement is generally not recommended for postmenopausal patients who have had a prior diagnosis of breast cancer.[95] Low-dose estrogen such as would be used for replacement can feed a cancer, whereas high-dose estrogens have actually been used to treat advanced breast cancer. Tamoxifen, given to treat postmenopausal breast cancer, has been shown to decrease osteoporosis, decrease cholesterol, and decrease HDL-cholesterol—in short, an estrogen-like effect.

Thyroid Supplements

Thyroid supplements used in the treatment of hypothyroidism in women do not increase the risk of breast cancer.[96]

Androgens

Athletes' use of anabolic androgens to increase muscle bulk and performance carries a major risk. Not only do androgens cause cardiovascular illnesses, but they also have been implicated in the development of prostate cancer, liver cancer, and osteosarcoma, as well as benign liver disease. Because of their serious health risks, these agents must be severely restricted and not used.

SEXUAL-SOCIAL FACTORS

We have seen that a person's lifestyle can increase that person's risk of developing cancer. Sexual-social behavior is another example of lifestyle's influence on cancer risk.

Cervical Cancer

Women who start having sexual intercourse before age 16 with multiple male partners, particularly those who are uncircumcised, have higher incidence of cervical cancer. Oral contraceptives and tobacco have also been shown to be risk factors for cervical cancer. Passive smoke exposure for three hours/day increases the risk of developing cervical cancer by a factor of three. A woman has a higher risk of cervical cancer if her husband had previously been married to a woman with cervical cancer. Fortunately, increased awareness of the importance of early cancer detection has led to increased Pap smears over the past two decades. As a result, cervical abnormalities have been detected in their early stages and treated earlier.

AIDS and Cancer

AIDS now rivals cancer as the most feared disease in the nation, and many Americans believe that almost everyone is susceptible to this deadly incurable disease (Media General—Associated Press Poll). The number of cases of Kaposi's sarcoma, anal cancers, and tongue cancers (the three tumors associated with AIDS) will probably rise accordingly.

CONCLUSION

All the studies reviewed suggest a consistent theme: If a woman tampers with Mother Nature's hormonal milieu by taking hormone pills, by disrupting reproduction, or by not reproducing at all, she has a high risk of developing certain cancers, especially breast cancer.

14
Air and Water

Mounting evidence suggests that our environment contains many carcinogens. The air we breathe, the water we drink, the radiation to which we are exposed, and the power lines that supply us with energy may pose threats to your health. It is important for you to understand what the dangers are so that you can work to modify them. As with many carcinogens, the time between exposure to environmental carcinogens and actual development of cancer may be quite long. Therefore, the cause of a cancer initiated by trace amounts of either airborne or waterborne carcinogens years before may be attributed to an unrelated or unknown factor at the time of diagnosis. This is why we must detect and clean our environment of as many carcinogens as possible.

OUTDOOR AIR

The American Lung Association estimates that air pollution costs the nation $40 billion to $60 billion a year. Since the mid-1950s, it has been shown that the air in large urbanized areas is a risk factor for lung cancer.[1-3] Collectively, the studies suggest that the increased incidence of cancer in cities is due to three factors: (1) more cigarette smoking by the people who live in cities; (2) increased exposure of nonsmokers to side-stream or passive smoke from lighted cigarettes; and (3) occupational exposures.

Various occupations involved with ambient air pollutants are risk factors for certain cancers. Gas production workers, especially if they are exposed to the products of coal carbonization, have a greater risk of getting lung cancer than those who rarely work in the gas production area. Men working at coke ovens in United States steel factories have an excess of lung cancer compared to men working in other parts of the steel industry. This is directly related to exposure to the emissions from the ovens. Roofers who work with hot pitch are exposed to large amounts of benzo(a)pyrene (BaP). They, too, have a higher risk of getting lung cancer. The concentration of BaP is a significant factor in heavily polluted cities and contributes to a high incidence of cancer.

The numerous atmospheric contaminants are found in one of two forms: particulate form, in which the carcinogen adheres to small particles in the air; or vapor form, in which the carcinogen is in a gas form. The carcinogens found in particulate form are more important than those in vapor form because they can remain in the air from four to forty days and consequently travel very long distances. Carcinogens in particulate form originate mainly from the burning of fuels. Contaminants in vapor form are derived from the release of aerosols from industrial activities, from car exhaust, and from natural sources. A city's atmosphere contains more contaminants than the atmosphere of a suburb or rural area. Many of these contaminants have been shown to be carcinogenic in various animals.

City air pollution is derived from many sources. A large amount of the particulate carcinogens comes from the burning of any material containing carbon and hydrogen, including petroleum, gasoline, and diesel fuel. A list of more than one hundred different particulates containing detected carcinogens has been compiled.[4] A great many more exist, but detection of additional carcinogens in low concentrations is difficult because existing instruments are incapable of measuring them.

Many studies indicated that tiny particulate air pollution in cities may be linked to higher mortality rates, but none showed this link to be conclusive.[5] But a large study, involving over eight thousand adults in six large United States cities, demonstrated that even though the air pollution was well within federal standards, there was a definite higher mortality related to tiny particle air pollution. People's lives were shortened by years rather than less significant periods.[6-8]

The carcinogens found in the vapor phase include benzene, carbon tetrachloride, chloroform, and vinyl chloride, among others.[9] Most of these chemicals are strong human carcinogens. Vapor phase carcinogens are derived from car emissions, industrial activity, burning of solid waste, forest fires, and evaporation of solvents.[10]

Asbestos, a potent carcinogen, can also be airborne. Persons working with the following may inhale high concentrations of asbestos: asbestos roofing and flooring, car brakes and clutches, dry walls, home heating and plumbing. Family members of persons who work with asbestos or asbestos products are exposed to very high levels of asbestos also. High levels of asbestos are found near asbestos waste dumps; near asbestos mines, mills, and manufacturing plants; near braking vehicles; at demolition areas; and in buildings that were sprayed with asbestos.

Asbestos as a risk factor for lung cancer is well established for those who work with the substance and for their family members. Cigarette smoking acts synergistically with asbestos to greatly enhance the risk of lung cancer. It is *extremely* rare for lung cancer to develop in an asbestos worker in the absence of exposure to tobacco smoke.

Diesel Exhaust Exposure

Animal studies in rats and mice show a link between exposure to whole diesel exhaust and lung cancer. The lung cancer is associated with diesel exhaust particulates and diesel exhaust gas.

Several human studies have also been done and show an increased risk of death from lung cancer in workers who have been exposed to diesel engine emissions.[11] This, too, is another controllable risk factor, especially emissions from vehicles that are obviously polluting the air.

ACID RAIN

Acid rain is a direct consequence of polluted air. Because of air pollution, in many parts of the world, rain can no longer be regarded as a beneficial occurrence; rather, it is thought to be a deadly acidic agent. Acid rain results when sulfur dioxide and nitrogen oxide are released into the atmosphere and converted into sulfuric acid and nitric acid. The evidence shows that fossil fuel combustion and power plant emissions contribute significantly to the production of acid rain.[12]

Next to carbon dioxide, acid rain ranks second as the most serious global pollution problem in modern times. Many natural habitats in the United States, Norway, Sweden, Scotland, and Canada, and some areas of the Netherlands, Denmark, and Belgium, have been reported to be severely hurt by acid rain. Because of the increased acid in the atmosphere, there has been a decrease in the fish population and in other forms of animal life and vegetation in the lake areas of Canada, Eastern United States, Sweden, and Norway.[13] Vegetation and some animal forms are affected first; later, fish suffer the harmful effects of acid increases. Acid rain has also decreased the amount of fir, spruce, and beech trees in the forests of central Europe.

Normal rain water is slightly acidic. But the higher acidity of acid rain is devastating to human, animal, and plant life. During the past thirty years, there has been a substantial increase in the amount of acid precipitation. Three important changes that have enhanced the production of acid rain are : (1) higher chimneys, (2) control of particulate discharge, and (3) a change from seasonal to year-round emission. Two of these were designed by environmentalists to control pollution. The tall chimneys allow the oxides of sulfur and nitrogen to stay longer in the atmosphere and, thereby, convert more efficiently to the acid.

The lethal effects of acid rain are due not only to the acidity but also to the aluminum and other toxic metals that are mobilized from the soil by the acid. Aluminum is toxic to fish and other life forms.[14] Zinc, nickel, lead, manganese, and cadmium are also increased in water after acid precipitation. Zinc, nickel, and mercury are toxic to aquatic forms of life. The direct toxic effects to man are still being reviewed. Aluminum poisoning is recognized in patients with impaired renal function and in patients with certain neurological diseases like Alzheimer's and amyotrophic lateral sclerosis in Guam.[15,16] Amyotrophic lateral sclerosis is prevalent in areas of Guam, where there is a high acid rain content. Consequently, there is a high aluminum concentration and low calcium level in the drinking water in Guam. Low calcium levels in the body lead to increased absorption of aluminum, which then gets deposited in the brain, causing the neurological disorder. The addition of calcium to the diet can help reverse this problem of increased aluminum absorption.

Another heavy metal of major concern is lead. Most of the lead that enters our bodies comes from food, dust, and air. Combustion of petroleum products is a main source of lead in the air and dust. Acid rain is also a culprit, leaching lead from the soil and putting it in our drinking water. Also mobilized by acid rain is mercury, which is consumed by fish that we, in turn, consume. And finally, acid rain reduces the selenium content of the soil, leading to deficiencies of selenium, which is important in cancer prevention.

Acid rain may also be deposited on the human skin, but there have been no harmful consequences from this. However, people can inhale the sulfuric acid and nitric acid, which inhibit normal functioning of the lungs.

Findings of the United States National Acid Precipitation Assessment Program confirm the following:

- Acid rain adversely affects aquatic life in about 10 percent of Eastern lakes and streams.

- Acid rain decreases the number of red spruce at high elevations.
- Acid rain contributes to the corrosion of buildings and materials.
- Acid rain and other pollutants, especially fine sulfate particles, reduce visibility in the Northeastern states and in parts of the West.

There seems to be no direct correlation between acid rain and the etiology of cancer in humans; however, studies are ongoing. The key regions in the United States affected by acid rain are the Northeast, Midwest, and West. Lakes in the Northeast are being acidified by acid rain produced by the high-sulfur coal burned in the large power plants of the industrial Midwest. To control acid rain, we should remove the sulfuric and nitric acids at their source by switching to fossil fuel with a low sulfur content. Low-sulfur fuel can almost completely obviate the production of acid rain, eliminating it as a risk factor for many illnesses.

DEPLETION OF NATURAL UPPER ATMOSPHERIC OZONE

The naturally occurring ozone layer in the upper atmosphere is crucial to the protection of living organisms because it absorbs harmful ultraviolet radiation. About 3 percent of the sun's electromagnetic output is emitted as ultraviolet radiation, but only a fraction of this reaches the surface of the Earth. Wavelengths of 240–290 are eliminated, and only a portion of the wavelengths at 290–320 penetrate to the Earth. The lower-range ultraviolet light wavelengths destroy DNA, which is the genetic material of all life forms.

Chlorofluorocarbons, commonly known as CFCs, are chemical compounds that have been shown to damage the protective ozone layer. Of major concern now is the appearance of an actual hole in the ozone layer over Antarctica.[17] The concern here is obvious: What happens if there is a hole in the ozone layer above more densely populated areas of the globe?

Ultraviolet exposure is highly associated with melanoma, basal cell carcinoma, and squamous cell carcinoma of the skin. People with fair skin, blond hair, and blue eyes who also sunburn easily are at highest risk for the development of these skin cancers. Not only does ultraviolet exposure cause cancer, but in most people it causes severe skin damage and ages the skin dramatically. The U.S. Environmental Protection Agency calculates that a 1 percent decrease in the ozone concentration will increase the incidence of most skin cancers by 3–5 percent. The EPA further calculates that for every 2.5 percent increase per year of chlorofluorocarbon, an additional million skin cancers and 20,000 deaths will occur over the lifetime of the existing United States population. In fact, in 1990 the incidence of skin cancer increased markedly: squamous cell carcinoma rose 3.1 times in women and 2.6 times in men; and melanoma rose 4.6 times in women and 3.5 times in men. By the year 2000, 1 in 75 will develop melanoma.

Effects on other living organisms may be far more important than the actual risk to man. Certain organisms, in particular phytoplankton, zooplankton, and the larval stages of fish, are very sensitive to small increases in ultraviolet exposure. The resultant decrease in the food chain and in the oxygen output from the oceans' plants will have serious and dramatic repercussions on all human life.

Addressing the Problem

A research model indicates that the global ozone will be 6 percent lower in the year 2030 than it was in 1970.[18] This will increase the incidence of nonmelanomatous skin cancer by 12–36 percent and melanoma mortality by 9–18 percent. An assessment by the U.S. National Aeronautics and Space Agency indicates that ozone depletion is occurring globally and is progressing faster than previously realized. We need to minimize the use of chlorofluorocarbons. CFCs are in aerosols, foam blowers for items such as hamburger cartons and drinking cups, refrigerants and cooling systems, and solvents for computer circuits. In most instances, nonchlorinated substitutes are available or can be developed. Some countries are recommending a 20 percent reduction of CFCs; the United States is recommending a 50 percent reduction. However, some CFCs remain in the air for over a century. Halones, used in fire extinguishers throughout the world, are synergistic with CFCs. Once use of these chemicals is stopped and once the ozone depletion has stopped, it will be many decades before any useful improvement is seen.

If pentane is used instead of chlorofluorocarbons as the blowing agent to produce foam products, *ozone is produced* both in the stratosphere and at the ground level. Now let's assume that pentane is used to produce a polystyrene drinking cup. Which do you think costs more to your pocketbook and the environment, a paper cup or a polystyrene cup? The paper cup costs more by far. A paper cup costs more to make from the standpoint of raw materials (wood, bark, petroleum fractions), finished weight, wholesale price, utilities needed to produce it (steam, power, cooling water), waste products produced, and air emissions (chlorine, chlorine dioxide, reduced sulfides, particulates).[19] The polystyrene cup is easier to recycle and ultimately to dispose. Here again, we have the proper technology; we simply need to do something about it.

We can all do something about this major problem. We can write to our senators and congressmen to encourage them to completely ban all chemical compounds that will further deplete the ozone layer. Again, the solution to this problem is totally within our control.

OZONE POLLUTION

Ozone at ground level is different from the naturally occurring protective ozone layer in the upper atmosphere that shields the Earth from harmful ultraviolet rays. Ozone at ground level is the most widespread air pollutant in any industrialized country and is formed when car exhaust and other emissions from industries react with sunlight.

Ozone forms when certain compounds react with sunlight. These compounds include nitrogen oxides and volatile organic compounds. Nitrogen oxides are derived from motor vehicles as well as industrial plants. Volatile organic compounds come from things like backyard barbecues and dry cleaners.

Smog is derived predominantly from ozone as well as from volatile organic compounds, carbon monoxides, nitrogen oxides, sulfur oxides, and other particulates. These compounds are derived from bakeries during the fermentation process; dry cleaning chemicals; paints; wood-burning stoves and starter fluid used to ignite charcoal; and industries and motor vehicles using fossil fuels. However, ground level ozone is clearly the most widespread air pollution problem we know today.

In a study involving children in a summer camp, researchers found that there was enough ozone pollution in the air at ground level to cause significant impairment of lung function in about 70 percent of the campers. The effects of this ozone pollution at ground level persisted for about eighteen hours after exposure, and the suspicion is that even small changes in the lungs' capacity may lead to cell damage and ultimately to chronic respiratory illness.

Ozone pollution is a health hazard, particularly for those with respiratory illnesses and those who exercise out-of-doors. Ozone at ground level has been linked to cancer, lung disease, heart disease, and many other chronic illnesses. In healthy people, ozone impairs the ability of the lungs to absorb oxygen. Repeated exposure to ozone leads to early stages of lung damage similar to that seen from smoking. Respiratory infections are quite common in people who breathe more ozone at ground level than others. People who are asthmatic do much worse when the ozone level is high. Cardiac patients do worse because the amount of oxygen in the air is reduced. The incidence of mortality also is increased in older people who have respiratory illnesses in areas with high levels of sulfur oxides in the air.

The Environmental Protection Agency conducted a study involving nonsmoking men in a room where ozone was close to the federal maximum. After five hours of walking and then bicycling, 80 percent of these men began to cough and feel chest pains. In a study of men who exercised for only two hours while breathing ozone that was below the federal maximum but still above the ambient air in very rural settings, 80 percent experienced serious symptoms of the lower airways. The airways were inflamed, and biochemical changes occurred with a subsequent impaired immune response at the local sites of the lung.

Most cities exceed the federal ozone standard. Los Angeles has the most and other cities that have a large amount of ozone smog include New York, Philadelphia, Trenton, Baltimore, Hartford, Chicago, and Houston. Some national parks like Acadia, Shenandoah, and Sequoia national parks have higher ozone levels than some cities because of their proximity to the major cities with smog and/or the air currents around them.

Ground level ozone can be controlled. We must insist again that the fuels burned are better and cleaner so that less volatile organic compounds, nitrogen oxides, and other ozone-producing compounds are emitted. And although the 1990 Clean Air Act is thought to be the most expensive environmental legislation ever passed in terms of attaining the new standards, enforcement of these standards must also be rigorous.

ULTRAVIOLET SUNLIGHT

There are two major forms of ultraviolet light emitted from the sun, ultraviolet A (UVA) and ultraviolet B (UVB). The UVB is the more harmful of the two and has wavelengths between 290 and 320 nanometers, whereas UVA has wavelengths between 320 and 400 nanometers, which is where the visible light spectrum begins.

The current package labeling on a sunscreen product states its ability to protect against UVB, the form responsible for causing sunburn and skin cancers. UVA can also cause skin cancer but, in addition, causes skin damage and premature aging of the skin. New labeling regulations by the FDA will reflect the UVA protection as well. You need to have protection from both forms of ultraviolet light.

Sunglasses should be used to protect your eyes from the harmful ultraviolet rays of the sun. People frequently ask whether the cost of the sunglasses reflects the protection they afford. Thirty different makes and prices of sunglasses were tested for ultraviolet transmission. Each of the sunglasses completely filtered all UVB radiation, hence no danger to the eye would be anticipated if sunglasses were worn. With respect to transmission of UVA to the eye, the results varied greatly but had no relation to price.[20] Hence, when you see a person with a pair of sunglasses costing $200, you can laugh quietly knowing that your $2 sunglasses give you just as much protection.

INDOOR AIR

Indoor air pollution has become a major problem, causing both specific illnesses and the minor complaints that now constitute the "sick building syndrome."[21] Indoor accumulation of radon (a gas formed by disintegration of radium), passive smoking pollutants, combustion pollutants from stoves, chemical emission from plastics, and insulation materials are just a sample of the indoor pollutants that are hazardous.

When radon is present in the soil below buildings or in surface water or construction materials, particularly granite, the indoor radon concentration will exceed the acceptable standard as set by the Environmental Protection Agency at 4 pCi/liter ("pCi" are pica Curies).[22] Some homeowners have spent $1,000 to $2,000 to comply with this standard. In 1988, however, Congress passed the Indoor Radon Abatement Act, which forces the EPA to set the standard of indoor radon equal to that of outdoor radon. The average cost to homeowners to comply with the newer standard could be close to $10,000.

Radon has now been implicated in up to 20,000 deaths from lung cancer in the United States.[23] A person living in a house with an indoor radon level of 4 pCi/liter has the same risk of developing lung cancer as a person who smokes half a pack of cigarettes per day.[24] The risk of lung cancer is increased if people smoke cigarettes and are exposed to radon, as in the case of coal miners.[25]

Freestanding stoves without chimneys increase the indoor air concentration of nitric oxide, benzo(a)pyrene, and sometimes even sulfur dioxide. These pollutants increase respiratory disease. Kerosene stoves also produce many pollutants, several of which are carcinogenic. Heat exchangers, cooling towers, and leaky shower heads provide favorable culture media for many microorganisms. These bacteria and other organisms disperse in droplets and remain airborne via mechanical or thermal air movements. *Legionella premophilia* (Legionnaires' disease) and many other organisms have been detected airborne in closed indoor situations.

Passive smoking is a serious problem in indoor air pollution. Passive smoking is responsible for doubling the lung cancer rate in persons exposed to it as compared to those not exposed to passive smoking.[26] In past years, it has been up to the individual to avoid such passive smoking, but things have changed. A nonsmoking Swedish office worker was awarded damages for a lung cancer he developed from breathing other people's tobacco smoke in the office. Now in the

United States, there are many laws to protect the passive smoker in certain public areas and on domestic airline flights. Hopefully, more and more such laws will protect us in *all* public areas.

Other indoor pollutants come from materials that are used in the construction of modern buildings, such as formaldehyde, isocyanates, solvents, and volatile synthetic organic compounds. These are used in the manufacture of insulin, decoration, and equipment. We know that formaldehyde is associated with human cancer.

To protect ourselves against indoor pollutants, we simply need to have adequate ventilation. Studies show that one or more air changes per hour should be provided, and that the carbon dioxide concentration should not exceed 0.5 percent. As we move toward a service-oriented society in America, with more people working in offices, this problem is everyone's concern. However, it can soon be eliminated if we work to modify the environment.

WATER POLLUTION

In 1960, W.C. Hueper warned that the drinking water in the United States was contaminated with natural and manmade pollutants and that some of these were potentially carcinogenic.[27] In addition, other reports in the past ten years have shown that there are carcinogens in the drinking water and that, in some areas, contaminated water has been associated with an increased cancer risk and other medical problems.

There are several groups of drinking water contaminants that may be carcinogenic. Synthetic organic chemicals comprise the first group, the carcinogenic potential of which is of greatest concern. The U.S. Environmental Protection Agency has found over 700 organic chemicals in our drinking water,[28] and that number probably represents a small fraction of the actual number that exists. Forty of these are carcinogens, and three (benzene, chloromethyl ether, and vinyl chloride) are associated with cancers in man.[29] Drinking polluted water is said by the EPA to be one of the top four health hazards to Americans, but enforcement of existing laws has been poor at best, and enforcement of additional laws and standards will be difficult. The standard set by the EPA allows municipalities to average their water toxicities over a year. For example, much more chlorine is added to water during summer months to hold down microorganisms. In some cities, the tap water level of chlorine carcinogens exceeds the standard by 20 percent during these months. The same spike of toxicity holds true for nitrates and pesticides, both used seasonally for lawn beautification and farming.

Water chlorination produces chemical compounds called trihalomethanes, which are the most common organic compounds found in drinking water. These compounds, which include chloroform and bromohalomethane, are associated with a high incidence of gastrointestinal cancers and urinary bladder cancers.[30,31] In fact, a study from the U.S. National Cancer Institute involving 3,000 people suggests that chlorine may double the risk for developing urinary bladder cancer. The EPA's safety limit of chlorine and its harmful associated carcinogens is based on the consumption of two liters of water a day, and this does not take into account increased consumption in summer, for example, or the fact that these compounds can be absorbed during bathing.

Fewer organic chemicals are found in drinking water that comes from ground water sources than from surface water sources.[32] Chlorinated drinking water from surface sources is linked with gastrointestinal cancers as well as urinary bladder cancers.[33-35]

The second group of water contaminants consists of inorganic chemicals. These are needed for normal biological processes and are found in all natural waters. Some, however, are carcinogenic. Arsenic, chromium, and nickel, each a known carcinogen to man, are found in our drinking water; these can either increase or decrease in concentration during water treatment.[36] Nitrate ions are found in surface or ground waters, and their concentration is not affected by water treatment. As you may recall from Chapter 10, nitrates can be converted to nitrosamines, which are powerful carcinogens. Nitrates are used for fertilizers, and in the early summer, the Corn Belt states' water supply sometimes has a 50 percent higher nitrate content than what is acceptable.

Lead also is a big problem. Lead can impair a child's IQ and attention span. One in six people in the United States drinks water with higher than acceptable levels of lead. Chicago has one of the worst lead water-pollution problems in the United States. Suppliers were still using lead pipes there until 1986. Lead pipes were used in antiquity in Pompeii; those people later realized that large numbers died until their lead pipes became calcified with calcium from the water.

The amount of calcium and magnesium in water determines water "hardness." It appears that soft water, water containing lesser amounts of calcium and particularly magnesium, is correlated with a higher incidence of all cardiovascular diseases.[37,38] Low calcium levels are also linked to osteoporosis, hypertension,[39] and even colon cancer.[40,41] No definite conclusions can be made yet as to whether all drinking water should be made "hard" with the addition of more magnesium and/or calcium to modify the risk for cardiovascular diseases and cancer, as well as other illnesses.

Radioactive materials constitute the third group of drinking water contaminants. Their concentration varies with geography, geology, industrial wastes, pharmaceutical use, and nuclear power generation.[42] So far there are no reported cases of human cancer related to different radioactive compounds in drinking water.[43] However, radon gets into ground water, especially in New Jersey, the New England states, and the Rocky Mountain states. Excessive levels of radon are seen in water supplies used for drinking and bathing by more than 17 million people.

Living organisms make up the fourth group. They include bacteria, viruses, and protozoa. Water purification has been effective in removing them from our drinking water. Some microbes resist current water purification, and these are responsible for 33 percent of all gastrointestinal infections in the United States. Microorganisms are not believed to be waterborne carcinogens; however, certain viruses cause human cancers.

The last group of water contaminants is solid particulates. Clays, asbestos particles, and organic particulates comprise this group. Clays absorb and bind carcinogenic agents and, hence, protect them from water treatment. Asbestos fibers are found naturally in water in many regions of Canada and some parts of the United States. In addition, some asbestos fibers are found where cement and other construction products are made, since asbestos is used in their production. Asbestos fibers can also get into the water supply by release from cement pipes and by processes associated with mining of iron ore. Many studies of the association between waterborne asbestos and human cancer are inconclusive because so many other variables may be interacting. However, one study by M.S. Kanarek has shown that measured concentrations of asbestos in drinking water are associated with lung cancer, gallbladder cancer, pancreatic cancer, and several other cancers.[44]

Our drinking water contains a number of carcinogens, including asbestos, metals, and synthetic organic compounds. Asbestos and nitrates are associated with gastrointestinal cancers; arsenic is associated with skin cancer; and synthetic organic chemicals, especially trihalomethanes, are associated with cancers of the gastrointestinal tract and the urinary bladder.

Who is to blame for the shambles of the water supply? Probably everyone. The standards issued by the EPA in the late seventies doubled in 1992. James Elder, commissioner of the EPA, says that forty-eight to forty-nine states do not comply with existing standards, or comply by way of loopholes. For example, a loophole permits water suppliers to flush lead-filled water out of plumbing before testing tap water. This loophole will be closed, but the EPA will allow twenty years more for compliance. On the other hand, the EPA has been lax. Studies show that radon increases cancer risk, and more to the point, drinking water with radon increases the risk for certain kinds of cancers. However, the EPA just recently imposed restrictions starting in 1996 for radon in the drinking water. Monitoring and removing radon is simple and inexpensive to do, but still no action will be taken until 1996.

Eighty percent of the top 1,000 superfund sites, that is, those designated as containing toxic waste and chemical contaminants, are leaching these toxic substances into the ground water. In many geographic sites in the United States, well water has been contaminated. About 10 percent of all underground tanks, which store gasoline or other hazardous chemicals, leak. Too many pesticides and fertilizers are used by farmers and homeowners. Industries dump chemicals and other harmful pollutants into our water supply, and homeowners dump chemicals into household drains.

Addressing the Problem

One of the major obstacles to our cleaning up America's underground toxic wastes is the unrealistic requirements that have been set by state and county authorities throughout the nation. Although the intentions may often be laudable, the effect of these laws has been to create such enormous costs, for most projects, that the clean-up effort is moving at a snail's pace. For example, a toxic site in Houston has a toxic-waste concentration of, say, 2,000 parts per billion. The local rules require a reduction of 99.99 percent. The problem is that there is no technology available at the present time that can accomplish this without digging up an enormous area of the earth and either processing it on the surface or moving it by rail to some remote location. These are expensive and disruptive operations, which are invariably fought by the agencies that are supposed to pay for them. The result is that litigation goes on for years while the people who live in the area are left to their toxic diet. The project, even if completed, will absorb excessive funds that might otherwise be available for many other projects.

The problem is that the objectives are simply too difficult to be accomplished by existing technologies. If the requirement had been to reduce the contaminants from 2,000 parts per billion to, say, 10 parts, it is possible that an in-ground vacuuming technology could have been used, reducing the health hazard by 99.5 percent and leaving limited funds available for twenty or thirty more of the same type of clean-up projects. The trick here is to promote the use of low-cost, in-ground technologies and increase the clean-up rate by

2,000–5,000 percent of the current rate without having to wait for the seemingly impossible dream of getting more funds from government and industry. The most promising development in this area is a new patented vacuuming technology that can "clean" far greater areas than the existing vacuuming technologies for the same cost. This device will be an advance if it can reduce the toxic chemicals to 0.6 parts per billion or less. If it cannot, then we must reexamine the standards set. It is better to clean up all the toxic sites by a significant factor like 99.5 percent than only a few sites by a factor of 99.99 percent and thereby propagate endless litigation.

A number of cities refuse to build costly processing plants and instead choose to pay less expensive fines. The EPA observes that small utilities tend to violate regulations the most, falsify documents, and even wash away evidence because of a thirty-day window given them by the state.

Bottled Versus Tap Water

Many people want to know if bottled water is safer than tap water. Recent findings indicate that many bottled waters derived from domestic or international springs or from other water sources contain microorganisms, and/or have contaminants. If you prefer bottled water, look for water derived from such processes as reverse osmosis, distillation, or a combination of reverse osmosis and deionization, which yields the purest form of water. This combined process gets rid of everything in water except H_2O; therefore, you should supplement your diet with certain nutrients already discussed in Chapter 5.

CONCLUSION

There are documented airborne and waterborne carcinogens. It is essential for us to detect and clean our environment of as many carcinogens as possible.

15
Electromagnetic Radiation

The electromagnetic radiation spectrum includes gamma rays, X-rays, ultraviolet light, visible light, infrared, microwaves, FM radio waves, AM radio waves, and long radio waves. Electromagnetic radiation with wavelengths longer than the color red (ranging from infrared to radio waves) or shorter than the color violet (ranging from ultraviolet to X-rays and gamma rays) is not visible to the eye but can be detected by other means. Radiation exposure is another risk factor for developing breast cancer.

DIAGNOSTIC AND THERAPEUTIC RADIATION

There are a number of real concerns concerning mammogram use, radiation therapy, and many other situations in which radiation exposure may increase the risk for developing breast cancer. The concern of increased risk is based on the many studies showing a high rate of breast cancer among women in Japan who were irradiated during the atomic bombings. More women who had exposure during ages 10 to 25 developed breast cancer from the radiation fall-out than women who were younger or women who were older.[1] Women with tuberculosis who had multiple serial chest X-rays to follow the course of the disease also had substantially increased rates of breast cancer.[2]

Mammogram

In 1980, FDA data showed that there were 4,000 mammography units of which only 19 percent met federal performance standards. In 1990, there were about 10,000 mammography units in use in the United States. Until recently, mammography screening had been promoted as safe and reliable for early detection of breast cancer; however, the radiation dose from current mammographic two-view examination techniques is extremely damaging to the glandular tissue (0.1-0.8 rad or 1-8 mGy).[3] Exposure today is much less than it was because the technology is much improved.[4]

The National Academy of Sciences and the National Cancer Institute estimate that for every 100,000 women at age 40 who are screened using mammography, there will be 10 more cancers than are normally seen in that age group due solely to mammograms. The estimate of 10 excess cases is based on the delivery of 1 cGy per mammogram per woman—the amount of radiation delivered by a technically good mammogram unit. However, as more radiation is delivered with older units or poorly calibrated units, this number will be higher based on the higher dose delivered to each patient.

Therapeutic Radiation for Cancer

Patients who had radiation therapy for various diseases have a higher incidence of breast cancer if the radiation therapy was delivered to or near the breast. Patients with Hodgkin's disease have a higher risk for developing a second malignancy from treatment. Patients who received chest radiation therapy for the treatment of Hodgkin's disease had a much higher risk for developing breast cancer than the normal population.[5] The women who did develop breast cancer secondary to the radiation for Hodgkin's disease were all under the age of 40 and on average had the radiation about ten years prior to the diagnosis of breast cancer.

Four patients of 910 survivors of childhood cancer developed infiltrating breast carcinoma after having had radiation delivered to the chest for the treatment of Wilms' tumor (bone sarcoma).[6] Three of these people were women and one was a man; they had received radiation between the ages of 8 and 13. The calculated dose delivered to the breast was about 300 cGy in this particular study. The number of breast cancer cases in this group of patients exceeds the expected number; hence, these breast cancers are attributed directly to the radiation therapy.

With more and more women becoming aware of breast-conserving surgery followed by radiation therapy to treat early stage breast cancer, there is a concern that primary radiation therapy delivered to the breast can, in fact, induce another cancer in the treated breast or in the opposite breast that receives scatter dose. The following studies, indeed, provide persuasive evidence that radiation increases the risk of breast cancer on the opposite side. A large Connecticut population was reviewed from 1935 to 1982. The risk of developing a second breast cancer was found to be almost 4 percent in the radiation-treated group versus 2.8 percent in the group treated by surgery alone.[7]

In a study done in Denmark from 1943 to 1980, the relative risk of developing breast cancer in a radiated patient after 9 years was 2.6 versus 2.0 for the nonirradiated patients.[8] Most of the other studies done, however, have shown no statistically significant increased risk in developing breast cancer in the opposite breast after having radiation therapy for breast cancer treatment.[9-16]

On balance, it seems that the risk is not substantially higher for developing breast cancer in the opposite breast when the patient receives radiation therapy for primary breast cancer treatment. But these patients obviously should be under close surveillance.

Therapeutic Radiation for Noncancerous Lesions

In the past, therapeutic doses of radiation had been given for benign lesions. This is generally no longer done.

There was a time when radiation was given to shrink the thymus gland in young babies because it was thought that this enlarged thymus gland was not normal. However, today we do know it is normal. Over 1,200 women were given radiation treatment in infancy for an enlarged thymus gland and they and their 2,400 nonirradiated sisters were studied. After a follow-up of about 36 years, there were 22 breast cancers in the radiated group and only 12 in their nonirradiated sister group. It was calculated that for every 100 cGy of radiation given, an excess of 3.5 breast cancer cases per 10,000 people was observed.[17]

Among children who received radiation therapy to the scalp, those who were exposed between the ages of five and nine had an increased risk for breast cancer.[18] And Stockholm women who received massive doses of radiation therapy for benign breast infections between the 1920s and 1950s, also had a higher risk for developing breast cancer.[19]

Summary

The data demonstrate that women are at high risk for developing breast cancer if they have been exposed to radiation at particularly critical times in their life—early childhood and teenage years. The exposure that puts a woman more at risk is low-dose radiation as with chest X-ray and perhaps mammography. High-dose radiation, therapeutic doses for treatment of breast cancer for instance, *generally* does not allow a cell to repair itself and the cell generally dies. There are a number of studies that show high-dose radiation can increase the risk for breast cancer.

In general, however, as with anything else in life, you must weigh the risk versus the benefit of getting a chest X-ray, of obtaining a mammogram, or of obtaining therapeutic radiation. When the risk is very high and the benefit low, you should consider not doing it. However, if the reverse is true, risk being low and benefit being quite high, go ahead with the test or treatment.

ELECTROMAGNETISM

Nonionizing electromagnetic radiation has become very important and is generated largely through electrical and magnetic fields that surround us. This kind of radiation includes infrared rays, microwaves, radiowaves, and alternating electrical currents. All of these, except for infrared rays, penetrate the body readily. Such radiation is found in household wiring, appliances, high-tension wires, radio transmitters, television screens, video display terminals, electric blankets, and even the Earth, which has its own electromagnetic field. In fact, this electromagnetic field is responsible for making a compass needle point in the direction of north. However, the Earth's electromagnetic fields do a flip flop, the North and South Pole fields trading places at intervals of hundreds of thousands of years. Beside vague symptoms of fatigue, nausea, headache, and loss of libido associated with electromagnetism,[20] there is now great concern over whether it can cause cancer.

An electromagnetic field is created along wires when electricity flows. The strength of the electromagnetic field is measured in gauss. The electromagnetic field is made of two components: the electric field made from the strength of the charge that starts the flow, and the magnetic field that results from the motion of the alternating currents.

Many countries like the United States use alternating electric currents that flow back and forth at a frequency of 60 cycles per second. This is within the extremely low-frequency range of the electromagnetic spectrum.

The energy needed to make electricity flow is called voltage. More voltage is needed to make electricity go farther. Depending on where electricity is needed to be delivered, voltage is either stepped-up or stepped-down along transmission lines by transformers at substations or on utility poles near homes. Most studies concerning the effects of electromagnetic fields on humans focus on the strength of the field.

All electrically driven products have electromagnetic fields. The closer you are to a given appliance or other source, the higher is the strength of the electromagnetic field. Table 15.1 lists electromagnetic field strength of common appliances from least to greatest.

Evidence shows almost a direct link between electromagnetic fields and cancer in rats. Researchers at Battell Pacific Northwest Laboratory in Richland, Washington, have shown that electromagnetic fields suppress the levels of a certain hormone called melatonin. Melatonin is produced by the pineal gland in the central part of the brain. It is a regulatory hormone and also modifies the functioning of the immune system. Low levels of melatonin have been linked to breast cancer as well as prostate cancer. Animal studies showing that exposure to electromagnetic fields lowers melatonin levels have been repeated and corroborated in multiple centers throughout North America.[21]

High- And Low-Voltage Wires

Many studies of the effects of electromagnetic fields on humans have also been conducted. Children and adults in Colorado living close to high-tension wires had a definite increase of all cancers. The likelihood of getting cancer is twice as high for children who live near the power lines.[22-24] A number of other investigations have corroborated these findings and have shown that men exposed to electrical and magnetic fields at work have an increased risk of leukemia (especially acute myeloid leukemia), brain tumors, and breast cancer.[25-29] Researchers at the University of California in Riverside confirm these results and say exposure to common sources of low- and high-energy electromagnetic radiation from overhead power lines probably promotes the growth of malignant tumors.[30] Many of these studies involve high-tension wires with 60 Hz (60 electromagnetic cycles per second).

It had been thought that low-voltage power lines, which have low frequencies and thus low energies, are too weak to have any biological effects. However, epidemiological studies show that low-frequency electromagnetic fields produce weak electric fields in our bodies, affecting such biological factors as hormone levels, the binding levels of ions to cell membranes, certain genetic processes inside the cell such as RNA and protein synthesis, and calcium ions. Calcium ions in the cell play a major role in cell division, which, in turn, has an important role in cancer promotion.

A study done by Savitz at the University of North Carolina in Chapel Hill measured the proximity of homes to power lines and also

Table 15.1   Electromagnetic Fields Of Various Appliances[22]

Source	Electromagnetic Field Strength* (measured in Milligauss)
Coffee makers	0.7–1.5
Crock pots	0.8–1.5
Refrigerators	<0.1–3
Clothes dryers	0.7–3
Irons	1–4
Toasters	0.6–8
Garbage disposals	8–12
Dishwashers	7–14
Televisions	0.3–20
Washers	2–20
Desk lamps	5–20
Blenders	5–25
Fans	0.2–40
Portable heaters	1.5–40
Fluorescent fixtures	20–40
Ovens	1–50
Ranges	3–50
Microwave ovens	40–90
Hair dryers	<1–100
Shavers	1–100
Mixers	6–150
Vacuum cleaners	20–200
Can openers	30–300
Electric lines on telephone poles	10–600
High-tension transmission electric lines	50–10,000

*At a distance of 30 centimeters

the low voltage of electrical and magnetic fields within homes. There was a positive correlation between childhood cancers, including leukemias and brain tumors, and the magnetic fields generated by the power lines. This study is important because it investigated high-voltage lines as well as low-voltage lines, which are on "telephone" poles in our cities. All the childhood cancer studies are significant because they are consistent and have been corroborated. They show an increased incidence of malignancies among people with long-term exposure to electromagnetic fields.

Higher rates of breast cancer in women in industrialized societies is, in part, due to electromagnetic fields and also the use of electric lights at night, which decreases melatonin that otherwise would decrease breast carcinogenesis.[31] Women who use electric blankets, especially postmenopausal women, also have a higher risk of breast cancer.[32]

Computer Monitors

A concern that has commanded major media coverage in the last several years is computer video display monitors and their potential to cause health problems. The "extremely-low-frequency" magnetic fields produced by these monitors have been linked to cancers, breast disorders, and other health problems. A review of sixteen studies shows that the preponderance of evidence links video display monitors with a risk of spontaneous abortion.[34] The U.S. Environmental Protection Agency recommended that the extremely-low-frequency radiation fields produced by such display monitors be categorized as *probable* human carcinogens. The EPA states that "the findings show a consistent pattern of response that suggests, but does not prove, a causal link" between radiation levels and cancer in people.[33] In March 1990, Dr. William Farland, director of the EPA's Office of Health and Environmental Assessment, ordered that the researchers' recommendation be deleted.

The magazine *MACWORLD* conducted a study of monitors manufactured by different companies and found certain uses to be hazardous. Color monitors produce more electromagnetic radiation than do monochrome monitors. The amount of radiation, it was discovered, is always higher at the sides, back and top of the monitor. The more powerful the monitor, the more radiation is emitted. Several precautions were suggested: Workers should sit at least two feet away from the front of the monitor and stay at least four feet away from the back or sides of a coworker's monitor. The same precautions should be applied to laser printers.

Some American computer makers already have low-radiation monitors for sale in Europe, where standards set by the government as well as by unions are very strict. IBM sells low-radiation monitors here in America but does not advertise them, perhaps fearing that these would create concern and anxiety about other terminals that the company produces.

Magnetic Resonance Imaging Scans

In the last ten years or so, there has been widespread use of magnetic resonance imaging scans (MRI scans). In many instances, MRI scans show more detail and, hence, give more information on a patient than conventional CT scans. Up until now, MRI scans have been thought to be without risk to the patient, that is, no radiation exposure or other harm. However, the newest and fastest MRI scanners may not be entirely safe.

Patients undergoing MRI scanning are exposed to three types of electromagnetic radiation: static magnetic fields, pulsed radiofrequency (RF) electromagnetic fields, and gradient (time-varying) fields. Atoms of all tissues resonate at specific frequencies within an electromagnetic field and produce radiofrequency signals, which are converted into images by MRI scanners.

The newest and fastest MRI scanners rely on the time-varying fields to obtain large amounts of information in milliseconds compared to the ten minutes or more needed by the conventional MRI scanners. The tremendous speed with which the newest MRI scanners acquire information results in a clearer image—one that is not distorted by patient movement or heartbeat—and a reduction in time for the patient to be in the magnet, which may also reduce the incidence of claustrophobia. However, time-varying fields, unlike static fields used in conventional scanners, produce electric currents in the body. These currents can cause cardiac arrhythmias or peripheral nerve stimulation, the latter of which has already been reported in three patients. There is, then, a potential for problems in patients with existing heart disease or seizure disorders. Only further research will help delineate the potential for harm to the body with the use of these very fast MRI scanners.

Electromagnetic fields have been used therapeutically for years to increase cell activity and heal bone fractures. Researchers report that cancer cells reproduce faster after exposure to electromagnetic fields and that these electromagnetic waves increase the activity of a certain enzyme called ornithine decarboxylase, which is involved in DNA synthesis and cell growth.[35] Certain cancer-promoting chemicals also stimulate the activity of this enzyme, and prior exposure to electromagnetic fields potentiates this effect. Exposure to the electromagnetic fields may alter the cancer cell membranes and make them more resistant to the immune system.[36]

Electromagnetic fields have other health consequences. Microwaves affect our circadian rhythms, which in turn affect our sleep patterns, growth, and repair mechanisms. The waves also affect the results of IQ tests in animals. Still other studies show that electromagnetic fields alter cortisol output; when secreted in larger amounts, cortisol suppresses the immune system.

The demand for electricity will increase by about 40 percent by the year 2000. To accommodate increased demand, there will have to be more high-tension wires. Given the fixed amount of land, more people will be living near the wires. Utility companies may also choose to increase the voltage of the power lines to meet this growing need. Larger power lines will generate stronger electromagnetic fields and, hence, pose a greater cancer risk.

Addressing the Problem

Some simple steps can be taken to minimize exposure to electromagnetic fields. Some computer monitors already have reduced electromagnetic radiation. Some electric blankets are made with reduced electromagnetic field strengths. Or you can simply use electric blankets only to preheat the bed. Redesign home appliances to minimize or eliminate fields. Move electric alarm clocks as far away from your bed as is practical. New transmission lines should be routed to avoid developed areas and increase the distance from the lines to the houses. Some utility companies are arranging their high-voltage transmission lines to reduce the magnetic fields. The problem is that little can be done to reduce the electromagnetic fields from the low-voltage lines within our cities.

Electromagnetic waves do, in fact, have health consequences and are probably associated with the development of cancer. We obviously need to be wary about where we live, avoid high-tension wires, and take other common sense precautions.

16
Sedentary Lifestyle

For quite some time, we have all accepted that a sedentary lifestyle or lack of exercise is a risk factor for the development of cardiovascular illnesses. Doctors preach it and people generally are aware of it, sometimes even putting on their sneakers to do something about it. Sales of exercise equipment have risen over the past few years, but more often than not, these treadmills, stationary bicycles, and other very expensive devices remain unused in most people's basements. Now, however, consider this: Exercise has been shown in animal studies and in human epidemiological studies to decrease the incidence of cancer.

BENEFITS OF EXERCISE ON THE IMMUNE SYSTEM

There have been a number of human trials looking at the effects of exercise on the immune system.[1-9] Most of the subjects in the studies were men. The studies included unconditioned people, people who were trained under supervision, and also highly conditioned marathon and cross-country skiers. The amount of time spent exercising varied in these people, as did the degree of strenuous activity. Because these studies examined patients before and after exercise, the patients served as their own controls for the experiment. In most cases, exercise produced a higher number of white blood cells, specifically the granulocytes that are needed to fight off infections and tumors. The higher count remained elevated for about forty-five minutes. The killing capability of the cells was not much different from that of sedentary individuals. There was no increase or decrease in the amount of antibody or in complement protein levels.

The lymphocyte count also was elevated in people who exercise. Both the B and T cell counts were increased, but the T cell count more so. Again, this elevation was transient and returned to normal. The functioning of the B and T cells when elevated seemed to be no different than when they were at resting levels.

In addition, exercise raises a person's temperature slightly. Accompanying the rise in temperature is the production of something called pyrogen.[10,11] Pyrogen, now known as part of the interleukins,[12,13] is an important protein produced by white blood cells that enhances lymphocyte functions. Fever has been shown to enhance the survival of animals infected with bacteria. High temperatures can also kill viruses—that's one of the major reasons you run a fever when you have an infection—and high temperatures have also been shown to kill cancer cells.

A significant number of animal studies have shown that exercise can actually inhibit cancer growth.[14,15] Many corroborate these findings. Rats were injected in their hind legs with tumors that were allowed to grow. One group of rats was not permitted to exercise; however, the other did exercise. The group that did exercise rejected the tumors uniformly.

EXERCISE AND WOMEN'S CANCERS

One of the largest human studies looking at the relationship between exercise and cancer was done at the Harvard School of Public Health in Boston in 1985. Almost 5,400 women were involved, all of whom graduated college between 1925 and 1981. Their ages ranged from 21 to 80, and more than half of them had been college athletes. To be classified as an athlete, the woman had to have played for at least one year in intramural or varsity sports, which included basketball, field hockey, softball, tennis, volleyball, dance, and other sports, or she had to have earned a college letter. This study showed that women who did participate as college athletes had a lower incidence of cancers of the breast, ovary, cervix, vagina, and uterus than did their classmates who had not participated.[16] The study showed that the risk of developing breast cancer was 1.86 times higher for nonathletes than it was for athletes, and the risk of developing cancers of the reproductive system was 2.5 times higher for nonathletes than it was for athletes.

A similar study at the University of Southern California also showed that regular vigorous physical activity leads to a reduced risk of breast cancer in women. Women who trained regularly, such as runners who ran at least two miles a day, five times a week, were deemed to be athletes. The investigators of this study suggest that longer menstrual cycles, characteristic of these physically active women, confer a protective effect against the development of breast cancer. Other studies confirmed these findings: Female athletes have been found to have lower breast cancer rates than their nonexercising colleagues. Females who begin training in ballet, swimming, or running before puberty are more likely to begin menstruating at a late age and have long and intermittent menstrual cycles than other girls. Earlier studies showed that women with breast cancer have significantly shorter menstrual cycles than women without cancer. Women with shorter cycles also have fewer days between menses and ovulation, the time period when breast tissue is least active and at least risk for cancer development. Longer cycles imply more days during the low-risk interval.

EXERCISE AND COLON CANCER

Colon cancer, the second most common cancer, has also been studied in relation to exercise.[17] It was found that men who have sedentary jobs have a 1.6 higher risk of developing colon cancer than their colleagues who have more active jobs. Workers considered to have sedentary jobs included accountants, lawyers, musicians, and bookkeepers. Those who were classified as having active jobs included carpenters, plumbers, gardeners, and mail carriers. It was found that men who have sedentary jobs have more cancer in parts of the large intestine further away from the rectum and sigmoid area, such as in the cecum, the ascending colon, and the transverse colon, whereas the active employees have a low rate of cancer in those anatomical areas. The sedentary individuals have a threefold increase over their active counterparts in cancer of the descending colon. The decreased incidence of colon cancer in men with active jobs is probably related to the fact that increased physical activity causes more motility of the gastrointestinal tract and more frequent evacuation of the colon. The longer the stool remains in the colon, the longer a carcinogen in the stool called fecapentaene has to exert its effect on the colon. Consequently, the higher is the risk for cancer in the various parts of the colon with which the stool is in contact.

The same relationship between colon cancer and a sedentary job was examined at the State University of New York at Buffalo. The risk of developing colon cancer increased significantly with time spent in jobs that involved sedentary or very light work. The risk of getting colon cancer was seen to be twice as high for people who work at a sedentary job for more than 40 percent of their work years than it was for those who never work at a sedentary job.[18]

A Swedish study involving nineteen years of follow-up and over 1.1 million men confirmed the two preceding studies. The risk of getting colon cancer was 1.3 times higher for those in sedentary jobs than for those in active jobs.[19]

What will happen to future generations as our jobs become more service related?

FUTURE PROJECTIONS

Children of today are much less physically active and physically fit than their counterparts of twenty or even ten years ago. Forty percent of children aged 5–8 exhibit signs of obesity, elevated blood pressure, and high cholesterol levels, according to a survey conducted by the American Alliance for Health, Physical Education, Recreation and Dance. The physical fitness of American public school children has shown no improvement in the last ten years and, in many cases, has greatly deteriorated according to a nationwide survey conducted by the President's Council on Physical Fitness and Sports. Part of the responsibility of getting our children into shape rests with the schools. However, only four states require all students to take a specific amount of physical education in all grades, kindergarten through twelfth: Illinois, New Jersey, New York, and Rhode Island. Only Illinois requires that all students take physical education classes every day. With a decrease in exercise, an increase in obesity, an increase in junk food, and the other risk factors that we have already discussed and will discuss, the incidence of cancer will continue to spiral with each succeeding generation unless we dramatically alter our lifestyles.

BEGINNING AN EXERCISE PROGRAM

A number of human studies have been done which show that increased physical activity promotes health with less disease in general, and a longer life.[20] The United States Preventive Services Task Force has shown that exercise and physical activity is helpful in cardiovascular disease, hypertension, diabetes, osteoporosis, obesity, mental health, musculoskeletal disorders, cancer, and immunological abnormality.[21] Everyone, young or old, should be on an exercise program; however, you must begin your exercise program slowly and cautiously work up to the desired level. You should not start a heavy physical exertion program particularly if you have been sedentary because you can have a heart attack.[22]

The main risk of beginning an exercise program is sudden death. Most reported cases of sudden death are older persons who had several cardiac risk factors. Among the non-life-threatening adverse effects of jogging and running are those ranging from blister formation to bursitis, Achilles tendonitis to stress fracture, and possibly early osteoarthritis (a wearing-out of bones). Other problems associated with jogging include heat stroke and problems related to breast connective tissue support. Long-distance runners can transiently have blood in their urine.

Because of the risk of sudden death associated with beginning to exercise, anyone 35 or older, or under 35 with cardiac risk factors, should be medically screened. This screening should include a full history and physical examination by a physician, and a resting electrocardiogram (ECG). An exercise electrocardiogram is indicated if the person has symptoms of heart disease.

An exercise program should be individualized for each person because abilities and motivations differ. Activities that offer constant and sustained exertion, like fast walking, running, and swimming, may offer physiological advantages over activities with varying levels of exertion, like volleyball and tennis. Your exercise program should start slowly and then gradually build up to the desired level. Your heart rate should be monitored. The safest training program is one in which training lasts twenty to forty minutes per day, three to four times a week, while maintaining the heart rate during exercise at 50 percent of the predicted maximum heart rate for your age.[23] Of course, you should be warned to stop exercising immediately if you experience chest pain, severe shortness of breath, palpitations, or other cardiac symptoms. You should contact your physician at once if any of these occur. And finally, it is well known that people who continuously engage in a heavy exercise program, like marathon runners, are more susceptible to getting upper respiratory infections. Heavy exercising can suppress the immune system and hence should be avoided.

About how many people are engaged in an exercise program? The Perrier Survey interviewed 1,510 adults at random and found that 59 percent of them were actively exercising in one form or another, but only 15 percent spent more than five hours per week exercising— equivalent to about 1,500 calories per week. Running was ranked sixth in popularity behind walking, swimming, calisthenics, bicycling, and bowling. Not all would be likely to improve cardiovascular fitness. Only about 5 percent of the adults were doing meaningful exercises that would actually improve cardiac fitness. The survey concluded that the one most important factor likely to initiate and increase a person's physical activity was his physician's recommendation.[24]

The new athlete often consults with his physician about matters that are related to exercise and nutrition. Young and old athletes alike realize that proper nutrition plays a big role in their performance. Over 7 million high-school athletes are in an age group that has the highest risk of nutritional deficiencies. An adequate diet, with the proper vitamin and mineral supplementation if necessary, is a must for all athletes. Athletes who are their ideal weight may require additional calories for the extra energy they need. They can monitor this by weighing themselves regularly to see if their daily dietary intake meets the needs of routine activities plus training requirements. Athletes must not increase muscle mass by taking any hormones like testosterone, which is a risk factor for cancer. Exercising the muscles will increase muscle mass.

Research from an important study shows that even a modest improvement in fitness among the most unfit people confers a very substantial health benefit.[25] The same study showed that people who were exercising routinely or only moderately did not have a corresponding "health gain" if they increased their exercising a little bit more. However, people who did not exercise and then started to exercise only a little bit increased their health benefit markedly. In this study, lower mortality rates among exercisers were seen for cardiovascular disease as well as cancer sites. High levels of physical fitness appeared to delay mortality from all causes, primarily due to the lower rates of cancer as well as cardiovascular disease.

Here again, people who are exercising even moderately are subsidizing the health-care costs for those who do not exercise. Fewer than 10 percent of Americans older than 18 meet the criteria for exercise proposed in the 1990 objectives for physical fitness and exercise.[26] These guidelines state that 60 percent of Americans between 18 and 65 should engage in regular vigorous physical exercise. An inactive individual should find walking a very acceptable form of exercise. Brisk walking will afford this person a substantial health benefit. Women walking at a pace that would generally not greatly benefit cardiorespiratory fitness, do experience favorable changes in the cardiovascular profile.[27] And it has been demonstrated that a home-based exercise program is as effective as group-based program in providing fitness for the elderly.[28] People are more likely to engage in low-intensity activities since they are more comfortable, convenient, and affordable, as well as safer. A minimal exercise program alone has been shown to reduce borderline or mild hypertension.[29]

You have already learned that exercise can reduce your risk for breast cancer, colon cancer, stroke, and hypertension, and assist in the management of diabetes, depression, and obesity. My recommendations for your exercise program are simple: brisk walking and stair climbing. There can be no excuse for not doing these—they require no fancy warm-up suits, no fancy leotards, and no membership fees. In inclement weather, you simply go to a shopping mall to walk. Virtually everyone can walk. With recent findings about the health benefits of lifelong exercise, walking should be done on a daily basis. It is used to improve aerobic capacity as well as to lose weight, and few injuries, if any, are ever incurred. You can burn more calories while walking if you carry weights on the extremities and swing the arms up high. Brisk walking has also been shown to reduce anxiety and tension, and is an adequate training stimulus for young and old.[30] Both age groups benefit from brisk walking as long as they increase their heart rate by 50–60 percent of their normal resting heart rate.[31]

Stair climbing is another simple but very beneficial exercise. Provided you do stair climbing for 15–20 minutes at a time, you will derive benefit. Going up one flight of stairs and then performing a task on that floor without continuous exertion is better than nothing, but it simply does not give you the cardiovascular benefit seen with continuous and repetitive stair climbing. During repetitive stair climbing, each individual step increases life by about four seconds.[32]

Four decades ago, people were amazed by the idea of cardiac patients' exercising, but now rehabilitation programs are common for these patients. The same should be true for patients with cancer. Cancer patients should ask their physicians about the types of activities that might be beneficial, as well as the recommended duration of exercise. In most instances, walking can be tolerated by all.[33]

TAKE CONTROL

The benefits of exercise are numerous. As mentioned, exercise is associated with a lower incidence of cancer for a number of reasons. The immune system is enhanced. There is an increase in gastrointestinal motility, resulting in quicker elimination of stools and carcinogens. And importantly, the person who is exercising is also aware of other risk factors and tends to be less obese, to eat more high-fiber foods, to eat less fatty foods, and to consume vitamins and minerals, in addition to not smoking or drinking. Exercisers also tend to be of better mental health[34] and have a lower risk of developing other diseases like diabetes[35,36] and cardiovascular illness.

There is no excuse for not walking or stair climbing. Check with your physician first and work into an exercise program gradually and slowly, but do exercise four times a week, at least twenty-five minutes at a time so that your heart rate gets up to about 50 to 60 percent of its normal resting level. Again, this is another risk factor over which you have absolute control. If you are not currently exercising, you can easily modify your life to include walking, stair climbing, or other forms of exercise.

17
Stress

As early as the second century, Galen, the physician who systematized medical learning, said that psychological factors contributed greatly to the development of cancer. He believed that melancholic women were more likely to develop cancer than those who were not. A number of physicians of the eighteenth and nineteenth centuries stated that there was a relationship between emotional trauma and the development of cancer. In fact, highly respected cancer specialists of that time, who were not quacks or charlatans, considered this relationship between stress and cancer to be very real. They based their conclusions on clinical observations.[1]

Over the last seventy-five years, many reports—some anecdotal, others more rigorously scientific—have suggested that psychological factors, such as stress, influence a person's immune response and, hence, susceptibility to infectious disease as well as cancer.[2] Until recently, there was a missing link needed to explain how the nervous system and immune system communicated. Special neuroendocrine cells have been found in all important immune structures, and specialized T cells have been found at the ends of large peripheral nerves.[3]

We now know not only that the nervous system can influence the immune response but also that the immune response, in turn, can alter nerve cell activities. Cells from the immune system can act as sensors to send messages to the brain, relaying information about invading microorganisms or other problems that might not otherwise be detected by the classical nervous sensory system.

The nervous system sends fibers to the thymus gland, the immune organ in which T lymphocytes are matured. The nerve fibers form a very specific pattern in this organ.[4] The spleen, lymph nodes, and bone marrow also contain very specific patterns of nerve fibers. The nerves follow the blood vessels into the organ and branch out into the fields of lymphocytes. Interestingly, the ends of the nerve are in regions containing T cells and not in areas that contain B cells.

The nervous system can modulate the immune system with nerve chemicals and also with its influence on specific areas of the brain. Likewise, the immune system has the potential to influence the nervous system. Work done at the Swiss Research Institute has shown that the firing rate of brain nerves is altered during immune responses. It is thought that the brain is informed by the immune system about the invasion of foreign invaders. Several cellular products that lymphocytes manufacture, such as interferon and interleukin, are probably responsible for informing the nervous system about these kinds of changes. One of the hormones produced by the immune system, called thymosin alpha 1, acts on the hypothalamus and pituitary gland to increase production of cortisol. Cortisol depresses the immune system by decreasing the number of lymphocytes, decreasing the mass of the spleen, and decreasing the size of the peripheral lymph nodes, among other things.[5] Early in life, thymosins are important because they protect T lymphocytes from the immunosuppressive effects of cortisol and allow them to mature. This mechanism is a normal regulation of the immune response.

EFFECTS OF STRESS ON IMMUNE RESPONSE

Other immunological parameters including those of lymphocytes have been studied. Lymphocytes are one of the front line defenses against tumors, among other things. In 1977, lymphocytes from twenty-nine patients whose spouses had died six weeks earlier were studied. In this group of patients, lymphocytes did not function properly.[6] This study has since been repeated several times in hospitalized patients admitted for depression with very similar findings.[7-10] These studies reveal that regardless of the other aspects of a patient's condition, depression alone is enough to produce abnormal lymphocyte testing.

Even mild forms of stress and loneliness can depress the immune response. A study of medical students both a month before final exams and on the day of the exam itself was conducted at Ohio State University School of Medicine. Multiple changes in cellular immunity were seen the day the exam was to be taken, especially in those who were most distressed and unable to cope well. Medical students more than other students should be well accustomed to taking tests, but immunological changes occurred in them nonetheless: a reduction in the helper T cell, and decreased activity of the natural killer cell, which is the immune cell needed to destroy cancer cells. Although these changes were more prominent the day of the test, they were also abnormal one month prior to the test, indicating that a generally higher stressed life or loneliness can lead to the development of these abnormal immune parameters.

Natural killer cell activity was also found to be depressed in other students who experienced stress but were unable to handle it effectively. These students subsequently had a great deal of distress and poor coping mechanisms. Natural killer cell activity was normal in good copers—those who had high levels of stress but low levels of distress.[11] In another study of college students, those who perceived themselves to be psychologically unhealthy also had depressed natural killer cell activity.[12]

Antibody production in those who experience stress has also been measured and studied. It has been found that dental students produced less antibodies during the more stressful parts of their academic year than at other times.[13]

A curious set of findings evolved from the University of Rochester School of Medicine in 1975.[14] The researchers were studying conditioned taste aversion in rats. Animals were first given a saccharin solution to drink and then the drug called cyclophosphamide, a commonly used chemotherapeutic agent today that also has immunosuppressant properties. In the experiment, however, the drug was used to induce nausea. The rats learned to avoid drinking the saccharin and hence avoided the nausea from the cyclophosphamide. Cyclophosphamide was not given to the animals in the later phases of the experiment. The rats forgot the taste aversion but were dying at a very high rate. The unconditioned animals, the control group, which preferred the saccharin solution to plain water did not die. The researchers concluded that the experimental rats were conditioned to associate the taste of the saccharin with immunosuppression and were, in fact, suppressing their own immune responses when they drank the saccharin solution.

Stress + Inability to Cope = Depressed Immune System

It has been clearly documented that emotional stress from whatever cause accompanied by poor coping ability is associated with the depression of animal and human immune systems. Human immune responses have also been depressed by hypnosis[15] and meditation.[16]

The largest groups of studies linking cancer to psychological stress are retrospective studies. These studies show that stressful events frequently precede several forms of cancer.[17,18] Children who developed cancer had a significant stressful change a year before, including personal injury and/or change in the health of a family member. In adults, the incidence of cancer was higher among people who experienced the loss of a loved one.[19,20] The incidence of cancer is also higher in people who are widowed, divorced, or separated;[21-23] individuals who have expressed a sense of loss and hopelessness; and those who have an inability to cope with the stress of separation. A higher incidence of cancer is seen in people who are unable to express negative emotions and who also have reduced aggressive behavior.[24-26] Sometimes, it is seen in those with masochistic personality as well.

Detection of a cancer occurs several years after the first cell changed into a cancer. When a person is asked about a past stressful event after being told that she does have cancer, her perception of that stressful event may be very different from what actually happened. However, prospective studies show the same relationship: an inability to cope with stress leads to a higher incidence of human cancer.[27-29]

Using several psychological tests to define the patients' inability to cope, a number of investigations have predicted subsequent development of cancer in people who had precancerous conditions,[30] or recurrence in patients having difficulty adjusting to their illness prior to surgery.[31] In other studies, patients who expressed high levels of anger toward their disease survived longer than those who did not.[32] There are clear psychological differences between women with benign breast tumors and those whose tumors are malignant. Their psychological reaction to the diagnosis of breast cancer was strongly predictive of the survival for the next five years.[33,34]

A prospective randomized epidemiological study of 2,020 middle-aged men followed for seventeen years found that those labeled "depressed" by the psychological test MMPI had a twofold greater chance of dying from cancer. In this study, all other cancer risk factors, like alcohol consumption, tobacco use, family history, and occupation, were controlled. Another interesting study reported surprising lack of closeness to parents among male medical students in their late twenties and early thirties who later developed cancers, primarily in their forties.[35] In Sweden, people who endured serious aggravation on the job had a 5.5 times greater risk of colorectal cancer than those without such pressure. People who work in high pressure situations, over which they have little control, face the highest risks.[36] This and other prospective studies indicate a good correlation between stress and cancer and are compatible with such an effect via the immune system.[37-40]

The medical community regards stress as a risk factor for cardio-vascular illness, and hopefully will soon regard it as a risk factor for cancer as well. I am convinced that stress is also one of many risk factors for the development of cancer. By itself, stress causes immu-nological depression; coupled with other risk factors a person might have, it can contribute to the development of cancer. We are all confronted with stress on a daily basis. Some stresses, however, present us with a feeling of distress or of being unable to cope.

Is there a cancer-prone personality? The evidence suggests that a person who is unable to cope with stress may have a higher risk for the development of cancer. Those who can cope better have less of a risk. Therefore, learn to cope, learn relaxation techniques (see inset on page 194) and techniques like meditation and biofeedback, and use any other techniques that you think will make you better able to cope and deal with stress.

A PERSONALITY PRONE TO BREAST CANCER

One of the earliest observations that there may indeed be a personality prone to breast cancer was a study of women with breast cancer who were found more likely to control feelings of anger than an age-matched group of women with benign disease.[41] Two other investigators inde-pendently confirmed these results.[42,43] A review of over eighteen sepa-rate studies shows that emotional control is implicated as a real risk factor in either carcinogenesis or disease prognosis.[44]

Breast cancer patients in particular show a behavioral type; many breast cancer patients are characterized by suppression of emotional reactions, especially anger, and by conformity and compliance. Pa-tients with breast cancer are also characterized as having poorly organized neuroses or psychoses, excessive self-esteem, hysterical disposition, and unresolved recent grief.[45] Emotional suppression is probably a real risk factor for developing breast cancer and not simply a reaction to having breast cancer. It is quite clear that emotional suppression in particular is linked to symptoms of depression and anxiety among breast cancer patients.[46]

Most of the studies demonstrate that stress and the above emotion-ally suppressed personality is, in fact, a risk factor for the develop-ment of cancer and specifically breast cancer.

PSYCHOSOCIAL INTERVENTION AND SURVIVAL

Breast cancer patients who have had at least one confidant have a better seven-year overall survival than those who have not had any confidants. After seven years of follow-up, breast cancer patients who

Relaxation Technique

Get into a very comfortable lounging position. Concentrate on "feeling" every part of your body with your mind. You can begin by thinking about your right foot, then your right ankle, right leg, right thigh, then left foot, etc. Then move from your hands up to your shoulders and neck, and so on. Now, start to tense specific muscle groups as hard as you can, hold them tense for twenty to thirty seconds, then relax them. Again, start with your foot muscles (tense, relax), the leg muscles (tense, relax), and so on. You can repeat the entire sequence once or twice. While you are doing this, tell yourself that you are tightening your muscles each time you do so, and, provided that your effort is exhausting, you will look forward to relaxing each muscle group. While this is happening, you can also think of a pleasant place that invokes fond memories. This sequence should produce relief and relaxation, and decrease your anxiety levels. Stress is another risk factor over which you have a great deal of control. Seize control of stress!

had at least one confidant in the three months following surgery had an average reduction in mortality of 42 percent compared with women who had no confidants at all. There was an even greater reduction in mortality (55 percent) if the breast cancer patient confided in a nurse or physician.[47] These mortality reduction figures are larger than ones considered to be medically significant in trials of adjuvant hormone therapy or chemotherapy of breast cancer patients.

Social support was the subject of another study involving breast cancer patients. Home interviews were conducted three months and eighteen months after initial breast surgery on 224 women with breast cancer. All the patients, 60 percent of whom were married, were followed for seven years. All of these women had confidants except 14 percent. This study found: (1) social support appears to be a significant factor that favorably affects a patient with breast cancer; and (2) survival is increased if breast cancer patients confide in a health professional.

The National Institutes of Health conducted a psychosocial immunological study on ninety women with stage I or stage II breast cancer.[48] Psychosocial factors, like depression and stress, were more strongly predictive of disease progression for those who did have a recurrence. Immunological status correlated well with psychological factors.[48] Women who were not depressed or stressed had a better immune system. The conclusion of the seven-year study was that mood and psychosocial factors contributed more to overall outcome than other factors. The more "up" the person is emotionally, the better she does.

In other studies concerning breast cancer patients, there is strong evidence to conclude that psychosocial support has great survival value, independent of all other factors.[49,50] Eighty-six patients with metastatic breast cancer were studied prospectively. All had routine oncological care. One group (fifty patients) had one year of psychosocial intervention consisting of weekly supportive group therapy with self-hypnosis for pain. The control group (thirty-six patients) did not have this psychosocial support. After ten years of follow-up, only three of the control patients were alive. Survival in the group that had weekly supportive therapy and self-hypnosis was almost double the time (36.6 months) compared to the control group that had neither supportive group therapy nor self-hypnosis (18.9 months). This intervention was most important in the early months of the disease.

In this study, breast cancer patients with stage I or stage II disease who responded with fighting spirit or denial were significantly more likely to be alive and free of recurrences (45 percent) than were women showing other responses (17 percent).[51] All the variables of breast cancer were identified and used in the study including age, menopausal status, clinical stage, type of operation, administration of postoperative radiation therapy, tumor size, histological grade, and psychological response. When each of the prognostic factors was examined individually, psychological response was the most important factor in the analysis of death from any cause, or death from cancer, or first recurrence. Psychological response was the most important factor affecting survival in this fifteen-year study. Histological grade of tumor was the second most important factor. Psychological response was not related to clinical stage, amount of cancer in the body, histological grade, or mammographic appearance. This study demonstrates that the patients' psychological response to their breast cancer definitely affects their outcome.

Survival is also linked to what the patient believes to be true. One study examined the deaths of over 28,000 adult Chinese-Americans and over 400,000 randomly selected "white" patients. Chinese-Americans, but not whites, die significantly earlier than normal (one to five years) if they have a disease, and their birth year is considered ill-fated by Chinese astrology and medicine.[52] The more strongly a group is attached to Chinese traditions, the more years of life are lost.

This study holds true for nearly every major cause of death that was studied: breast cancer, female genital urinary cancer, leukemia, all other cancers, heart attacks, diabetes, peptic ulcer, pneumonia, kidney disease, etc.

CONCLUSION

Constant depression and anxiety are risk factors for developing a cancer. Uncontrollable stress is another risk factor for developing cancer. Psychological factors, like stress, depress the immune system and increase the opportunity for cancer cells to grow unabated. If you develop a cancer and believe that you will do badly, studies show that you *will* do badly. If you develop a breast cancer and think that you will do well and you deny that you have the illness, studies show that you *will* do well.

You will learn in Chapter 24 that physicians are obligated by law to tell the patient the life expectancy for his or her particular illness. A significant number of patients who, after hearing that they have a finite period of time to live—three or six or nine months—go home, circle a day on the calendar, and proceed to die on that day. Since psychological factors have a tremendous influence on overall survival, perhaps a physician should not precommit a sentence for a patient based on the survival of thousands of similar patients who were simply treated "conventionally." Based on many studies, a modified lifestyle that includes psychological support, as in our Ten-Point Plan, will give a patient a better quality of life and increased survival.

18

Genetics and
Breast Implants

Only about 5 percent of all breast cancer patients have an inherited basis for this disease.[1] There is no genetic basis for all other breast cancer patients. Breast cancer in these other people is due to the risk factors that we have discussed. Chance alone may account for some clustering of breast cancer cases seen in some families because breast cancer is a very common malignancy, affecting one in eight women. However, in other families, clustering of several cases of breast cancer may be related to an inherited mutation in a specific gene.

ONCOGENES AND THE HOST

Every person has a set of oncogenes and of tumor suppressor genes. Oncogenes promote tumor growth only when they are turned on. Tumor suppressor genes actually inhibit tumor formation when they are turned on. What activates these genes? Certain vitamins and minerals turn on tumor suppressor genes and, at the same time, suppress oncogene activity. Many other factors—like dietary fat, tobacco, alcohol, etc.—activate oncogenes. The individual person and what that person does to himself or herself determines whether oncogenes will be turned on or off.

However, certain people may have a predisposition to having the oncogene turned on more quickly than the tumor suppressor gene.

For example, some people who smoke do not necessarily develop cancer. Hence, some exposed individuals may genetically resist the carcinogen effect. Other people, however, may show an increased susceptibility to a given carcinogen. The majority of people are in between those who are resistant and those who have an increased susceptibility. This situation, therefore, is not based on true genetics but simply on a predisposition for activating existing genes that can promote or suppress tumors. Many carcinogens require enzymatic activation and each person manufactures a different amount of enzymes.

HEREDITARY CANCER

There are six features that characterize most hereditary forms of cancer:

1. Early age when the cancer is found.
2. Multiple cancers occurring in the same individual at the same time with specific patterns and combinations within families or patients.
3. Certain physical signs and biomarkers in certain hereditary cancer syndromes.
4. Characteristic pathological features.
5. Longer survival when compared to people who develop the same cancers without a hereditary basis.
6. Mendelian inheritance patterns of cancer transmission.

These features do not all apply all the time to a specific patient because there are variable expressions and penetrance (degree of expresion as time goes on) of the affected genes. In any event, these six features will help guide the clinician in identifying a hereditary variant of many hereditary cancer syndromes.

Besides strict Mendelian genetics, traits can be passed along by non-Mendelian genetics and by genomic imprinting.[2,3] Genomic imprinting is the phenomenon whereby the expression or nonexpression of a gene is determined by the parental origin of that gene. It has long been known that many factors can actually modulate genomic imprinting, non-Mendelian traits and genotypes like: dietary factors including antioxidants, free radicals, fats; hormones, including estrogens and androgens; environmental pollutants, and other factors.[4] Other than strict Mendelian genetics, all the other forms of genetic influences on disease are esoteric and have little influence on the majority of our diseases.

Breast Cancer Genetics

As has been stated, about 5 percent of all breast cancer patients have an inherited basis for the development of the disease.

BRCA1

The first breast cancer gene, BRCA1, was discovered in a patient who had early onset breast cancer and was also seen in patients with breast and ovarian cancer. This gene is linked to a region on chromosome number 17q21.[5–7] In 23 families with the 17q21 chromosome, there were 146 cases of early onset breast cancer, in both breasts, or in male family members who had the 17q21 chromosome. All these patients were less than 45 years old. Another study shows the same 17q21 linkage in 5 families with breast and ovarian cancer.[8] The cancer associated gene in the 17q21 region of chromosome 17 has been called the BRCA1 gene for breast cancer 1 gene. If a person has the BRCA1 gene, risk of developing breast cancer by age 50 is 59 percent compared to about 2 percent in the normal population for this age. The risk for developing breast cancer in a patient 70 years old with the BRCA1 gene is 82 percent whereas it is only 7 percent in those aged 70 who do not have the gene. This shows that the gene is highly penetrant, which means that it is expressed more forcefully as time goes on.

The breast cancer gene can be carried either by the mother or the father; however, male carriers generally go not develop breast cancer. Both male and female carriers are at an increased risk for developing colon cancer and male carriers are also at an increased risk for developing prostate cancer.[9–11]

As was mentioned, the BRCA1 gene has been seen in older onset familial breast cancer but much less often than in younger onset disease. The data from the Breast Cancer Linkage Consortium include 121 families whose average age was over 45 with the diagnosis of breast cancer. But the majority of all cases with this gene are much younger women.

p53 Gene

On the same chromosome number 17, there is another area called the p53 region. When the p53 gene has been *mutated or changed or altered,* cancers develop. The p53 gene is the most commonly altered gene in human cancer. It is one of the most important members of the tumor suppressor oncogene family. Of the 6.5 million people worldwide who are annually diagnosed with cancer, about half of them have the p53 mutation in their tumors.[12,13] An altered p53 or mutation of p53 is found in about 25 percent of all breast cancer, 12 percent of brain cancer patients, 12 percent of soft tissue sarcomas, 6 percent of leukemias, and 6 percent of osteosarcoma patients. In 1993, it was voted "Molecule of the Year" by the journal *Science* because of its involvement in so many different cancers and other illnesses.[14]

The *p* stands for protein but really denotes prevention because the action of p53 is to help prevent cancer by acting as a tumor suppressing gene. The p53 protein or suppressor gene simply puts breaks on cell growth and division so when a cell starts to grow too rapidly or divides too many times, it will push that cell into a program of self-destruction and prevent multiplication of the cell. The p53 gene normally binds to other genes and thereby controls their expression.

When the p53 gene is mutated, it simply does not act as a preventor any longer, and cancer cells may grow without worry that the p53 gene will squash and suppress them. Newborn experimental animals bred to eliminate the p53 gene look quite normal, but after several weeks they began to develop tumors, and after six months all the mice either had cancer or had died of cancers. The p53 protein is the leader in the body's antitumor army. When the p53 protein is mutated or changed, rapid cell death/rapid cell proliferation can occur and can actually spur on abnormal cell growth.

The normal p53 can push cells into a suicidal mode that is called apoptosis. Apoptosis is part of normal cellular development and is triggered by DNA damage from radiation, chemicals including chemotherapy, and free radicals. When DNA is damaged, the level of p53 protein rises dramatically. All the experiments conclude that p53 in its normal state controls the development and growth of cells. The mutant p53 stops the usual programmed cell death.

When free radicals attack any protein including p53, a mutation occurs: p53 is no longer the same and no longer can control cellular growth as a tumor suppressor gene.

Cancer-Related Genetic Syndromes

The Li-Fraumeni Syndrome

An *inherited defect or altered* p53 gene, i.e., a mutation found at birth, can lead to a variety of malignancies at an early age including breast cancer, brain cancers, soft tissue sarcomas, osteosarcomas, leukemias, adrenal cortical carcinomas, and many other cancers. The early onset breast cancer and all the subsequent cancers that develop from a mutated p53 gene were first described by Dr. Li and Dr. Fraumeni.[15] If a person has a mutated p53 gene, that person is destined to develop a cancer. The Li-Fraumeni Syndrome is an inherited disorder in the form of an autosomal dominant trait (a single gene acting alone to produce an outcome) that obeys strict genetics. The early age of onset and the very high frequency of second cancers in a single individual were observed in the families that Drs. Li and Fraumeni described and are quite consistent with features of hereditary forms of cancer.

Cowden Syndrome

Women who have Cowden Syndrome have a higher frequency of developing breast cancer. Cowden Syndrome is a rare disorder that is characterized by multiple sores and other changes (hamartomas) of the mouth and skin. People with Cowden Syndrome also have a higher rate of thyroid problems including goiter and carcinoma of the thyroid.

Muir Syndrome

This genetic disorder is characterized by many skin tumors in addition to polyps and adenocarcinomas of the large bowel, small intestine, and stomach. This very rare syndrome is inherited as an autosomal dominant trait. Women with this syndrome have a higher rate of developing breast cancer.

Proliferative Breast Disease (PBD)

Researchers looked at the incidence of proliferative breast disease—a benign (not cancerous) proliferation of epithelial cells in the ducts of the breasts—in women who had no cancer but whose relatives did. Women who had relatives with cancer had a much higher incidence of proliferative breast disease (35 percent) than did their counterpart women who had no relatives with breast cancer (13 percent). Proliferative breast disease may be a precursor to breast cancer in genetically predisposed individuals or in those people who, through the free radical mechanism, develop a change in their p53 gene. Of course, the fact that a woman has proliferative breast disease, unlike the other genetic disease we have talked about above, does not mean that this woman will develop breast cancer.[16]

Genetic Counseling

Currently, women who are in high-risk families should:

- Examine their breasts routinely beginning in their late teens.
- Have a physical exam twice a year starting at age 20.
- Perhaps have annual mammograms starting between the ages of 20 and 25.
- Perhaps have ovarian cancer screening with ultrasound and possibly serum CA-125 levels.
- Above all, maintain an excellent lifestyle to decrease risk factors.

In addition, patients in high-risk families may consider being tested for the BRCA1 gene and the mutated p53 gene.[17] Some investigators think it is prudent for a patient at high risk to have prophylactic mastectomy and/or prophylactic oophorectomy (removal of ovaries).[18]

Prophylactic surgery simply minimizes but does not completely eliminate the risk for developing breast cancer or ovarian cancer even if both ovaries or breasts are removed. Patients who have the BRCA1 gene or the mutant inherited p53 gene may elect to postpone an oophorectomy until after they have children. I recommend intensive surveillance, strict modification of lifestyle factors, and the program in my Ten-Point Plan (see page 319).

Whether family members are genetically affected or unaffected, they experience tremendous psychological consequences. Unaffected family members often feel relief but, at the same time, tremendous guilt. After affected or nonaffected patients receive genetic information, they require intensive psychological support. In addition, once this information is known to the patient, insurance companies may use the information to deny that person life and health insurance.

After a breast cancer is apparent, other oncogenes become evident in the bloodstream as well. Many investigators have used these as markers and also attempt to use them as predictors of outcome and survival. They include erB, erB2, erB3, H-ras, neu-oncogene, and many others. So far they have not been very good predictors of outcome. One thing that has been shown is that when the short arm of chromosome number 17 is lost, the tumor behaves in a very aggressive mode in a patient with breast cancer.[19]

Summary

Strict inherited genetics has very little to do with adult cancers.[20] Strict genetics is involved in about 5 percent of the patients with breast cancer. The true Mendelian genetic syndromes have been outlined and, so far, little can be done about them. In all other patients who develop breast cancer, however, free radicals that are produced by a variety of risk factors previously outlined cause alterations or mutations in existing normal genes like the p53, among others. Once these genes change, once the tumor suppressor genes no longer work, or once the oncogene gets turned on, a tumor cell can grow uninhibited. It is important to modify lifestyle early enough in life so that these changes in the oncogenes and tumor suppressor genes never result from free radical formation. It is important, further, to modify lifestyle in a patient who has a breast cancer so that no further free radicals are formed and tumor promotion does not occur. Change your lifestyle factors now.

BREAST IMPLANTS

In the past twenty years, the number of breast augmentation procedures has undergone a dramatic increase year by year. During this time, about 150,000 to 170,000 American women have undergone augmentation mammoplasty yearly. About 80 percent of these are purely for cosmetic reasons and the rest for reconstruction. Approximately 2 million women in the United States have had breast implants.[21,22] Augmentation procedures have included: simple injections of liquid silicone not encapsulated, implants of various materials, and self-tissue transplantation.

There has long been a concern as to whether breast implants can lead to the development of cancer. Breast implants or injections of silicone *can* obscure breast abnormalities on mammography. Positioning the augmented breast on the mammogram machine so that only the breast tissue around the implant or injections is viewed is a major challenge.[23] Breast implants may cause pain and hardening of the breast tissue around the implant. There have also been reports that implants have been associated with cases of lupus or scleroderma, or other autoimmune diseases.[24] One study examined eleven children who were breast-fed by mothers with silicone implants and developed esophageal dysmotility seen commonly with autoimmune diseases.[25] Various mechanisms for this have been proposed.[26] European physicians have recommended that mothers with silicone implants refrain from nursing their infants.

But when it was learned that animal studies showed a relationship between implant material and cancer, the FDA issued a warning to all makers of breast prosthesis to prove that the devices were safe and clinically effective or remove them from the market. For thirty years, there had been no regulation of breast implants. And usually a product must be shown to be safe and effective before it is released on the market. Then on April 16, 1992, the FDA's policy was that implants would be available only through controlled clinical trials for breast cancer patients who wanted implants for reconstruction purposes.

Soon after that announcement, a study showed that there was little or no risk for breast cancer after breast augmentation with silicone implants.[27] However, when the data were critically reviewed by other physicians, various fallacies were seen in the study and the following conclusions were drawn :

- Patients who were turned down for augmentation had risk factors for the development of breast cancer or had breast masses at initial evaluation; hence, the numbers were biased in favor of people less likely to develop any breast cancer subsequent to augmentation;
- Eighty-five percent of the people who did undergo augmentation

in that study were under age 40 and at much less risk of developing breast cancer, and if the patient had a genetic linkage for developing breast cancer it would have already been obvious;

- Most of the women in the study had smaller breasts, less breast tissue, and therefore a lower risk of developing breast cancer;
- Forty-five percent of the women studied were under 30 years of age and generally had a maiden name at the time of the study with a subsequent name change after marriage that would impede the identification of patients and proper follow-up of records.[28]

The type of breast cancer linked to breast implants is specifically a sarcoma of the breast. It has been shown that the polyurethane coating on the implants can break down in the body and continuously release small amounts of a carcinogen called 2-toluene diamine (TDA). The polyurethane coating is used because it decreases the scar tissue around the implant. The estimated risk for developing breast cancer from breast implants is 1 in 50.[29]

The Council on Scientific Affairs adopted by the American Medical Association House of Delegates recommends that women who desire to have implants should have a right to choose as long as informed consent is obtained about the risks and that the informed consent is without bias.[30] Without being given this opportunity, women will leave the United States to have the implant procedure performed elsewhere. Much more testing needs to be done concerning all biological implanted materials to ensure their safety.

PART FOUR

Breast Cancer: Detection to Conventional Treatment

19

Breast Cancer Detection and Diagnosis

Breast self-examination, physical examination by a physician, and mammograms/ultrasound are the main modalities to detect a breast cancer.

BREAST SELF-EXAMINATION

Breast self-examination, as pictured in Figure 19.1, can be performed by every woman after being properly taught. About 90 percent of breast cancer symptoms are found by women themselves, either accidentally or by self-examination. Although 96 percent of women surveyed by the National Cancer Institute were aware of breast self-examination, only 40 percent actually did it. It is important to learn this technique properly; a woman who examines her breast incorrectly may have a false sense of security when she finds no masses. However, a study revealed that only 20 percent of women were proficient at detecting about half of the lumps in a model of a breast with seven lumps in it. An editorial review also indicates that breast self-examination is not very effective.[1] As you can tell, a woman who actually goes through the motions of breast self-examination every month may not be able to find the cancer mass in her breast. Therefore, breast examination should be done in conjunction with the yearly physical examination by a qualified physician.

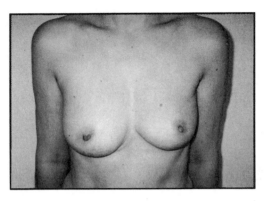

Before beginning, read the detailed instructions on page 210.

a. Stand in front of mirror and lean forward. Look for changes in size or shape of breasts, discharge, for pulling inward of nipples, for changes in appearance of skin.

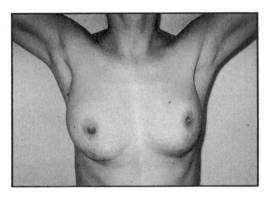

b. Place hands behind head. Repeat your observations.

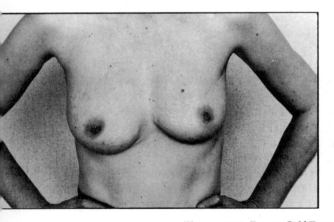

c. Push down on hips. Repeat your observations.

Figure 19.1 Breast Self Examination

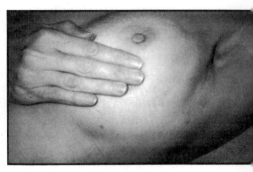

d. Lie on your back and examine each breast. Gently but firmly feel for masses.

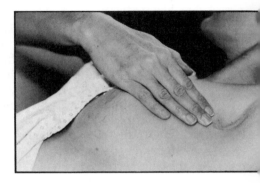

e. Examine axilla (armpit area) in the same manner, gently but firmly feeling for masses.

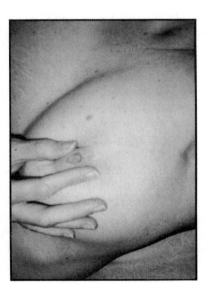

f. Squeeze nipple. Look for discharge, changes in shape, size, or skin of nipple.

Breast self-examination should be done a few days after the menstrual period begins because the breasts are not swollen or tender at that time. After menopause, you should pick a particular date each month, like the first Monday of the month, to examine your breasts.

The first step in breast self-examination is to stand in front of the mirror without clothing from your waist up and lean forward. You must look for any changes in the shape or size of your breast, for discharge from the nipples, for pulling inward of the nipples, or for changes in the appearance of the skin, like dimpling or an orange-peel appearance. Since changes in the breast may be accentuated by changing the position of your body and arms, you should next put your hands behind your head and observe your breasts; and finally, observe them after you place your hands on your hips, pushing inward on your hips with your hands.

The next few steps begin with lying on your back and placing a folded towel under your right shoulder if you have large pendulous breasts that hang off to the side of the chest. The towel acts to tilt the chest, allowing the breast to lie flat on the chest for easier examination. Now, put your right hand and arm behind your head. Use your left hand, elbow raised and fingers flat on breast. Move your fingers in a circular motion around your breast, working in from the outer edge of the breast to the nipple, in order to explore for masses. Do not pinch your breast between your thumb and fingers because this may give you the false impression of a mass. Feel gently but firmly. Thoroughly examine the area between your breast and axilla (underarm) because this is the location of some of the lymph nodes that drain the breast. Now, repeat the process on the opposite side with your right hand. If you think anything is abnormal, contact your physician.

Examine your breast monthly and try to memorize the location of your own lumps, if you have lumpy breasts. Also divide each breast into four imaginary quadrants. In this way you can easily "map" the location of the lumps. Since there is more breast tissue in the upper outer quadrant, the upper part of the breast located closest to the axilla, you will find more abnormalities in this area if they are to be found.

Some studies suggest that while breast self-examination may reveal breast cancers earlier, this has not led to a reduction in mortality from breast cancer itself. These studies include prospective, randomized trials from the World Health Organization[2] and two studies in England.[3,4]

Encouragement from the doctor or nurse practitioner increases the frequency at which a patient will practice breast self-examination. However, it has been shown that young women who find asymptomatic benign breast lesions by performing breast self-examination were exposed to unnecessary anxiety and unnecessary medical investigations, including invasive procedures and potential risks of false reassurance.[5] Also, patients who already had breast cancer did not practice self-examination often unless it was encouraged by the physician.[6]

Many elderly women do not perform breast self-examinations because of arthritis, poor eyesight, or loss of feeling in the fingers. A study demonstrates that these women can use the palm of their hands in the lying down position to feel for breast lumps. Also, they can use a hand-held magnifying mirror to look for lumps. Men should also examine their breasts from time to time because there are 1,400 cases of breast cancer each year reported in men.

You can write to the National Cancer Institute in Bethesda, Maryland, for information on free classes about breast self-examination in your area, or call toll free 1-800-638-6694.

PHYSICIAN EXAMINATION

Examination by a competent physician is the main defense a woman has in detecting breast lumps. This part of the examination is not foolproof and the proficiency of physicians to detect breast lumps has also been called into question.[7] Generally, physicians who spend the most amount of time doing the examination found the most lumps, and this was not linked to level of training or experience. OB/GYN physicians were less able to find lumps compared to internists, family practitioners, or any other physician who spent more time in doing the examination. It is difficult, however, to feel lumps that are less than 1 cm in size except if they are superficial (near the surface of the skin). And since mammograms can miss anywhere from 10 to 15 percent of all cancer lumps, some of which are quite large, physical examination is an integral part in the detection of a breast cancer.

A good examination, as shown in figures 19.2 and 19.3, can take anywhere from ten to fifteen minutes. It should be done in a well-lighted room because changes in skin texture and color tend to be quite subtle but significant. The physician should first check for symmetry of the breast, differences in size and shape, and ask the patient if any differences occurred recently. The breast surface should be inspected for dimpling or flattening, discoloration, ulceration, erosion, or dilated veins. Examination of the nipples should include determination of inversion, crusting or discharge, or deviation of one nipple compared to the other.

I first examine the patient seated on the examining table. With one hand underneath the breast, my other hand is pressing gently from the top of the breast and rolling the breast tissue back and forth to determine if there are any palpable masses in the breast between my two hands. The same type of examination can be done with hands on

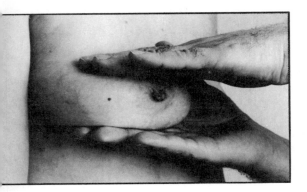

a. Physician rolls breast back
   and forth between hands.

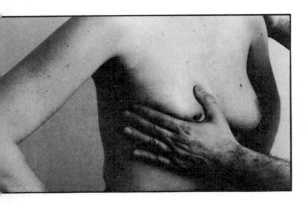

b. Breast mobility checked
   when patient pushes
   on hips.

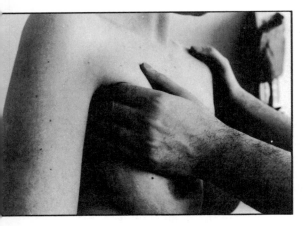

c. Axilla examined.

Figure 19.2 Physician's Examination of Seated Patient

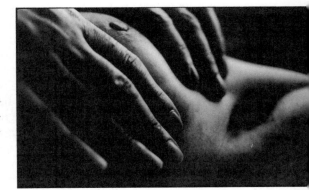

a. Physician examines breast with gentle, circular motion.

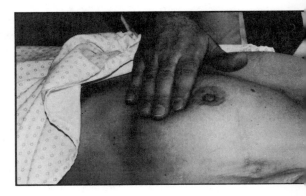

b. Physician examines areola. Fat and glands stop at margin, but ducts attach under it.

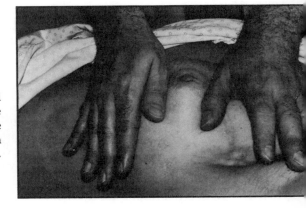

c. Physician examines ductal system by applying pressure with both hands. Possible discharge and its location on nipple are observed.

Figure 19.3 Physician's Examination of Reclining Patient

each side of the breast compressing together, again feeling for any masses that might be within the breast but between the two hands.

Next, the patient should put her hands on her hips and push down on her hips with force. If there is a malignant mass that is attached to the deep muscles, the mobility of the breast when the physician attempts to move it from side to side will be severely limited. For the next maneuver, the patient raises her arms above her head. The physician inspects the under portion of the breast, which is called the inframammary fold region. While in this position, the patient leans forward slightly so the physician can look for early nipple or skin retraction. Now, the patient puts her arms down along her sides in a relaxed position, and the physician examines the axilla. While doing this, the physician's fingertips should roll underneath the pectoralis muscle to ensure the examination of the lymph nodes underneath that muscle high up in the axilla. Examination of the supraclavicular region, that is the region above the collar bone and near the neck, should be done at this stage of the exam as well.

Now, the patient should be in a reclining position. The patient's arms should be over her head and, if the breasts are large and pendulous, one hand of the physician should hold the breast on top of the chest wall while the examination is being performed. The method I find best is to plant my fingers on one area of the breast and, without lifting my fingers, examine that area for lumpiness or masses by pulling the breast in a circular motion with those fingers. Examination must be done gently; hard palpation can obliterate any sensation of small lumps beneath the examiner's fingers. After this region of the breast is thoroughly examined, the physician's hand should be lifted, put on to another place on the breast, and the motion repeated until the entire breast is examined. If a lump is felt in the breast, it should be sequestered between two fingers and evaluated for hardness, buoyancy, and mobility. The inframammary fold area, the bottommost part of the breast, is sometimes difficult to examine because it normally is thickened and hardened in women who have larger breasts. Examination of this region must be thorough so that a small mass is not missed. Although breast cancers are infrequent in this region, time must be spent here.

Care and attention should also be given when the areola (the colored, circular area around the nipple) is examined since the consistency of the breast tissue is very different here. The fat and glandular material of the breast generally stops at the margin of the areola. Finally, the physician should examine the nipples for any discharge. To see if there is discharge, both hands should be used to form a concentric ring several centimeters away from the nipple and pressure should be applied. During the application of pressure, the physician's hands should roll toward the nipple, thereby expressing any discharge from the ductal glands if, indeed, there is one.

Physical examination, not mammogram, was the main reason for the reduction of breast cancer mortality in the Health Insurance Plan Study which compared mammography to physical examination as a screening tool (used when a patient has *no* symptoms or obvious findings).[8-10] In some studies, the physical examination is slightly more accurate than a mammogram in indicating a breast mass that turns out to be cancer.[11,12] Studies from various foreign countries including Japan and Belgium all support this information. Other studies show that the physician's physical examination is roughly equal to that of mammography for the detection of cancers.[13]

MAMMOGRAPHY

In this section, I review screening of asymptomatic patients with mammography. It should be noted that women who have genuine signs or symptoms suggestive of a malignant process in the breast are definitely candidates for mammography regardless of their age. In this situation, the mammogram is simply the next step in the diagnostic work-up to aid in diagnosis and determine when and how or whether to perform a biopsy.

Mammography employs X-rays to examine breasts. The objective of a mammogram is to detect a breast cancer before it has a chance to spread to other organs of the body. While this is certainly a noble pursuit, does it work? And, importantly, what age groups should be screened by mammography? This latter question is a subject of great emotion, anger, and tremendous anxiety for women in their 40s who have always thought that a mammogram is protection but are now being told there is no role for mammographic screening in this age group. So emotionally charged is this subject that every self-serving institution has jumped on one side or the other of the issue.

On December 3, 1993, the director of the National Cancer Institute of the National Institutes of Health proposed changing the guidelines and recommended that women between the ages of 40 and 49 *not* have routine screening mammography by issuing the following statement: "Experts do not agree on the role of routine screening mammography for women ages 40–49. To date, randomized clinical trials have not shown a statistically significant reduction in mortality for women under the age of 50."[14]

This statement was made after much scientific discussion and review of data that had begun in October 1991[14] when Dr. Anthony Miller, author of the Canadian study (below), presented in closed session to the Board of Scientific Counselors of the NCI's Division of Cancer Prevention and Control a preliminary analysis demonstrating that there is no benefit to routine mammogram screening of women aged 40–49. At that point, the NCI began planning an international workshop of scientists on breast cancer screening that convened in February 1993. The consensus of the experts in the workshop was: "The randomized trials of women ages 40–49 are consistent in show-ing no statistically significant benefit in mortality after 10–12 year follow-up. . . . For this age group, it is clear that in the first 5–7 years there is no reduction in mortality from breast cancer that can be attributed to screening. There is uncertain and, if present, marginal reduction in mortality at about 10–12 years. Only one study provides information on long-term effects beyond 12 years, and more informa-tion is needed."[14]

The NCI endorsed the workshop results after they were reviewed by both NIH and non-NIH researchers and, during October 1993, disseminated draft revisions for mammography guidelines for women aged 40–49. The director said during his March 9, 1994, Senate testimony: "Two principles need to guide us whenever possible: the consensus of scientific peer groups and clinical trials as the instru-ment for consensus."[14]

But so politically charged is this subject that when the director of the National Cancer Institute was interviewed, he stated, "What I would do as an individual is recommend annual mammograms, but I can't recommend it to the public because I don't have the facts."[15]

But guess what: Just a few weeks later, under great emotional and political pressure from many groups, including the National Cancer Advisory Board, the National Cancer Institute caved in and did a complete about-face even though Dr. Peter Greenwald of the Na-tional Cancer Institute's Division of Cancer Prevention and Control said, "In a meta-analysis of eight randomized studies done in differ-ent countries at varying screening intervals, one sees remarkable consistency in showing no statistical benefit in mortality after 10 to 12 years of follow-up.[16]

In late November 1993, the National Cancer Advisory Board (NCAB), composed of many nonscientists, told the NCI to "defer action on recommending any changes in breast cancer screening guidelines at this time."[14] Then on February 23, 1994, the Board told the NCI: "Inasmuch as cancer research is the primary mission of the National Cancer Institute, the NCAB recommends that the NCI not involve itself independently in the setting of health care policy."

The NCI director was summoned to the Senate to explain the NCI's flip-flop position. Shamelessly, the director of the NCI in his March

9, 1994, testimony to the U.S. Senate said, "I want to put to rest the concern that the NCI's position is influenced by political considerations or expediency."[14]

He also said that the "current NCI position is in close alignment with positions of several public and private organizations—e.g., the National Women's Health Network, the U.S. Preventive Services Task Force, the American College of Physicians, and the American Association of Family Practitioners."[14] This is simply *not true* for some of them. In fact, many organizations have cried out for a change in the guidelines because the scientific data show absolutely no benefit for the 40–49 year old group.[17] The U.S. Preventive Services Task Force states that screening should only be for 50–75-year-old women every one to two years.[18] The American College of Physicians says screening should begin at age 50.[18] And the American Academy of Family Practice—annual screening for women 50 to 75 years of age.[18]

A good physician-scientist must dispassionately examine the scientific data as it evolves. Let us now do that in a historical perspective. As I have previously mentioned, the mortality rate, or life span, for patients with breast carcinoma has remained unchanged since 1930, which means there has been no progress in the treatment of breast cancer. That shouldn't be very startling to most people, but it is because most people hear from the news media that the medical profession has one triumph after another, one miracle breakthrough after another. These "breakthroughs" are reported to the media by basic scientists, cancer charities, and organizations that continually ask for your dollars, either from you directly or from the Congress. They say that with a few more dollars, they will hand you the real cure to this illness, to this cancer; just look at all the triumphs to date. Hearing all these marvelous accomplishments from the media, a typical person wonders who the heck can be dying of breast cancer these days. What we have done is improve the quality of life, somewhat, for patients with breast cancer. So the oncology community has had to turn its attention to another area—early detection using mammography, which was portrayed as the next ray of hope. However, it takes approximately eight years of growth before a breast cancer can be found on a mammogram. During those eight years, many things happen, including the dissemination of those cancer cells to other organs by way of the bloodstream.

Let us now review the scientific data which leads to the conclusion that routine screening mammography affords no benefit whatever to women aged 40–49. In New York in the 1960s, a randomized controlled trial began that indicated for the first time that screening for breast cancer using mammography resulted in benefit.[19] However, there were skeptics[9] and international committees recommended the study be repeated before any mass screening took place around the world.[20,21] Consequently, clinical trials were begun in Sweden,[22] Canada,[23] Scotland,[24] England,[25] the Netherlands,[26] and Utrech.[27] An analysis of longer term was conducted by the New York HIP (Health Insurance Plan of Greater New York).[28] All the studies concluded that over a short period of time, breast cancer patients benefited marginally by early detection through the use of mammography. However, *the overall survival or mortality was unaffected* even when detection as determined by mammography was earlier. Each one of these studies, however, had its problems with design and absolute conclusions.[29] Furthermore, none of these studies looked at specific age groups and thus could not comment upon whether screening was useful in one group or another.

A group of investigators[30] analyzed the New York Health Insurance Plan study, the Swedish study, the Netherlands study, and a study from Florence, Italy,[31] to see if women aged 40 to 50 benefited from regular screening mammography. As was already stated, these studies were not designed to specifically look at different age groups. No statistically significant results were discovered. Looking specifically at the Health Insurance Plan study at eighteen years, there was a difference of six deaths favoring mammography. This is not statistically significant nor is it biologically plausible that a difference should first appear long after the screening in the fifth decade of life.[32]

Then, the media was given explosive information. In 1991, the Canadian National Breast Screen Study demonstrated that women aged 40 to 49 and other groups who had undergone routine mammography and physical examination had a higher death rate from breast cancer than women who had undergone only a single physical breast examination.[33-35] And even though there was severe criticism of the poor quality of mammogram technique and equipment (mammography technology substantially improved after 1985 but many of the films in this study were done much prior to that),[36,37] the preliminary results of the Canadian study demonstrated no benefit to women aged 40 to 49.

A retrospective study of another group of women did suggest a five-year survival benefit for women under age 50 who were screened by mammography,[38] but this study was flawed in a number of ways, and the data are not given much credence because it was a nonrandomized study.

Although the Canadian study had faults, the combined results from all published randomized controlled trials showed that the cumulative mortality rates from breast cancer after seven years are not reduced in women who are 40 to 49 years old but are reduced by one-third in women who are 50 to 65 years old.[39]

About one-third of all breast cancers occur in women under the age of 50, another third, between the ages of 50 and 64, and the last third over the age of 67.[40] The youngest and the oldest age groups are not benefited at all by routine mammogram screening.[41,42] Premenopausal women have more fat in their breasts and it appears much more dense on mammograms. Mammography detects different sorts of lesions in younger and older women and is worse at detecting clinically important breast cancers in younger women.

The Swedish two-county trial revealed that two additional cancers became evident clinically for every ten that were detected at first screening in women aged 40 to 49. For women aged 50 to 69, less than one additional cancer was picked up after the first year of screening.[43] Cancers are more difficult to see mammographically in young women and they grow faster in that population.[44] Another significant problem was that the cancers that were detected in the first screen in women aged 40–49 were *in situ* carcinomas and other lesions of low malignant potential. Less than half of these would develop into invasive cancer compared with more than 95 percent of the lesions picked up in women aged 50–69.

Another Swedish study based on an eleven-year follow-up suggests that women aged 40–49 may, in fact, benefit from early screening.[45] But when the data were looked at critically, there was no statistical significance for this finding. Since the benefit was seen after eleven years of follow-up at a time when this group was over 50 and would ordinarily have annual screening, the nonstatistically significant finding is probably related to the age, at which screening has been found effective.

Hence, these and other scientific medical data[46–49] demonstrate no benefit of a routine mammogram screening for asymptomatic women aged 40–49. These are simply the facts and no emotional lobbyist or marches, no vested interest groups can change the facts. Better mammogram technology is needed: a dual track rotating anode and selection of three filters that permit the optimum anode filter combination for almost any patient, particularly patients who are young with dense breasts. Also, a newer technology must reduce the radiation dose delivered to the breasts; as you have read, the radiation exposure from mammograms is cumulative and slightly increases the risk for the development of breast cancer. But more importantly, patients aged 40–49 should be screened with the use of the questionnaire on page 42. The resulting risk assessments should be combined with a pathological breast biopsy report if available to make an overall assessment of risk. If the overall combined risk is high, there might be a real benefit in screening such women on mammogram machines

Table 19.1 Screening Mammogram Guidelines

Age	Current	Aborted 1994 NCI	My Recommendations
35–40	Baseline	None	None
40–50	Every 2 years	None*	None**
50	Annual	Every 1–2 years	Annual (age 50–65)
65			None**

*"Talk with physician about appropriateness of screening mammogram, taking into account family history and other risk factors."
**Determine Breast Cancer Risk Assessment with the use of self-test risk assessment (Chapter 3) combined with pathology report of breast biopsy, if available.

that can "see through" dense breasts.[44] And by providing women with such an overall risk assessment, which can be utilized by all women, there will be more participation in screening, particularly for those aged 50–64.[50–52]

A very revealing study looked at the rate of false alarms for breast cancer. Over 2,900 consecutive patients complaining of some breast disorder were reviewed. Almost 400 of these women were found to have breast cancer: 57 percent of these by accidental discovery, 15 percent by breast self-examination, 24 percent by physician's physical examination, and only 4 percent by screening mammography. The extent of disease found by accident was not different from that found by actual screening intervention. And the percentage of false alarms was not that different either when compared to cancers found by routine screening. For instance, 87 percent of the cases thought to be breast cancers proved to be false alarms with all detection techniques: breast self-examination, physician's examination, routine screening mammography, and accidental discovery.[53] The investigator suggested 20 percent of all false alarms could have been avoided if routine physical examination before the age of 45, breast self-examination before the age of 35, and screening mammography before the age of 60 had been *discouraged*. Breast pain and nipple discharge are usually not symptoms of breast cancer, and this accounted for another 30 percent of the false alarms.

The following questions and answers were developed by John M. Lee, M.D.[54] to simplify the morass of statistical information concerning the use of screening mammography in women aged 40–49:

Question: What are a 40-year-old woman's chances of getting breast cancer in the next ten years?
Answer: 13 per 1,000.
Question: Of these 13, how many would survive without screening?
Answer: 5. Some cancers are so slow-growing that mortality is not increased by waiting for the appearance of symptoms. A cancer detected by screening does not always equal a life saved.

Question: Of the 8 per 1,000 destined to die without screening, how many do controlled studies indicate would be saved by screening consisting of an annual physical examination plus mammography?

Answer: One-quarter or 2.3 per 1,000. False negative results account for a portion of the unavoidable deaths as do aggressive cancers that develop and metastasize between screenings.

Question: How many false positives (from both the physical exam and the mammography) will have to be evaluated to save 1 life in this age group?

Answer: 150.

Question: What is the cumulative 10-year risk of a false positive screening result?

Answer: 13 percent at 3 percent per year. The woman must be aware of the possible medical and psychological harm of a false positive result.

Question: After submitting to an annual physician's examination, how much does a 40-year-old woman increase her chance of dying of breast cancer by not getting an annual mammogram screening?

Answer: By 1 in 1,250.

Question: By skipping mammography 1 year?

Answer: By one in 12,500.

Question: How much extra life can the average 40-year-old woman expect if she adds mammography to an annual physical examination for the next 10 years?

Answer: 7 days.

50-to-65-Year-Old Age Group

There is no question, however, about the benefit of mammographic screening of women aged 50–65. However, the Swedish studies suggest that a screening mammogram every thirty-three months is probably sufficient to reduce breast cancer mortality in this age group.

65 and Older Age Group

There are no reliable data to suggest that routine mammographic screening can reduce the death rate or mortality in the age group 65 and above.[41,55] Medicare, the United States' medical reimbursement system for people age 65 or older, reimburses for mammograms only every twenty-three months.

In 1992, health departments in forty-eight states and in the District of Columbia participated in the Center for Disease Control's Behavioral Risk Factor Surveillance System.[56] In this survey, a standardized questionnaire was given to women aged 18 and up. It was found that 32 to 60 percent of those age 50 or older reported having had a mammogram, 38–73 percent reported having had a clinical breast examination, and from 23–55 percent had had both examinations. Overall, about 40 percent of the women said that they had had both examinations during the year before the interview. More women had had a physician's breast examination than a mammogram (58 percent versus 46 percent). The more educated and higher socioeconomic status the women were, the more often they reported having either a mammogram or physician's examination, or both. The most important factor to influence a woman to have a mammogram was encouragement from her physician to do so. This study also concluded that women in this older age group who have a high risk for breast cancer and will receive the most benefit from such screening are the least likely to receive breast screening when compared to women under age 50.

Cost of Mammogram Screening

There have been several cost estimates of routine mammographic screening in women age 40 or more. If all the women over age 40 in the United States were screened with mammography and each mammography cost $50 per examination, then the total annual cost would be close to $3 billion.[57] Another group of investigators estimate that if only 25 percent of all the women in the United States aged 40–49 were screened in the year 2000, and assuming the cost of mammography was $80, the cost for the screening would be over $408 million.[58,59] The estimated expense per year of individual cancer is estimated to be $22,350. This has been reviewed elsewhere as well.[60] The overall cost for a year of earlier detection by adding mammography to the physician's physical examination for women aged 40–49 is $134,000 per year. The two major contributors to the cost are the work-ups of patients with false positive results and also the number of mammograms that must be done before one person's cancer is detected early, approximately 8,000 to 11,000 in women aged 40–49. Keep in mind that early detection by screening mammography in this age group does not change a woman's mortality or life span.

Mammogram of an Augmented Breast

In 1993, it was estimated that 150,000 American women underwent augmentation mammoplasty, 80 percent for cosmetic reasons and the remainder for reconstruction. With standard mammography, silicone gel implants obscure between 20 and 85 percent of the breast tissue, making the detection of a cancer very difficult. There is a higher rate of false negative mammogram diagnoses in breast cancer patients who have implants. This increased rate of false negative mammograms is 41 percent. There is also a higher rate of axillary nodal metastatic disease in patients with augmented breasts.[61,62]

The standard two-view screening mammogram is not adequate, and another view is required where the implant is pushed toward the back of the compression plate and the breast tissue is pulled forward to improve the visualization of the breast tissue.[63] Some patients have silicone that has been displaced from the implant. In this case, mammogram is of limited value, and cancer screening must rely heavily on the physician's clinical breast examination.[64,65]

Mammography and the Spread of Cancer Cells

Based on many studies, compression of a cancer mass, as with screening mammography, may spread cancer cells.[66,67] In 1980, a study showed a two-fold higher mortality rate among women with breast cancer who had dense breasts compared to women whose breasts were not dense.[68] Women with dense breasts required a five-fold increase in compressive force for the mammogram in an attempt to flatten the breast and thereby have more visualization on the X-ray picture.[69] The Swedish trial demonstrated more deaths occurred in the group of breast cancer patients who had a comparatively high compression force ("as much as the women could tolerate") than in the group with less compression.[70] After nine years, the number of deaths was equal in each group; life span is the same no matter what the treatment is, but early deaths may be avoided with less compressive force. More studies need to be done.

OTHER DIAGNOSTIC TOOLS

Tools other than mammography can be used to diagnose breast cancer. These tools include:

Ultrasound

Ultrasound of the breast also is quite important to diagnosis. High frequency sound waves produced electronically pass into the breast and reflect off tissue structures back to the instrument. No radiation is produced in this method of evaluation and ultrasound is best used for detection of fluid-filled masses. Ultrasound should not be used by itself but rather in conjunction with either physical examination and/or mammography. Ultrasound cannot identify malignant lesions less than 1 cm in diameter or microcalcifications. This method can be used to differentiate cystic from solid masses especially in women with a palpable breast mass that cannot be aspirated by the clinician's palpation alone but rather needs the guidance of ultrasound.

Thermography

Thermography is based on the fact that the temperature in the region of a breast cancer is elevated. Even though it has been used clinically for over twenty years, it is not a very reliable tool to diagnose a cancer. Thermography is risk free. But there are high false positive and high false negative rates.

Translumination

Translumination is a technique of shining light through the breast. Although this technique has been around since 1929, it has not been very efficient at detection of cancers. More recently, technology has improved the light source and, therefore, the detection rate. However, at this point, translumination should be considered quite experimental.

CT and MRI Scans

Computed tomography as well as magnetic resonance imaging, both of which can detect tumors, have been used. Both are expensive.

PET Imaging

Positron Emission Tomography (PET) is a noninvasive diagnostic imaging technique that will have a major impact on oncology practice. Accumulation of injected, inhaled, or ingested radioactive compounds provides the information about tissues and organs detected by PET scanning. PET scanning has been used to determine many aspects of tumors and tumor response to therapy. With regard to breast cancer, PET scanning has been used to make a diagnosis, localize the extent of disease, and monitor therapy. PET scanning may eventually eliminate the need for surgical removal of axillary lymph nodes because it will be able to detect whether lymph nodes are involved with cancer. PET scanning can also determine if other sites in the body are involved with the breast cancer.

SUMMARY

My recommendations for asymptomatic women are, in their order of importance:

1. Physician breast examination—all women starting at age 35.

2. Mammogram—women aged 50–65, annual.
3. Self breast examination—all women, all ages.

If overall breast cancer risk assessment is high (self-test on page 42 plus available pathological breast biopsy), then mammogram should be obtained based upon clinical judgment.

The physician's physical examination seems to be as good or better than a screening mammogram. The emotionally charged widespread use of screening mammograms has cut deeply into much needed health-care dollars for no gain. Clinical scientists should make recommendations and set policy based on scientific facts and not emotions or wishes. It is a disservice to give false hope to young women about the value of mammograms. Only the truth should be given to people.

A physician who is the director of cancer prevention, detection, and control research at Duke Comprehensive Cancer Center, co-chair of the international screening workshop, and a woman in her forties, best sums up the NCI statement:

> If mammography were a treatment, we would have to call it an unproven treatment for women in their 40s. I believe we owe the American woman the honesty of telling her the truth—that the benefit of this test for women in their 40s is not proven.[71]

20
Establishing the Diagnosis and Stage

To ultimately establish the diagnosis of breast cancer, a piece of the breast tissue in question must be brought to the pathologist for review and examination under the microscope. During this time period, a series of factors that predict outcome must be made: specific breast cancer type (pathology), axillary lymph node status, tumor size, estrogen and progesterone receptor status, and several others. The next step is to determine the "stage," i.e., find out with our limited technology if the cancer is confined to the breast or has already spread. All this information is used to predict prognosis and determine treatment options.

TECHNIQUES

Numerous techniques are used to establish the diagnosis and stage.

Needle Aspiration

A needle aspiration can be performed on any breast mass in the setting of a physician's office; a mammogram is not necessarily done first. Aspiration is done using a 20 or 22 gauge needle and a syringe and usually no local anesthesia.

A cyst can be silent or painful and, depending upon the amount of fluid within the cyst, it can either be soft and fluctuant with low pressure and a low amount of fluid, or tense and hard and may feel like a solid tumor if it is completely filled with fluid. If the palpable mass is cystic and needle aspiration removes fluid from it, the cyst will collapse. This generally precludes the diagnosis of cancer and biopsy is not required.

Although there has been a fear that repeated aspirations will increase the risk of future cancer or cause tumor cells from the aspirated mass to track along the needle tunnel, this has not been borne out in two studies.[1,2]

If the cysts are relatively new, the fluid that they contain is thin and straw-colored. If the cysts are older, the fluid may be thicker and darker in color, from brown to greyish green.[3] Unless the fluid is bloody, there is no value in sending fluid aspirated from the cyst to the laboratory for analysis.[4,5] There is no evidence to suggest that analysis of breast cyst fluid for electrolytes, androgen conjugates, or other elements could accurately predict the development of future breast cancer.[6]

If a cyst recurs, it may simply be aspirated again if indicated. About 20 percent of simple cysts will refill and less than 9 percent will refill after two or three aspirations. One should be suspicious of an intracystic carcinoma or another type of cancer within the cyst if the aspiration contains blood, or if a palpable mass remains when all the fluid is withdrawn, or if the cyst repeatedly refills, or if a mammographic density persists.[7]

Aspiration of a solid mass can be done by inserting the needle into the mass and applying a little more backward pressure on the plunger of the syringe. A "core" biopsy is thus obtained through the needle, and this tissue can then be sent to the laboratory for pathological diagnosis. However, the range of false negatives (anywhere from 1 to 35 percent) and false positives (up to 18 percent) is high and must be kept in mind when a report comes back. If, however, the pathological specimen results come back as nondiagnostic and the mass is still present, then an open biopsy of the lesion must be performed.

Incisional Biopsy

If the breast mass is very large and the physician is suspicious that the lesion is a cancer, an incisional biopsy may be performed. Local anesthesia is administered to the skin region, a small incision is made directly over the mass, then a portion of that mass is removed and sent to a laboratory. This incisional biopsy procedure is done only when the mass is too large to be totally removed or when the patient is inoperable for other reasons and a diagnosis must be made.

Excisional Biopsy

Excisional biopsies are also performed as outpatient procedures. The intent is to remove the entire mass lesion. If the mass is near the areola, then an areolar incision may be made and tunneled down to the mass. If, however, the mass is located more in the periphery of the breast, then a curvilinear (Langer's lines) incision should be made, as part of a small segment of a concentric circle around the breast. A radial incision, which would look like part of a spoke of a wheel, should not be used because it does not yield a good appearance. It is important that a small drain be put in any excisional biopsy to avoid the accumulation of a large amount of blood and hematoma that can cause scar tissue, possible dissemination of cancer cells that are left behind, and poor appearance. The drain used can be as small as a small rubber band. Many physicians who do excisional biopsies do not put in a drain and I have seen it take weeks to resolve a large hematoma that, ultimately, produces poor appearance. Margins of the removed specimen should be marked so that the pathologist may determine where tumor has been left behind in the breast, if at all. Approximately one-third of the time, cancer cells are inadvertently left behind by excellent surgeons. At this time also, the removed specimen should be sent for analysis of hormone receptors, DNA, and cell cycle, all of which will be discussed.

Biopsy of Nonpalpable Lesions

Since the use of mammography has increased dramatically, more and more small lesions have been detected that are too small to be detected by palpation. This entire subject has been thoroughly reviewed by Drs. Schwartz and Feig.[8,9] These authors offer the following criteria that mandates a surgical biopsy:

- The presence of a solitary mass, especially if spiculated or margins not well defined.
- The presence of a specific mass that is significantly different in size or contour compared to the others in the breast.
- Microcalcification clusters.
- Calcifications in or adjacent to a nonpalpable mass.
- A distorted area of breast tissue that is not seen in the other breast mammographically.

A surgeon is usually consulted when the reading of a mammogram comes back as suspicious, and the radiologist recommends biopsy intervention. The majority of lesions removed are benign. However, when a patient hears that there is a suspected lesion on the mammogram, her immediate reaction (and her attorney's reaction) is to have the lesion removed. However, if the mammographic findings are "soft," then it would be quite prudent to delay biopsy until another mammogram is obtained four to six months thereafter. By waiting, the woman can avoid a biopsy and scar tissue and still not jeopardize her medical situation. And, in fact, surgical scars that result from breast biopsies can give rise to breast cancers.[10]

However, the news media, consumer groups, cancer charities, and ultimately the attorneys, force immediate biopsy. But when mammographic findings are ambiguous or equivocal (soft) and a cancer is later proved, there are absolutely no data at all to show that the patient's breasts or her survival was at all jeopardized by waiting four to six months to repeat the mammograms to see if a change has occurred.[11] To go one step further, there has been absolutely no change in mortality for breast cancer since 1930, which means everything that we have done to date—screening programs, chemotherapy, radiation therapy, surgical techniques—has done absolutely nothing to increase the survival of any patient with breast cancer. So waiting six months to repeat a mammogram to ascertain whether an equivocal mammographic lesion has progressed, represents little or no time at all and, in fact, has absolutely no impact on survival.

No mammogram should ever be thrown away; the patient should always hand carry her own films to various physicians. All old films should be given to the radiologist for comparison, and if possible, serial mammograms should be done in the same radiology office as long as there is technically good quality and proficient radiologists to read them.

If a patient feels strongly that six months is too long to wait, she can have a film done at the third or fourth month; however, she must realize that the six-month film is the most important one because it takes about six months for a radiographic change to manifest itself by mammogram. If the six-month film is stable, then the next set of films should be done on both breasts six months thereafter.

As Dr. Schwartz points out, breast biopsies are not emergencies. However, once a biopsy has been recommended and a woman has made the decision to go ahead with the biopsy, somehow, emotionally, it had to be done yesterday. But waiting two or three weeks has absolutely no bearing on the ultimate outcome. And a biopsy for a nonpalpable lesion requires scheduling and planning.

The nonpalpable breast lesion is localized using a needle in the breast, which is guided by mammographic films. The needle is inserted while the patient is in the mammogram suite. She is then taken to the surgical suite so the surgeon can make an incision by following the needle to the lesion identified.

Many devices like grids have been developed to help the radiologist identify the region of the breast involved. Once the needle or wire is inserted, there is no need to inject a dye to pinpoint the region. The dye (methylene blue dye) may interfere with the measurement of hormone receptors or stain more tissue than what is needed to be removed.

An excisional biopsy may be performed to remove a margin of tissue around the lesion in question. The incision should be curvilinear, i.e., parallel to the areolar margin. There is no need to remove the skin overlying the lesion because the breast ultimately will be treated with radiation or mastectomy if, in fact, a cancer is determined. If the lesion in question is composed of calcifications, then excised tissue must be analyzed by X-ray to ensure that all those calcifications are in the removed tissue. Both the radiographic specimen (specimen that was X-rayed) and the actual tissue specimen should be sent to the pathology laboratory. A frozen section, which calls for an immediate diagnosis from the pathologist, and also has inherent flaws, is not at all indicated in this procedure for many reasons.

The biopsy site is closed using a drain. No sutures are in the breast; sutures are to close the skin only.

About 20 to 30 percent of nonpalpable lesions as shown on mammography turn out to be cancer.[8,12] Once the diagnosis of cancer is established, the patient can come back with her partner to the physician and review all her options, allowing her time to think about them before the next steps are taken.

Keep in mind that about 80 percent of all breast lumps detected are benign. Generally, your doctor will recommend that you observe the lump through one menstrual cycle and if it reduces by day four or five of menses, it is usually a benign cyst. If it does not reduce in size, see your physician.

I have had a number of patients "who knew their bodies"; even though the lump did reduce completely after menses, they thought something was still abnormal. Listen to the patient and pursue the work-up if indicated.

On the other hand, my own cousin, while caring for her husband who was being treated for prostate cancer and for her son who is mentally handicapped, came to see me for routine examination. I found no clinically abnormal lumps but only a dime-size area of the breast skin that did not feel just right—it felt a little leathery. I sent her for a mammogram, which was negative; ultrasound also was negative. She wanted to stop there. I did not. With great reluctance, she and her husband came with me to a competent breast surgeon who did not want to perform a needle aspiration. At my insistence, and to the grumbling of all involved, it was done and was found to be nondiagnostic. All wanted to end the investigation there—all but me. Yes, there were some expletives about me; I almost had to find another surgeon. It is true, physical findings were negative except for the small leathery skin, and the rest of the entire work-up was negative. Medically there was no reason to proceed. To make a long and frightful story short, an excisional biopsy was performed and was positive for cancer. My cousin ultimately did well with conservative breast cancer management.

The bottom line—if you have a good reason to pursue a work-up in spite of initial negative findings and attitudes, keep pushing to establish a diagnosis.

DETERMINE IF CANCER HAS SPREAD

Once the diagnosis of cancer has been established from the biopsy specimen, it is now important to determine if the cancer has spread or metastasized to other areas of the body. A chest X-ray, bone scan, and liver function tests are necessary. It is also important to include clinical examination of the axilla prior to biopsy. Even though the clinical examination may be negative, one-third of these cases ultimately will be shown to have cancer in the lymph nodes. If the liver blood tests are normal and clinical examination does not reveal an enlarged liver, it is extremely unlikely that liver metastases will be detected by computed tomography scanning (less than 1 percent).

The tumor has metastasized from the breast to another organ if any of the above tests are positive and the work-up may be stopped at that point. There is no need for surgical intervention other than the initial biopsy, and the patient can then be considered for systemic and/or local treatment depending on the circumstances.

If the metastatic workup is negative, the patient should be referred to a radiation oncologist to see if she is eligible for primary radiation therapy of the breast before any further surgery is done.

A full discussion of a biopsy report on page xxx includes a discussion of estrogen receptor, progesterone receptor, cellular phase fraction, DNA ploidy status, etc.

PATHOLOGY—THE MICROSCOPIC CLASSIFICATION OF CANCER

There are basically two groupings of breast cancer, one that invades tissue, which is referred to as invasive or infiltrating, and one that does not invade tissue, which is called *in situ*. The classification that we will discuss is the one that has been adopted by the Armed Forces Institute of Pathology (AFIP) and the World Health Organization (WHO).

Carcinoma *In Situ* (Non-Invasive)

This cancer is the expression of abnormal cellular growth changes before invasion. Carcinoma *in situ* has an eight- to tenfold risk of developing a subsequent invasive carcinoma. It may involve the ducts or the lobules.

■ *Ductal carcinoma in situ*

This is regarded as an early stage of a breast cancer. One or more mammary ducts are filled and distended with malignant cells but these cells have not invaded the basement membrane. Theoretically, these malignant cells should not gain access to lymphatic channels and, therefore, not produce metastases. However, when patients with ductal carcinoma *in situ* have a mastectomy, 60 percent of their disease is ductal carcinoma *in situ*, and 15–25 percent is invasive carcinoma. With more mammograms being done, the detected number of ductal carcinomas *in situ* has increased.

Although men rarely get breast cancer, about 5 percent of the male breast carcinomas are ductal carcinoma *in situ*. These men generally present with nipple discharge that is usually bloody whereas women do not present in this manner.

Clinical Presentation

Fifty percent to 65 percent of women who had ductal carcinoma *in situ* presented with a palpable breast lump. Ductal carcinoma *in situ* is also suspected if a woman has no palpable breast mass, or has Paget's disease of the nipple, or has a bloody nipple discharge.

Pathological Types

There are several pathological types for this ductal carcinoma *in situ*:

- Comedo carcinoma—produces firm masses involving multiple ducts.
- Ductal carcinoma *in situ*.
- Predominant intraductal with an invasive component.
- Medullary with lymphocytic infiltrate.
- Mucinous (colloid).
- Papillary.
- Tubular.

Prognosis

Approximately 15–20 percent develop a local recurrence in five years;

20–50 percent of these will develop invasive breast cancers that need to be treated accordingly.

Treatment

Until recently most patients with ductal carcinoma *in situ* were treated with mastectomy. In only about 1 percent of these patients was there tumor recurrence or death due to breast cancer. More recently, patients with ductal carcinoma *in situ* have been treated with excisional lumpectomy, axillary node dissection, and then primary radiation therapy. In some patients who had only an excisional biopsy, the frequency of recurrence of cancer in that breast varies from 24 to 70 percent. However, when microscopic ductal carcinoma *in situ* was found, some patients were treated with or without wide excision and with or without whole breast radiation therapy. Observation alone might be prudent in the elderly woman because of the long period of time for the development of an invasive cancer. If the ductal carcinoma *in situ* is palpable by clinical examination, it can be treated either with mastectomy or by having lumpectomy, axillary node dissection, and radiation therapy.

■ Lobular Carcinoma In Situ

Lobular carcinoma *in situ* never forms a palpable cancer and is considered a premalignant process. It is found primarily in premenopausal women and may involve multiple areas of the same breast. If a mirror image biopsy is performed in the other breast, about 25 percent of the time, you will find lobular carcinoma *in situ* as well. Calcifications are rarely found on mammograms. (See Table 20.1 to compare this diagnosis with ductal carcinoma.)

Pathological Types

Only lobular carcinoma *in situ*.

Prognosis

It usually takes ten years for lobular carcinoma *in situ* to progress. About 20 to 25 percent of all patients who have an initial diagnosis of lobular carcinoma *in situ* will have developed an invasive carcinoma in one or both breasts after twenty-five years. The second cancer is usually ductal carcinoma *in situ*, invasive ductal carcinoma, or both. Whereas the progression of lobular carcinoma *in situ* is about 1 percent per year to an invasive cancer, the risk for progression of ductal carcinoma *in situ* is about 2–3 percent per year. So lobular

Table 20.1 Comparison of Ductal vs. Lobular Breast Carcinoma *In Situ*

Comparative Features	Ductal Carcinoma	Lobular Carcinoma
Age at diagnosis	Pre- or postmenopausal	Premenopausal
Physical findings	None (microscopic form)	None
	Mass (gross form)	
Mammographic findings		Microcalcifications
	(80% of cases)	No specific findings
Multicentric or bilateral	Occasionally	Frequently
Metastases	None (microscopic form)	None
	Possible in axillary	
	lymph nodes (gross form)	
Malignant potential	Risk in biopsied breast,	Bilateral risk
(invasive breast	usually at biopsy site	
carcinoma)		

Source: Deckers and Ricci. 1991, "Evolving strategies in operable breast cancer. Noninvasive or occult malignancies." *Hospital Practice.* September 15:103–126.

carcinoma *in situ* is really an indication that the woman will have an increased risk for developing invasive cancer in the future.

Treatment

There are three treatment possibilities offered to a patient with lobular carcinoma *in situ.*

1. Careful and close observation.
2. Mastectomy with biopsy of the opposite breast.
3. Bilateral mastectomy—should rarely be considered in a minority of patients who are extremely uncomfortable about having a higher risk for developing a cancer in the future.

There seems to be no role for radiation therapy in the management of this disease. Just one final note: Remember this diagnosis is only an incidental finding when a breast biopsy is done for another reason altogether since nothing on a mammogram can reveal a lobular carcinoma *in situ.*

■ Paget's Disease

Paget's disease represents an *in situ* carcinoma of the nipple that may be associated with either a noninvasive or an invasive breast carcinoma.

Clinical Presentation

The patient usually notices redness, crusting, discharge, or eczemoid changes of her nipple, which brings her to a physician who makes the diagnosis of Paget's disease. Over 50 percent of the cases may have a palpable breast mass as well.

Pathological Types

Only Paget's disease.

Prognosis

The five-year survival data are related to whether there is nipple involvement, a breast mass, or positive lymph nodes. (See Table 20.2.)

Treatment

Traditionally, a mastectomy was performed if only the nipple was involved. If the nipple was involved and the breast had a palpable mass, a modified radical mastectomy was done. More recently, patients have been treated with breast-conserving surgery with or without radiation therapy.

■ Cystosarcoma Phyllodes

This is an extremely rare breast cancer that is generally benign and does not spread to lymph nodes. However, about 25 percent of these cases are malignant.

Presentation

It usually presents as a large and bulky tumor mass that is smooth, multinodular, and rounded. When it grows to a very large size, it usually does so rapidly. Prominent veins on the breast's skin surface are usually part of the clinical picture.

Table 20.2 Five-Year Survival Data for Paget's Disease

Nipple Involved	Breast Mass	Positive Lymph Nodes	Five-Year Survival
Yes			85%
Yes		Yes	46%
	Yes		68%
	Yes	Yes	22%

Pathological Types

- Benign cystosarcoma phyllodes.
- Malignant cystosarcoma phyllodes.

Prognosis

Benign cystosarcoma phyllodes recurs locally 20 percent of the time, probably because the tumor was not completely removed initially. One-half of patients with recurrences have aggressive metastasis to the chest wall and chest cavity.

Because the malignant form of cystosarcoma phyllodes is treated aggressively from the outset, only 8 percent have local recurrences. Spread to the regional lymph nodes is rare, occurring in about 15 percent of all cases. Spread to lungs and bone occurs in 66 percent and 28 percent of metastatic cases, respectively.

The average survival time is thirty months for all cases. The longest survival time recorded for someone with metastatic disease is fourteen and one-half years.

Treatment

Cystosarcoma phyllodes is treated with a very wide excision. Most patients are cured in this manner, but if the margins of the surgical specimen are not free of disease, the risk of a local recurrence or metastases is high. The risk of metastases is also related to how much of the connecting breast tissue (stroma) is involved, and how aggressive the cells look microscopically. But, generally, this lesion is treated by a wide, local excision or, simply, mastectomy.

Invasive Cancers

Invasive cancers cover a broader spectrum than do *in situ* cancers. Diagnosis, staging, prognosis, and treatment of invasive cancers are discussed at length in chapters 19 through 22. The following is an overview of the general characteristics of invasive cancers:

■ *Invasive or Infiltrating Ductal Carcinoma*

About 80 percent of all cancers of the breast are invasive or infiltrating ductal carcinoma. The terms invasive and infiltrating are synonymous. These cancers are quite hard and commonly metastasize to the axillary lymph nodes. Patients are usually women in their mid-fifties who generally present with a thickening or a swelling in the breast in contrast to a very prominent lump that is characteristic of the ductal carcinomas. Invasive lobular carcinoma accounts for only about 5 to

10 percent of all invasive carcinomas. However, both invasive lobular and ductal carcinomas have similar prognoses. Invasive ductal carcinoma metastasizes more frequently to bone or other organs like lung, liver, and brain but lobular invasive carcinomas metastasize mainly to the surfaces of organs.

■ Tubular Invasive Carcinoma

Constituting about 2 percent of all breast cancers, these carcinomas are generally small, less than 1 cm or so in diameter. Tubular invasive carcinoma has a much better prognosis than invasive ductal carcinoma. Patients present with a palpable breast mass and skin retraction or fixation in about 15 percent of the cases. Metastasis to the axilla is quite rare. Importantly, this tubular carcinoma must be distinguished from a benign condition such as sclerosing adenosis or microglandular adenosis. There are two treatment possiblities: (1) mastectomy; or (2) excisional lumpectomy, axillary node dissection, and radiation therapy. Recurrences have been reported in less than 5 percent of the patients. Only a few patients have been reported to have metastatic disease outside the local regional area of the breast.

■ Medullary Carcinoma

About 5–7 percent of all breast carcinomas are medullary. This type of cancer also has a better prognosis than invasive ductal carcinoma. It can metastasize to axillary lymph nodes. Sixty percent of patients who have medullary carcinoma are younger than fifty. Medullary carcinoma is the fastest growing of all breast cancers. Patients with atypical medullary carcinoma have a less favorable prognosis than patients with regular medullary carcinoma.

■ Mucinous or Colloid Carcinoma

About 3 percent of all breast cancers are mucinous or colloid carcinomas. These carcinomas are extremely slow growing and become quite bulky. The initial finding for a woman is a breast mass. She may also have nipple discharge, fixation, and skin ulceration. Prognosis for a patient with mucinous carcinoma also is more favorable than with invasive ductal carcinoma.

■ Inflammatory Carcinoma

Inflammatory breast carcinoma is a diagnosis made by the physician when he or she clinically observes and examines the breast. The breast looks as if it is inflamed because it is red and warm. The skin has ridges and it appears pitted because of its edema and swelling. The skin's edema is called *peau d'orange*. Skin induration (thickening and hardening) is present with or without a palpable breast mass. The breast is reddened in either one section or in its entirety. Oftentimes, this condition is mistaken for an infection and may initially be treated as such by physicians. There may be a discrete mass in the breast or no mass, or a very indistinct mass when the breast is actually sectioned pathologically. To reiterate, this is a clinical diagnosis although a biopsy will support the diagnosis if the tissue specimen has cancer cells in the small lymphatic channels of the skin. The signs and symptoms of inflammatory breast carcinoma are actually due to the tumor invading these lymphatic channels in the skin or to capillary congestion.

Inflammatory breast carcinoma has the poorest survival of all the breast cancers. In the past, with radiation therapy or mastectomy, less than 10–15 percent of the patients survived and over 80 percent of them had distant metastases. Now, however, chemotherapy is given as the initial treatment, and some studies show an improvement in the disease-free survival, which means that there are less cancer events during the period of time that the patient is alive. There is an 80–90 percent response rate with chemotherapy, but despite a clinical complete response, i.e., disappearance of all the initial signs and symptoms, the majority of all pathological specimens have residual tumor in them. When various modalities are combined—chemotherapy first, then preoperative radiation therapy, then mastectomy, and then maintenance chemotherapy—a 40 percent five-year survival rate is obtained. For those who have inoperable inflammatory breast cancer after initial chemotherapy and radiation therapy, experimental protocols involving high-dose chemotherapy and autologous bone marrow transplantation (see page 274) are being investigated.

There are other invasive carcinomas that occur with much less frequency and they include: papillary carcinoma, metaplastic carcinoma, apocrine carcinoma, adenoid cystic carcinoma, squamous carcinoma, secretory carcinoma, and several others.

PROGNOSTIC FACTORS
(FACTORS THAT PREDICT OUTCOME)

The prognostic factors that are considered standard and predict a patient's outcome are axillary lymph node status, tumor size, pathological classification, nuclear grade, estrogen and progesterone receptors, and DNA ploidy, and S-Phase Fraction, etc. These factors combined with the ultimate stage (extent of the disease spread) will determine the patient's treatment options as well as the patient's prognosis. We know, however, that by the time we can actually detect a breast cancer, tumor cells have probably been spread to other parts of the body through the bloodstream.

Axillary Lymph Node Status

Patients who have negative lymph nodes have an 85 percent five-year survival compared to less than a 40 percent five-year survival for patients with four or more positive lymph nodes in the axilla. However, about 30 percent of all patients with negative axillary lymph nodes will have a recurrence and die of their disease. So other factors are important as well. About 9 percent of the patients who have been found to have negative lymph nodes by routine pathological examination, were found to have micrometastases after special preparation for the pathologist. These patients had a poorer prognosis compared to the truly node-negative patients.

Best Prognosis: Negative axillary lymph nodes (see Table 20.3).

Cancer Size

The diameter of the cancer is one of the most important prognostic factors, especially in patients who have negative lymph nodes at time of dissection. As seen in Table 20.3, the five-year survival rates are directly correlated with the diameter of the cancer for patients who have negative axillary nodes. The larger the size of the cancer, the lower is the survival rate. The twenty-year recurrence rate is only 14 percent in patients who have less than 1 cm in diameter of cancer.

Best Prognosis: <1 cm cancer diameter.

Pathological Classification

Prognosis also varies according to the different pathological subtypes of breast cancer that were reviewed above. Long-term recurrence rates of less than 10 percent are seen for patients who have ductal carcinoma *in situ*, pure tubular, papillary, and medullary cell types. When the size of the tumor is combined with the special pathological subtype, a decision to treat or not to treat with systemic therapy in patients with negative axillary lymph nodes is clear-cut. For instance, approximately 25 percent of all patients who have tumors less than 1 cm in diameter or whose tumor is either ductal carcinoma *in situ*, pure tubular carcinoma, papillary carcinoma, or typical medullary carcinoma have recurrence rates ranging anywhere from 1–10 percent. There is no need to use systemic therapy in these patients as determined by the National Institutes of Health Breast

**Table 20.3 Five-Year Survival in Patients
With Negative Axillary Nodes and Various Size Cancers**

% Patients	Diameter of Cancer	Five-Year Survival
8%	<1 cm	99%
64%	1–3 cm	91%
28%	3 cm	85%

Cancer Consensus Conference of 1990. An additional 25 percent of patients have tumors larger than 3 cm in diameter and have a recurrence rate greater than 50 percent. Systemic therapy is generally given to these patients. The majority of the patients (50 percent) have tumors ranging from 1–3 cm in size with recurrence rates, generally, of 30 percent. And the majority of these patients are "cured" without ever having any systemic therapy. There may be some other prognostic factors that help the clinician decide whether systemic therapy in these patients with negative lymph nodes should be given or not.

Best Prognosis: Ductal carcinoma *in situ* or
Pure Tubular carcinoma or
Pure Papillary carcinoma or
Pure Medullary carcinoma.

Histological or Nuclear Grade

The grading system is pretty subjective and is based upon the pathologist's scoring of a number of factors when looking at particular cancer cells. However, if the system of grading is reliable, then knowing the grade is important. For instance, grade 1 affords the best prognosis, and grade 3, the worst prognosis.

Best Prognosis: Grade 1.

Breast Lymphatic Vessel Cancer Invasion

The finding of cancer cells in the lymphatic channels of the breast tissue of patients whose lymph nodes in the axilla are negative heralds a very high recurrence rate and eventual death from the disease.

Best Prognosis: No cancer cells invading the breast lymphatic vessels.

Breast Blood Vessel Invasion

Here again, recurrences and deaths from breast cancer are significantly more frequent in patients whose blood vessels in their breast tissue were invaded with cancer cells.

Best Prognosis: No breast blood vessel invasion.

Estrogen Receptor (ER) and Progesterone Receptor (PR)

Generally, but not always, patients with estrogen receptor negative tumors have a higher rate of recurrence independent of nodal status or size of tumor. A positive progesterone receptor is more important to predict the time of recurrence for patients who have positive axillary lymph nodes. However, estrogen status and tumor size are the most important factors to predict disease-free survival in patients with negative axillary lymph nodes. The most important reason to know the estrogen and progesterone receptor status in patients is to predict whether the patient will benefit from using hormonal manipulation such as tamoxifen (an estrogen-blocking hormone) systemic therapy.

Inaccuracies are inherent in measuring the receptors, however. False negative results will occur if:

- The breast specimen is not frozen within 15 minutes;
- The breast specimen is not large enough to be tested;
- The body has mounted a defensive reaction of normal cancer-fighting cells around the cancer thereby decreasing the number of cancer cells in the specimen;
- The cancer is *in situ*;
- The patient is taking exogenous hormones (pills) or producing enough estrogen in her body to bind the available receptor sites so they cannot be detected in the lab assay.

Best Prognosis: Positive estrogen and progesterone receptors (>15 femtomoles/mg)

Ploidy and S-Phase Fraction

The determination of the DNA content of cancer cells and the rapidity with which they grow is important. Tumor cells with the normal amount of DNA are called diploid tumors. An abnormally high DNA content is called aneuploidy, and the prognosis is usually poor. Aneuploidy is seen in about 60–70 percent of all early breast cancer patients. Some studies, however, do not confirm that aneuploidy is linked to poor prognosis.

The S-phase fraction, which denotes how quickly the cells turn over, is a more important prognostic factor to determine survival than ploidy status or nuclear grading. The higher the S-phase number, the more quickly the cancer cells are turning over and forming, the more likely the patient is to have recurrent disease and die earlier. In other words, patients who have fast-growing tumors have more frequent events and earlier death. A high S-phase fraction is also linked to a high expression of certain oncogenes and the loss of the p53 tumor suppressor gene (see page 199). This also may be one of the reasons the high S-phase fraction can predict early recurrence and earlier death.

Best Prognosis: Diploid status
DNA index = 1.00
S-phase fraction <7%

Cathepsin D

Cathepsin D is an enzyme manufactured in lysosomes, tiny organelles within cells in the body. It is manufactured in higher amounts than normal in patients who have breast cancers. Cathepsin D may have a direct role in cancer cell invasion and ultimate metastases. A high level of Cathepsin D is correlated with an increased recurrence rate and also heralds an earlier death in the patient. Breast cancer patients who have negative lymph nodes in the axilla but whose tumors are aneuploid and have high levels of Cathepsin D have a recurrence rate of 60 percent in five years.

Best Prognosis: Low Cathepsin level (<50 units)

Other Potential Prognostic Factors

With newer technologies, many other factors have been detected in breast cancer cells. The list of them is quite lengthy and includes HER-2/*neu*, p53, pS2, Ki-67, epidermal growth factor receptor, stress proteins, NM23, plasminogen activators, markers of angiogenesis, and many others. Ki-67 is specific for all rapidly dividing cells in a cancer. This is an indicator of how aggressive a cancer is. With each one of these, there are a few studies involving only a handful of patients and extolling its virtues as a good prognostic factor. But until there are meaningful numbers of patients in these studies, we must rely on the prognostic factors that we have already discussed. Even with these accepted prognostic factors, we must be aware that different laboratories may have different quality controls and methodologies.

Circulating Tumor Markers

Circulating tumor markers include CEA (carcinogenic embryonic antigen), LSA (lipid associated sialic acid), and CA 15-3. These tumor markers have been reported in some patients who have progressive disease before the disease became evident. However, sometimes these tests are negative or low when there is obvious cancer in the patient. And sometimes when the patient is perfectly healthy, these tests may be elevated, which forces "million dollar work-ups" looking for the possible site of cancer recurrence. These tests now have fallen out of favor generally. Some people continue ordering them, especially the CEA. High CEA levels are correlated with late stages of the disease at which point, neither physician nor patient needs the CEA to tell how badly the patient is doing.

To summarize, the prognostic factors that are linked to low risk of recurrence are the following: ductal carcinoma *in situ*; tubular, papillary, or typical medullary types of cancer; tumor diameter size of less than 1 cm; low S-phase fraction; diploid tumor; nuclear grade 1; and a tumor diameter of 1–3 cm without high risk features. Those factors associated with a high risk of recurrence are the following: aneuploid tumor; high S-phase fractions; high Cathepsin D levels; absent estrogen receptors; and a tumor diameter greater than 3 cm.

STAGING OF BREAST CANCER

Once the diagnosis of breast cancer has been made by biopsy, other areas of the body must be evaluated to determine if the cancer has spread from the breast into other sites. This is called staging the patient. Treatment and prognosis are determined by the stage of the patient. Currently, oncologists use a TNM staging system, *T* denoting the size of the tumor, *N* denoting the presence or absence of lymph node involvement, and *M* denoting whether the disease has spread to other sites of the body. This TNM system may not be totally applicable to breast cancer, so for the purpose of this book, we will discuss the following stages in terms of an "English translation" of the TNM system.

Carcinoma *in situ*

Breast cancer *in situ* is an early form of breast cancer that accounts for about 5–10 percent of all breast cancers. These are found only in the one area of the breast tissue without going to any adjacent structures.

Stage I

The cancer diameter is 2 cm or less and has not spread outside the breast.

Stage II

Any one of the following sentences may be true:
• Cancer diameter is 2 cm or less and has spread into the axillary lymph nodes; or

- Cancer diameter is between 2 and 5 cm, and the cancer has either spread to the axillary lymph nodes or not; or
- The cancer diameter is larger than 5 cm but not spread to the axillary lymph nodes.

Stage III

This stage is divided into Stage IIIA and IIIB. In Stage IIIA, the cancer diameter is less than 5 cm and has spread into the axillary lymph nodes that have grown into each other or into other attached structures; or cancer diameter is larger than 5 cm and spread into the axillary lymph nodes. In Stage IIIB, the cancer from the breast has spread into nearby structures like the chest wall, which includes ribs and muscles of the chest; or, the cancer has spread to lymph nodes near the collar bone.

Stage IV

The breast cancer has spread to other organs of the body that may include the bones, lungs, liver, or brain, etc.

Inflammatory Breast Cancer

This classification has already been discussed and is considered inoperable initially.

CONCLUSION

Now that you have all the information about your cancer including tissue type, nodal status, prognostic factors, extent or stage of disease, you can explore the best treatment options available for your case.

21

"Conventional" Localized Treatment Options for Breast Cancer

Once the diagnosis of invasive breast cancer has been made, two areas of treatment must be considered. "Localized" treatment is directed to the breast and, in some cases, its draining lymph nodes. "Systemic" treatment, on the other hand, is directed to all parts of the body including organs to which breast cancer cells *may* have spread or places where breast cancer dissemination already is known to be, for example, the lungs, liver, brains, or bone.

Localized treatment is intended to remove or eradicate breast cancer in the breast itself or in its immediately adjacent structures, like lymph nodes. It was thought, until recently, that breast cancer spread only by way of lymph node channels. We now know that breast cancer can spread by way of lymph nodes and also *can spread by way of the bloodstream when the breast cancer cells invade the tiny blood vessels of the breast*. Hence, breast cancer cells may be taken by the blood to almost any site in the body.

Until 1970, all surgical therapy was governed by the concepts and teachings of cancer biology as established by a German pathologist, Virchow, in 1863. For over one hundred years, the paradigm that he established was followed and no one veered from it until the results of the National Surgical Adjuvant Breast and Bowel Project were published in 1970. Until that study was published, radical mastectomies were the norm. More recently, modified radical mastectomies have been done and, finally, lumpectomies and axillary node dissection. Let me define these terms:

Radical mastectomy, also known as Halsted radical mastectomy, is the removal of the entire breast, the chest wall muscles and its coverings, and all the axillary lymph nodes. The woman then has a flattened chest wall, the area below the collar bone site.

Modified radical mastectomy is the removal of the entire breast, some of the axillary lymph nodes, the lining over the chest muscles, and usually a small muscle of the chest wall. This is the usual surgery for the treatment of breast cancer when mastectomy is an option for the woman or man.

Total mastectomy is the removal of the entire breast plus the cover of the chest wall muscle but not the muscle itself. No lymph nodes are removed.

Lumpectomy is simply the removal of the breast mass and a little margin of tissue around it.

Axillary node dissection is the removal of the nodes from underneath the arm, the area called the axilla.

Because the old paradigm taught that breast cancer spread by way of lymph nodes alone, the radical mastectomy was performed routinely. The feeling was, the more you remove, the better. The Halsted modification of the mastectomy was designed to control not only the disease in the breast but also the regional lymph node disease. This Halsted radical mastectomy was applied to breast cancers both large and small. But in the late 1800s, some innovative surgeons were removing smaller parts of the breast but unknowingly leaving behind microscopic amounts of tumor (called positive margins). Hence, the tumor came back in almost 100 percent of the patients, and death occurred from the cancer. Using Halsted's radical mastectomy, the recurrence rate was reduced to about 25 percent, but for the next fifty years, the recurrence rate and cure rates remained about the same. And even in the 1950s, aggressive surgeons tried to improve the radical mastectomy by doing operations that took even more tissue away from the woman. The so-called extended radical mastectomy removed lymph nodes above the collar bone and also nodes in the central portion of the chest, but no survival benefit was demonstrated from this procedure.

The turning point toward less surgery occurred when the National Surgical Adjuvant Breast and Bowel Project (NSABBP) showed that after a Halsted radical mastectomy, the ten-year survival rate was only 36 percent in women who had one to three positive lymph nodes in the axilla and only 14 percent when there were four or more positive lymph nodes. It was then realized that women had cancer dissemination at the time of their mastectomies and did not die of a local chest wall recurrence, but of breast cancer that had spread into other parts of the body like the liver, lungs, brain, bone, etc.

Therefore, axillary lymph node dissection today is performed only to determine the prognosis and plan treatment and not as an attempt to cure the patient. If the patient has positive lymph nodes, we know that his/her survival rate is much less. Axillary lymph node dissection is still very "conventional," and it is still the consistent recommendation for all cases of breast cancer. How the breast itself is treated has nothing to do with whether an axillary node dissection is done or not. Obtaining only ten lymph nodes or less is an inadequate surgical dissection. PET scanning might help determine whether the lymph nodes are involved with cancer or not and, hence, obviate the need for any axillary node dissection at all.

Which patients are candidates for radiation therapy? Once the diagnosis of breast cancer is made by an incisional biopsy or excisional biopsy (lumpectomy) but before the axillary node dissection is done, the patient should be referred to a radiation oncologist. The radiation oncologist will determine whether the patient is a candidate for conservative surgical technique, which includes re-excisional lumpectomy and axillary node dissection followed by radiation therapy. Radiation therapy after conservative surgical procedure has two functions. First, radiation treats the entire breast in an attempt to kill any cancer cells that may be in another section of the breast. Secondly, and equally important, by so treating an intact breast, radiation preserves the appearance of the breast.

The *general* criteria for a patient to be considered for radiation therapy include:

- Breast cancer diameter of up to 4–5 cm; however, studies have shown that patients who have larger breasts and who have lesions larger than 5 cm may be adequately treated if the ultimate cosmetic outcome is acceptable to the patient.[1] But importantly, the cosmetic outcome must be good. There is no role for conservative management of the breast if the patient ends up with a mound of tissue on her chest wall rather than having a cosmetically pleasing outcome for her breast. Cosmetic outcome is critically important when a patient is considered for primary radiation therapy and conservative surgical techniques.
- A single breast cancer and no evidence of other disease elsewhere on the mammogram.

- No cancer remaining in the site from which the lump of cancer was removed, i.e., negative surgical margins.

The *general* criteria that would exclude patients from being candidates for radiation therapy include:

- A very poor cosmetic outcome that can be predicted before radiation therapy. For example, patients with small breasts who have very large tumor masses that when removed will leave a large defect in the modest-sized breast; or patients who have collagen vascular diseases such as scleroderma or lupus—these patients generally will have a poor cosmetic result.
- Clinical inspection of the axilla before axillary node dissection that reveals lymph nodes matted onto each other.

Radiation therapy is the use of high energy (megavoltage) X-rays to kill cancer cells and shrink tumors. The source of radiation may be a large machine that revolves around your body and sends radiation to a specific part of your body. This technique is called external beam radiation therapy. On the other hand, internal radiation therapy is treatment administered by putting a radioactive source or device inside a specific location of your body. Cells are killed immediately around the source of the radiation in this instance.

How do we know that conservative surgical treatment of the breast with radiation therapy is an effective alternative for women? First of all, studies had to determine that radiating lymph nodes was as effective as the surgical removal of axillary nodes. Randomized clinical trials demonstrated there was little or no survival benefit in women who had surgical removal of axillary nodes compared to women who had radiation treatment to their axillary nodes without the removal.[2,3] Hence, the only goal of treating the axilla is to prevent a local recurrence in that area, which is a very uncomfortable, debilitating, and sometimes a very messy event. Treating the axilla surgically or with radiation therapy has absolutely no effect on survival or local control. As was pointed out previously, the only reason for doing an axillary node dissection is to determine prognosis.

Is there any difference in local control or overall survival (life span) between a mastectomy or breast-conserving surgery, i.e., lumpectomy and axillary node dissection, combined with radiation? A mastectomy, as you remember, is the removal of the entire breast and some axillary lymph nodes while preserving the chest muscles;

whereas, primary radiation therapy involves conservative surgery (removing the bulk of the tumor surgically with axillary node dissection) and delivering moderate doses of radiation to eradicate any residual cancer that may be in the breast itself. Randomized clinical trials involving long-term follow-up with large numbers of patients demonstrated that survival was totally identical after a modified radical mastectomy in one group or lumpectomy, axillary node dissection, and radiation therapy in the other group.[5,6] Several other trials have shown similar survival rates.[7-9] Other long-term radiation therapy studies when compared to mastectomy show that the local recurrence rate is very low, cosmetic results are very good, and the complication rate is very low.[10-13] Indeed, the NIH Consensus Conference of 1990 agrees that breast conservation treatment is "appropriate and preferable because it provides survival rates equal to those of total mastectomy and axillary dissection while preserving the breast."[14]

How much tissue around the breast cancer should be removed in a woman who has elected to have conservative surgery and radiation therapy? For cosmetic reasons, only about 2 cm of apparently healthy breast tissue around the breast cancer should be removed. Otherwise, the cosmetic result, which is the most important reason for choosing this procedure, will not be optimal. Local recurrence rates were investigated in patients who had a lumpectomy (the breast cancer plus a margin of 2 cm or so) versus patients who had a quadrantectomy (almost one-quarter of the breast removed). Women who had a quadrantectomy had less recurrences in the local breast region than those who had lumpectomy after radiation.[4,5] However, there was no difference in survival between these two groups.[15,16] But a quadrantectomy really defeats the purpose of conservative breast care for cosmetic reasons. One of the ways to decrease the recurrence rate for patients who have lumpectomy is to make sure that the surgical margins of excision are negative for any cancer and to look closely for intraductal carcinoma, which is seen in about 10 percent of all patients. But again, quadrantectomy truly defeats the purpose of breast conservation treatment.

It must be noted that separate incisions have to be made for performing the lumpectomy (tumor excision) and for performing the axillary node dissection. This not only enhances the functional and cosmetic outcome, but also prevents "contamination" by cancer cells from one field into the other.

Radiation Therapy Dose

Using megavoltage radiation therapy, the entire breast should receive a total dose of 45–50 Gy at about 1.8 Gy per day. The cancer bed site from which the cancer was actually removed should receive a higher dose called a boost, and this dose can range from 10–15 Gy. The boost dose can be given by way of electron beam from a large machine that revolves around your body, or from an implant using radioactive seeds in the cancer bed site inside the breast itself. These seeds are removed after a certain period of time that has been calculated to deliver a certain dose. No radiation is delivered to the axillary lymph node site if the axillary lymph nodes are negative for cancer.

Can radiation be avoided in patients who receive just the lumpectomy and axillary node dissection? There is about a 40 percent recurrence rate in those patients who had only lumpectomy without radiation therapy compared to a 10 percent rate of recurrence for patients in whom radiation therapy was added.[3] This again had no bearing at all on overall survival. Patients who receive a quadrantectomy probably have the same rate of recurrence without radiation therapy.[16,17] Although those specific subgroups have been identified by the NIH Consensus Conference, trials currently underway may show that improved mammogram technology can help identify those patients who don't need to have radiation therapy.

Does an axillary lymph node dissection have to be performed? Even though the physician finds no evidence of clinical enlargement of lymph nodes in the axilla, there may be a 30–35 percent chance that some of those nodes are positive for metastatic disease. Several other things may guide the physician in making a decision about node dissection. If it has been determined that the patient will receive adjuvant systemic therapy like hormonal or chemotherapy, there may be no need at all for an axillary lymph node dissection. Systemic therapy is recommended for patients who have the following factors known at the time of lumpectomy: positive estrogen receptor in a postmenopausal woman, aneuploidy, high S-phase fraction, high Cathepsin D level, or a large-size tumor. In addition, cancers that have many microvessels in one field of examination under the microscope will increase the patient's risk for developing recurrent disease and/or metastatic disease to either axillary lymph nodes or other distant organ sites.[18]

Should a patient have chemotherapy prior to mastectomy or prior to lumpectomy, axillary node dissection, and radiation therapy? Chemotherapy has been given to patients with large breast cancer masses before any surgical intervention for the following reasons:

- To shrink the tumor so that conservative surgery, i.e., lumpectomy and axillary node dissection followed by radiation therapy, can be an option.
- To see if the chemotherapeutic agents are working in a particular patient by noting any change in the cancer breast mass.
- To use a systemic treatment when small numbers of cancer cells have spread away from the breast mass, which may be more responsive at this stage.[19]
- To decrease the *possible* stimulation of already disseminated cancer cells when the majority of the cancer mass is excised from the breast.[20,21]

Several studies have shown that preoperative chemotherapy reduced the breast mass to less than 3 cm in 77 percent of the women whose cancers had been larger than that.[22,23] And some studies are looking at the possibility of using chemotherapy and radiation therapy only, thus eliminating the need for any surgical intervention. However, the preoperative use of chemotherapy is considered experimental at this time and randomized clinical trials are ongoing.

Does the phase of the menstrual cycle at the time of surgery dictate the patient's survival? Animal studies first demonstrated a higher rate of recurrence in the breast if surgical resection was performed a few days before or during menstruation. The recurrence rate was lower if the surgery was performed during the mid-ovulation phase. A number of studies confirm this relationship in humans but only for those women who have positive axillary nodes.[24-27] A flurry of papers challenged this finding and, finally, when the subject was reviewed in four very large studies, no association between timing of surgery and outcome was seen.[28] Given the fact that the first several studies were simply retrospective reviews, the relationship between surgical resection and menstrual cycle may be spurious. At the moment, the scientific data suggests no specific optimal time when surgical resection should be done. If otherwise stated to patients, undue anxiety and no real benefit will make patients victims of misinformation.

Since conservative surgical procedures with radiation therapy produce the same outcome for recurrence rates and survival rates, is breast conserving surgery in widespread use now? A number of studies have shown a substantial geographic variation for the use of breast-conserving surgery with radiation therapy in the United States. It is most frequently used in the northeastern states and less frequently used in the southeastern states.[29-32] The most interesting finding was that primary radiation therapy with breast-conserving surgery was offered in the seventeen states that require physicians to inform breast cancer patients about all treatment options. Physicians have their own attitudes and belief system, particulary surgeons, and they clearly influence the ultimate decision made by the patient. The way information is presented to a patient can influence her decision. For instance, a physician may tell a patient, you can have either a mastectomy, "which will immediately get rid of the tumor," or lumpectomy, axillary node dissection with radiation therapy. . . . Or, the surgeon may say something like, "If it were my wife, if it were my mother. . ." Some studies show that physicians are more apt to offer the breast-conserving surgery to younger women rather than older women.[33] Also, because patients are not properly educated, there is a belief among them that if you remove the breast, you remove the problem forever. That is simply not true. The chance of recurrence to the chest wall versus recurrence to the breast if left intact is the same and the rate of long-term survival is identical between the two procedures. A woman *truly* has a choice if she is deemed to be a candidate for either.

It has been found that women who undergo breast-conserving surgery with radiation therapy have a better psychological outlook and quality of life in general compared to women who have modified radical mastectomies.[34] There may also be financial considerations for having a mastectomy versus breast-conserving surgery and radiation therapy. According to claims data, a modified radical mastectomy averages $6,160 across the country with New York reporting the highest total charge of $7,870 compared to the typical charge seen in Iowa of $4,100.[35] Charges for breast-conserving surgery, i.e., lumpectomy, axillary node dissection is about 60 percent of those costs. When radiation therapy costs are added to costs for breast-conserving surgery, the total costs can vary from $20,000 and $25,000.

If a patient has a mastectomy, should that patient receive radiation therapy? A patient who has a modified radical mastectomy with negative axillary nodes has less than a 10 percent chance of a recurrence on the chest wall or axillary area. However, when the lymph nodes are positive, the risk increases to 20–30 percent with the most common site of local recurrence in the chest wall as well as the lymph nodes above the collar bone (supraclavicular). The indications for having radiation treatment to the chest wall and some of the regional lymph node sites are the following:

- Breast cancer diameters greater than 5 cm.

- Four or more positive axillary lymph nodes.
- The breast cancer mass very close to the chest wall.

Once a recurrence becomes evident on the chest wall or lymph node draining sites of the breast, treatment is of little help. Surgical excision may be the best means of controlling the problem then, and in spite of excision, recurrence may come again. Chemotherapy does not control these recurrences and once a recurrence is manifested, radiation therapy fails to control it in 30–60 percent of the cases. Even when radiation therapy is combined with surgical resection or chemotherapy for the recurrence, the control rate does not improve appreciably. Once a chest wall recurrence manifests and continues to grow, other symptoms such as ulceration, bleeding, odor, pain, and weeping from the cancerous wound ensue. If the breast cancer recurs in one of the lymph node regions, local treatment is not effective and growth of the cancer there may lead to involvement of nerves, pain, and swelling of the arm in addition to erosion, ulceration, and all the other symptoms mentioned for the chest wall.

Hence, if a patient is deemed to be at high risk for a future local recurrence, the patient should be treated with radiation immediately after surgery to minimize the risk because recurrences are difficult to eradicate.[36]

BREAST RECONSTRUCTION AFTER MASTECTOMY

Patients may be offered breast reconstruction after mastectomy because:

- They were not suitable candidates for breast conservation.
- Women may desire a reconstruction several years after having had a mastectomy.
- A mastectomy had to be performed as the treatment for a recurrence in a breast originally treated with breast-conserving surgery followed by radiation therapy.

The most common way of doing a reconstruction consists of either inserting an implant or transferring a flap of tissue containing muscle and skin from another site of the body. The implants used are made of silicone or saline and put underneath the pectoral muscle. To improve the cosmetic outcome, a nipple and areola may be reconstructed on the skin of the reconstructed breast. Also, the opposite breast may need to be changed to make it symmetrical with the reconstructed one. Recently, machines have been developed to tattoo the reconstructed nipple-areola complex with nontoxic pigments and shade with the appropriate colors. However, this is not typically done. Implants are not without complications. A fibrous capsular contraction may develop that can cause pain and also alter the cosmetic appearance. Other complications include rupture of the outer shell of the implant, infection, leakage, and a possible increased risk of autoimmune disease. Complications associated with a flap reconstruction include infection and necrosis (death) of the flap tissue.

When is the best time to reconstruct a breast? If reconstruction is done immediately, patients feel "whole" and this decreases anxiety and depression. It also eliminates the problem of external prosthesis. But there is a down-side to immediate reconstruction. If a breast cancer recurs at all on the chest wall, it usually does so within the first two years of initial diagnosis. So a reconstructed flap or implant makes it more difficult to detect a recurrence by physical examination and by mammographic means. Given this problem, many physicians recommend waiting two years for reconstruction.

PROPHYLACTIC MASTECTOMY

Patients who are at high risk for developing a breast cancer have been considered for prophylactic mastectomy. Patients who are at high risk include those who: score high on the self test, or have a pathological breast biopsy diagnosis of a high-risk condition like atypical epithelial hyperplasia or premalignant lesion called lobular carcinoma *in situ,* or have an early stage of a malignant disease like ductal carcinoma *in situ.* Genetic analysis should be performed for the rare genetically inherited breast cancer syndromes that affect about 5 percent to 10 percent of women who are also in the high-risk category.

However, when all the studies are reviewed critically, *there is no benefit at all for doing prophylactic mastectomies.* Instead of prophylactic mastectomy, a patient at high risk must have good follow-up, practice breast self-examination, have an examination by a physician twice a year, and get a mammogram, depending on the indications.

Some patients, however, may consider the anxiety of close follow-up unacceptable and prefer to have prophylactic mastectomy. This group of patients should be assessed psychologically and thoroughly educated about the risks and about ways to modify those risks to have optimum breast health.

If prophylactic mastectomy is to be done, it must be done completely to avoid any residual breast tissue. Pectoral fascia, the nipple-areola complex, the axillary tail, and a sample of the lower axillary lymph nodes must be removed, otherwise the patient will be left with the same risk. The pros and cons of prophylactic mastectomy have been reviewed.[37,38]

SIDE EFFECTS OF SURGERY AND RADIATION

The surgical complications seen after breast cancer excisional biopsy or axillary dissection are hematoma (blood in a sac), seroma (fluid in a sac), or infection. During the third or fourth week of radiation therapy, a skin reaction may occur, particularly underneath the breast, that is very similar to a sunburn reaction. This is called desquamation, which may be moist or dry and should be treated as if it were a burn. Air circulation on the desquamated skin is important; hence, the use of a bra should be minimized at that time. Women who have large pendulous breasts are more apt to develop moist desquamation and should be forewarned to minimize the use of a bra from the third or fourth week of radiation therapy onward. The bra rubs against the skin and acts as sandpaper to an already sensitive area. I have told patients to use aloe vera gel, not the aloe vera cream, three or four times a day from the very first day of radiation therapy. Gel will get right into the skin and not be greasy. Oftentimes, patients are told by the radiation oncologist or radiation technologist not to put anything on the skin because this will make the reaction worse. They are concerned because the radiation dose is calculated so that the surface of the skin gets a certain dose. If something thick is placed on the skin, the dose will be higher on the surface of the skin for reasons that involve physics. A gel, which gets into the skin very rapidly, does not have this effect. The aloe vera gel will, in fact, help protect the skin. Certain antioxidant nutrients, as we have already discussed, also protect the skin.

Some patients complain about fatigue during radiation therapy. This is not due so much to radiation *per se,* but mainly to the fact that:

- They have been told they may experience fatigue during radiation therapy.
- They must travel to and from the radiation therapy unit every day, five days a week.
- The anxiety and depression associated with a newly diagnosed cancer also produces fatigue.

Adriamycin or methotrexate chemotherapy given concurrently with radiation therapy produces a poorer cosmetic outcome and increased risk of pneumonitis. For that reason, when chemotherapy is given concurrently with radiation therapy, only Cytoxan and 5-fluorouracil are given to avoid these complications.

A higher risk of rib fracture or pneumonitis may occur in 1 or 2 percent of people treated with radiation therapy. The pneumonitis may manifest with low-grade fever, shortness of breath, and sometimes a cough. In less than 5 percent of the patients, a chest X-ray may reveal fibrosis in the region of the lung that was partially treated underneath the breast. This, however, will never give the patient a clinical problem. Arm edema is found in 8–10 percent of all the women treated with axillary node dissection, chemotherapy, and radiation therapy. But this is generally related to how vigorous the surgical procedure had been as well as concurrent use of chemotherapy and radiation therapy. The arm swelling can be relieved with a compression sleeve and sometimes physical therapy.

Radiation is sometimes used to treat the chest wall in women who had mastectomies according to the criteria above. A piece of material is placed on the chest wall during radiation therapy to intensify the radiation dose on the skin surface. This will usually increase the likelihood of a skin reaction, which is handled in the same way as previously described.

Thrombophlebitis of Axillary or Breast Veins

A thrombophlebitis can develop in the axillary vein (vein in armpit) or a superficial vein on the intact breast surface approximately two to four weeks after a biopsy, axillary node dissection, or mastectomy. This condition is not common; hence, it is often not recognized or treated. This thrombophlebitis (Mondor's disease) causes severe pain and limits the arm motion. Proper treatment includes one aspirin daily and warm moist compresses (not dry heat) applied to the inflamed venous cord three to four times daily for twenty minutes at a time. Be careful not to burn your skin.

Second Malignancy Risk

The risk of developing another malignancy in the opposite breast, original breast, or chest wall has been reviewed and is higher if radiation is combined with chemotherapy.

Pain Syndrome

Patients complain about a pain syndrome that can manifest itself months or years after mastectomy. The pain is quite real and treatable although the syndrome is not often recognized by physicians including the surgeon, oncologist, or primary care physician. Pain is often described as radiating, shooting, burning, sharp, or constricting, and occurs in as many as 5–10 percent of postmastectomy and lumpectomy patients. Pain control can be effectively treated with a variety of analgesics, or if very severe, a TENS (transcutaneous electrical nerve stimulation) unit.[39]

HYPERTHERMIA

Hyperthermia treatment of cancer cells involves temperatures above 41–42°C (approximately 106°F). These temperatures have a direct killing effect on both normal and tumor cells. Killing cells is dependent not only on the temperature but also on the length of time the high temperature is applied to the tissue. Heat can sometimes be effective against cells that would otherwise resist the effects of radiation therapy. And heat also can make an otherwise radio-resistant cell more responsive and sensitive to radiation. High temperatures can also potentiate a variety of chemotherapeutic drugs like bleomycin, cisplatin, cyclophosphamide, melphalan, mitomycin C, and nitrosoureas.

Hyperthermia is effective for small and superficial cancers that can be implanted with heating elements. Recurrent breast cancer on the chest wall is an ideal setting for the use of hyperthermia and radiation therapy. When the two are combined, tumor masses decrease dramatically. The problem, however, has been technical difficulties in assuring quality control and adequate delivery of an even amount of heat for all the tissues. Only a few centers have efficiently performed hyperthermia because of these technical stumbling blocks.

CONCLUSION

Review this chapter with your own condition in mind. Next, turn to Chapter 22 to learn if you need systemic treatment.

22

"Conventional" Systemic Treatment for Breast Cancer

Until recently, the medical profession had been deluding itself for over a century in thinking that breast cancer was a surgical disease and the more tissue removed, the more women would be cured. We now realize that by the time a breast cancer is detected and then removed surgically, it has already disseminated to other parts of the body.[1]

Thus the notion of systemic therapy came into the picture. Systemic therapies are agents that enter the bloodstream and travel throughout the body to theoretically kill cancer cells anywhere. Systemic therapy includes hormonal therapy, chemotherapy, and treatment with biological response modifiers. Hormones, like estrogens, are important growth promotors for many cells including some breast cancer cells. The intent of hormone therapy, then, is to interfere with or stop any hormone that will allow the cancer cell to grow. Certain drugs block the action of your hormones; or certain organs, like ovaries, can be removed to stop the production of hormones such as estrogens. Chemotherapeutic agents are chemical drugs that can be taken orally, intravenously, or intramuscularly. Biological response modifiers are agents that try to enhance or re-direct your own immune system.

HORMONAL THERAPY

The intention of hormonal therapy is to kill cancer cells that depend upon hormones to grow. Breast cancer cells may have estrogen receptors that act as doorways for estrogen to enter the breast cancer cell and thereby feed it. There are also progesterone receptors on cancer cells. About 50 percent of all breast cancers are estrogen receptor positive, which means they depend on estrogen to grow. If estrogen is unavailable, those cancer cells will die. An estrogen receptor above 10–15 femtomoles/mg is considered positive, and below that is considered negative. Women who are still premenopausal, i.e., menstruating, have about a 30-percent chance of having positive estrogen receptors on their breast cancer cells. Postmenopausal women, those who have stopped menstruating, have about a 60-percent chance of having a positive estrogen receptor on their breast cancer cells. Women who are about to enter menopause, i.e., perimenopausal women, have the lowest estrogen receptor positive rate, less than 20 percent. The charcoal method of assay for these receptors, both estrogen and progesterone, is preferable over any other assay.

Organ Removal

Castration in premenopausal women refers to either surgical removal of both ovaries (oopherectomy) or removal of their function through radiation therapy or drugs. Castration was one of the first forms of systemic treatment for women with advanced breast cancer. Patients who have estrogen receptor positive tumors will have a 50–60 percent response with this procedure. All patients, estrogen receptor positive or not, will have a 30–40 percent response. Radiation directed to the ovaries will yield similar responses but takes about one to two months for an effect to become apparent. The dose of radiation required to render the ovaries ineffective is only 2,000 cGy and can be given over a course of three days to each ovary. Metastasis to bone, soft tissue, lymph nodes, and lung generally respond to hormonal manipulation like castration, but metastasis to liver or brain rarely respond. If a woman does respond to castration, she can have an additional response of 40–50 percent to another hormonal modality in the future. Patients who do respond to hormonal manipulation generally live about two years longer than those who do not. Surgical removal of the adrenal glands, independent of other procedures, produces about a 30–40 percent response in women who have metastatic breast cancer. Surgical removal of the pituitary gland from the brain has also been shown to give a 40–50 percent response rate in patients who had estrogen receptor positive tumors. If either or both of these procedures are done, the patient is then totally dependent on the daily administration of other vitally needed hormones that were produced by these organs. In an attempt to avoid technically difficult surgical procedures, a search was begun for chemical agents that would accomplish the same thing. A new drug, called aminogluthethimide, was developed. This was found to stop the production of hormones, including estrogens, by the adrenal gland and yielded a 35–50 percent response rate in estrogen receptor positive patients.

Individual Hormone Therapy

Estrogen

Postmenopausal women with advanced breast cancers have also been treated *with* estrogens. At high doses (premarin 10 mg three times a day) there is at least a 30-percent objective response lasting over a year, and when the estrogen receptor is positive, there is over a 50-percent response in some cases.[2,3] The mechanism of action at this high dose is totally unknown. Patients who initially respond to this estrogen therapy and then become resistant may have continued disease regression if the therapy is abruptly stopped. If further regression of tumor is obtained, which occurs in about 30 percent of all cases, a subsequent hormonal manipulation is predicted to work. And so the old wives' tale handed down in the last several decades that estrogen should never be used in patients with breast cancer has no basis. In fact, *high* dose estrogen is useful in the treatment of advanced cancers.

Androgens

About 20 percent of all postmenopausal women with advanced breast cancer respond to androgen therapy. Androgens are hormones that increase male physical qualities and include testosterone. There may be a brief response to androgens in premenopausal women if they had their ovaries removed. Here again, the mechanism of action is totally unclear.

Progesterone Agents

Megestrol (Megace), at a dose of 40 mg four times a day, exerts an antiestrogen effect. In patients who are resistant to tamoxifen, megestrol can produce remissions for about seven months in 30 percent of all patients. The mechanism of action is unknown. These three classes of hormones have largely been replaced by a safer and more effective antiestrogen, tamoxifen.

Tamoxifen

Tamoxifen is an antiestrogen that blocks the doorway, the estrogen receptor, to a cancer cell so that estrogen, which feeds the cell, may not enter. The usual tamoxifen dose is 20 mg a day and only occasionally is there any benefit from a higher dose. During the first few weeks of treatment with tamoxifen, a flare of "bone pain" and a transient high calcium blood level are noted in some patients who have extensive bony disease. This increased bone pain is a good sign and demonstrates that the drug is actually exerting its anticancer effects. Tamoxifen, generally, is effective for postmenopausal patients, patients who have positive estrogen receptors, or patients who had a prior hormonal manipulation that was effective. Tamoxifen, similar to the other hormones, produces about a 40 percent response rate, and this is slightly higher for postmenopausal women. Premenopausal women have a lesser response unless they have positive estrogen receptors, and then they can have up to about a 75 percent response. But castration seems to be superior to tamoxifen in premenopausal patients whose estrogen receptor is negative. Not considered a first line agent, tamoxifen is superior to androgen therapy and has largely replaced other individual hormones as well as adrenalectomy and hypophesectomy in postmenopausal women.

Hormonal Treatment for Premenopausal or Perimenopausal Patients With Metastatic Disease

Oopherectomy is the standard hormonal approach to this group of patients.[4] Other treatments include tamoxifen, aminoglutethimide, androgens, and megastrol (Megace).

Hormonal Treatment for Postmenopausal Patients

Postmenopausal breast cancer patients with positive estrogen receptors take 20 mg of tamoxifen a day. Once tamoxifen stops producing a response, aminoglutethemide can be used and a response is seen in almost half of the patients, whereas megastrol produces responses in 31 percent of these cases. These hormonal agents should be used in sequential order since there is no advantage in combining them.

CHEMOTHERAPY

Combination chemotherapy might be considered when tumors are rapidly progressive or there is rapidly progressive liver metastasis, or a patient has inflammatory carcinoma, or lymphangitic spread in the lungs. Additionally, chemotherapy may be used for a patient who is receiving hormonal treatment but has rapidly progressive disease.

Combining two or more chemotherapeutic agents as opposed to using single agents in the treatment of breast cancer is commonly done today. The drugs that have been approved for treating breast cancer are the following: aminoglutethemide, cisplatin, chlorambucil, cyclophosphamide, dactinomycin, doxorubicin (Adriamycin), estrogens of all chemical structures, etoposide, floxuridine, 5-fluorouracil, fluoxymesterone, goserelin, ifosfamide, leucovorin, leuprolide, lomustine, progesterones, megestrol, melphalan, methotrexate, testosterone, mitomycin, mitoxantrone, prednisone, tamoxifen, thiotepa, vinblastine, and vincristine.

Since the 1970s in the United States, combination chemotherapy has been the treatment of choice for premenopausal women with positive lymph nodes. Combination chemotherapy came into being in the mid to late 60s; hence, a new paradigm was established and everybody was eager to become involved in this new form of treatment. Combination chemotherapy initially produced remarkable results in otherwise extremely fatal and extremely rare tumors. So clinicians around the country jumped on the band wagon to see if combination chemotherapy could do spectacular things for all the other cancers. This occurred as the subspecialty of medical oncology went from its infancy to become a very dominant and major field.

The following are the most commonly used combinations of drugs for breast cancer treatment:

CMF (cyclophosphamide, methotrexate, 5-fluorouracil)
CAF (cyclophosphamide, adriamycin, 5-fluorouracil)
CMFVP (cyclophosphamide, methotrexate, 5-fluorouracil, vincristine, prednisone)

Combination chemotherapy as above is superior to individual single agents. In the above regimens, methotrexate, 5-fluorouracil, and adriamycin are given intravenously on days one and eight of a twenty-eight-day cycle. Cyclophosphamide is given orally on days one through fourteen. CMF and CAF are the most commonly used regimens. CMF, CAF, CMFVP generally produce about a 50 percent response rate in almost all sites of breast cancer metastases including liver, bone, soft tissue, and other organs. The duration of response varies from twelve to eighteen months. When patients relapse after receiving combination chemotherapy, second-line chemotherapeutic agents are not very effective. For the small number of patients who have a *complete remission* (complete disappearance of all tumor as detected by current technology) using combination chemotherapy, the average duration of this remission is sixteen to eighteen months; and the average length of survival is close to thirty months but only twenty-four months for those who did not achieve a complete remission from the outset.

Patients who have minimal amount of disease will do better than those who have more disease present in their bodies. A hormonal manipulation can be used in patients who have a recurrence of disease after combination chemotherapy because chemotherapy does not compromise a possible response to any subsequent hormonal manipulation.

Chemotherapy improves patient outcome mainly by reducing the number of relapses in the breast and/or draining sites and also in soft tissues like skin metastases. Chemotherapy has had little or no influence in diminishing the rate of bone or other organ metastases.[5,6] And no matter what combination of drugs is used, CMF followed by adriamycin or other agents, there has been no change in the response rate or survival rate.

Do the response rates and survival rates with chemotherapy look familiar to you? They are almost identical to rates in patients who simply have hormonal manipulations as reported on page 260. Some clinical researchers have advocated higher doses of chemotherapeutic agents to produce higher response rates and maybe increase survival. But no greater benefit is obtained with higher doses, which produce more morbidity and side effects.[7-9]

Is the timing of chemotherapy important for women who have positive axillary lymph nodes? Chemotherapy given immediately after surgery to women with breast cancer who have positive lymph nodes has shown some benefit in studies with regard to disease-free survival. Some studies have shown a minimal effect on increasing life span, i.e., the survival time, but the survival statistics are not statistically significant.[10-20] All these studies included patients who were premenopausal or postmenopausal with negative axillary lymph nodes. Other studies show that there may also be a benefit in giving chemotherapy immediately postoperatively while the patient is still in the hospital regardless of the status of her axillary lymph nodes.[21,22]

Is there an optimal time during the day to administer chemotherapy? During the twenty-four hours of a day, there is a rhythmic cycle to the body's activities. Many biological events exhibit such circadian rhythms. Many of you know, for instance, that body temperature rises in the afternoon. Human bone marrow cells, circulating white blood cells, enzymes, and DNA activity of normal cells and many cancer cells are particularly affected by these rhythms.[23-25] Chemotherapy given to animals during their nighttime hours has a positive effect on survival. Human repair mechanisms for normal cells peak during the night hours because that is when the body repairs itself from any damages incurred.[26] It follows, then, that if chemotherapy is administered during the night hours, normal cells will be best protected since they are already in a repair mode. Initial studies[25] show that tumors are more responsive at night. And in a study involving 118 children with acute lymphoblastic leukemia, survival was better and there was a lower relapse rate in those who received chemotherapy at night versus the group who received chemotherapy during the morning.[27] Although it is not very practical to give chemotherapy in the evening hours, animal studies and some human studies show a real benefit. If chemotherapy were given in the evening, there might not be a need to administer the very expensive new agents used solely for the purpose of keeping the white and red blood cells higher during the time of chemotherapy.

ADJUVANT SYSTEMIC THERAPY
FOR EARLY BREAST CANCER

The term adjuvant systemic therapy refers to a systemic therapy given to a patient who is free of any detectable cancer anywhere in her body. This therapy is administered at about the same time the primary site is treated by surgery and/or radiation therapy. All patients who receive adjuvant systemic therapy have a negative metastatic workup, which includes a normal bone scan, a normal chest X-ray, and normal liver function blood tests. This patient's status is "no clinical evidence of disease" (NED) because no disease is detectable with currently available technology. Adjuvant systemic therapy is generally given to patients with positive axillary lymph nodes (removed), and to some patients with negative lymph nodes who have several high-risk prognostic factors. For the last twenty to twenty-five years, patients with positive axillary nodes generally have been offered adjuvant systemic therapy. In patients who have negative axillary lymph nodes, it is not so well defined who should receive adjuvant systemic therapy.

Some general conclusions may be made now about systemic adjuvant therapy:

- The disease-free interval, the period of time in which there are no disease events, has been longer in women who receive adjuvant systemic therapy.
- Statistically, the overall survival, the life span of a patient from the time of diagnosis until death, has not changed significantly in patients who receive adjuvant systemic therapy no matter if it is chemotherapy or hormonal therapy.

- Ovarian ablation or castration, the removal or destruction of the ovaries, is more effective in premenopausal women and perimenopausal women.
- Tamoxifen is more effective in postmenopausal women.
- There is a greater benefit in using tamoxifen for two or more years.
- Combination chemotherapy is better than single-agent chemotherapy.
- Combination chemotherapy is more effective in premenopausal women than it is in postmenopausal women.
- There is no additional benefit in using chemotherapy for more than six months.
- Biological response modifiers or other immune system enhancers have shown no benefit at all.
- Patients who have positive estrogen receptors generally do better than patients who have negative estrogen receptors.

In 1992, the Early Breast Cancer Trialists' Collaborative Group published a report involving 133 randomized trials with 75,000 women who had early breast cancer.[28] There were 31,000 recurrences and 24,000 deaths among these women. Systemic treatments consisted of hormonal therapy, chemotherapy, or immunotherapy. Analysis of all these data revealed the overall survival benefit is quite small. For every 100 Stage II breast cancer women (positive axillary nodes) treated, about 12 women more than expected became 10-year survivors.

The benefit of adjuvant therapy depended entirely upon the patient's risk of dying from the disease. In this study, adjuvant systemic therapy lowered the relative risk of death by 25–30 percent, which means that the real benefit translates into about 4 percent for a person who actually has a 10–20 percent risk of dying from breast cancer in the first five years. Obviously, as her risk of dying from the cancer increases, i.e., if she has positive nodes and multiple high-risk prognostic factors that contribute to a poor prognosis, the real percent of benefit rises but only slightly. *Two-thirds of all the patients in the study had benefit from receiving hormonal systemic therapy compared to one-third of the group who had benefit from receiving combination chemotherapy.*

What these articles don't discuss is the fact that we are able to detect the breast cancers earlier with better mammographic technique compared to even ten to fifteen years ago. So if we can detect cancers earlier, we are simply starting the five-year clock or the ten-year clock sooner. The end point is always the same, but it simply appears that the patient is living longer. For instance, if breast cancer is a fifteen-year disease from start to finish, and we previously detected breast cancers by mammogram or clinical palpation around year eleven or twelve, patients lived only three years thereafter. Now we are detecting the cancers earlier—around years seven or eight—hence, it appears that the patients are living longer but this is not the case in reality. That is why statistical maneuvers with these 133 trials and other randomized trials have not shown any difference in overall survival benefit.

Ovarian Ablation

Postmenopausal women with negative estrogen receptors benefit from tamoxifen. Premenopausal women treated with tamoxifen alone show distinct risk reductions as well. And, intriguingly, ovarian ablation/castration (removal of ovarian function) achieves the same advantage in premenopausal women that combination chemotherapy does.[29] The long forgotten information of the fifties concerning ovarian ablation/castration has now been revived by meta-analysis of the 133 randomized trials showing that combination chemotherapy and ovarian ablation produce the same results in premenopausal women.

Until this analysis, prior reports of ovarian ablation in this group of women had showed different results.

- Some studies showed no significant delay in recurrence.[30-33]
- Some studies showed significant delay in recurrence but not in death.[34,35]
- Some studies showed significant delay in death but only in certain subgroups of patients.[36,37]

But in the Early Breast Cancer Trialists' Collaborative Groups study, ovarian ablation reduced the annual mortality by 25 percent. This exact reduction is seen in similar groups of women who received combination chemotherapy, which suggests that some of the benefits of combination chemotherapy in these younger women can be attributed to interfering with the hormones produced by ovaries. Women who receive chemotherapy become amenorrhoic (menstrual cycles stop), either temporarily or permanently. The older the woman, the more likely chemotherapy will permanently stop her menses. And several trials have shown that women who do become amenorrhic,[38,39] or who have positive estrogen or progesterone receptors,[40] have more benefit from combination chemotherapy than those who do not. In the review of 133 trials, there seemed to be further benefit by adding ovarian ablation to chemotherapy, but the benefit was small and the size of the patient groups was small. Two examples of such trials are those at the Mayo Clinic[41-43] and the Swiss Cooperative Group.[44] Postmenopausal women did not have significant benefit from combination chemotherapy but had a much larger benefit from hormonal systemic therapy. It is unlikely in premenopausal women, then, that all the benefit is obtained through hormonal mechanisms alone. There may be a small benefit from adjuvant combination chemotherapy. There were no estrogen receptor data to review in these trials because the studies were done prior to the availability of this laboratory test. From other studies, we know that people who do have positive estrogen receptors are more likely to respond to hormonal systemic manipulation.

After long-term follow-up in patients who had ovarian ablation, there continued to be a reduction in the annual mortality. This is seen also when tamoxifen is used. And this may suggest that a continuing hormonal manipulation will progressively increase the benefit even after a long period of time.

Should we recommend ovarian ablation/castration or combination chemotherapy to premenopausal women and perimenopausal women? Given the analysis of 133 randomized trials that both ovarian ablation and combination chemotherapy produce similar results, it seems prudent to recommend removal of ovarian function. In this way, the same result is achieved with many fewer side effects compared to the multiple acute side effects of combination chemotherapy with its attendent long-term morbidity. To be absolutely scientific, a randomized study can be done to investigate ovarian ablation versus combination chemotherapy versus both.[45]

ADJUVANT SYSTEMIC TREATMENT FOR BREAST CANCER PATIENTS WITH NEGATIVE AXILLARY NODES

In May 1988, the National Cancer Institute proclaimed an urgent Clinical Alert calling for the routine use of systemic adjuvant therapy for all patients with breast cancer who had negative axillary nodes. The "justification" for this was based upon the fact that about 15–20 percent of these patients relapse during the first five years after having had breast surgery and radiation therapy. The statement issued by the National Cancer Institute was that if all axillary node negative breast cancer patients were treated, "thousands of lives could be saved each year in the United States."[46] This Clinical Alert sent shock waves through the oncology community and was almost a mandate regarding treatment simply because of the statement issued by the National Cancer Institute. The implications of such an alert were far reaching. It meant that about 80 percent of the women would be unnecessarily treated. In addition, side effects of the chemotherapeutic agents were incalculable, the cost was monstrous, and there were even legal implications. If a physician decided not to treat such a patient, could that physician be held legally responsible with this Clinical Alert in place?

Studies then ensued that should have been conducted before such a Clinical Alert was issued. We know that about 70,000 women in the United States will develop breast cancer and have axillary nodes that are negative. About 70 percent of these women will be well treated simply with local surgery and radiotherapy or both. It is important to decide which patients should receive adjuvant systemic therapy based on scientific data and not emotional responses. Table 22.1 shows the results and relative cost of adjuvant systemic treatment in node negative breast cancer patients.

In each of the above studies, the control groups received absolutely no treatment at all. One study examined the use of chemotherapy within thirty-six hours of breast surgery; another study started a twelve-week course of four-week cycles of chemotherapy within a thirty-day period of the initial breast surgery; another study examined tamoxifen only; and the fourth study showed results from administering six cycles of chemotherapy. Looking at the column labelled "disease-free interval, treatment versus no treatment," you can see that there was very little difference between those who received a treatment and those who did not. Perhaps only 8 percent to 15 percent of the people may have benefited from being treated. That range is derived by subtracting the percentages in each group. You can also see that there was absolutely no survival advantage with any of the treatments, chemotherapy or tamoxifen, and that the patients who received neither did as well as far as life span as those who received chemotherapy or tamoxifen. Toxicity ranged from mild to quite high. In fact, a number of treatment-related deaths were reported. Toxicity brings with it emotional and physical side effects that cannot be calculated in terms of cost. When the actual costs are determined, however, the total direct cost for each treated patient ranges from $400 to about $6,000.

An analysis of the costs and the number of patients involved has been done.[51] It has been estimated that 5,040 of the 70,000 women with breast cancer who have negative axillary nodes would benefit from treatment with an improved disease-free interval, which means they will have less disease events during their life span, but no benefit in overall survival or life span. To achieve the benefit for these 5,040 patients, the other 65,000 would have to be treated with the various regimens outlined above. They will not and cannot have *any* benefit from treatment and the total cost of this is almost $340 million per year. The analysis does not consider toxicity and a possible 50–100 treatment-related deaths for these 5,040 women.

**Table 22.1 Results and Costs of Adjuvant Systemic Treatment
in Node Negative Breast Cancer Patients**

Year	Study Group	Four-Year Disease-Free Interval Treatment Vs. No Treatment	Survival Advantage	Toxicity	Cost
1989	Single course of CMF within 36 hours of breast surgery[47]	77% vs 74%	None	High	$ 400
1989	Twelve 4-week cycles of MF+L within 30 days of breast surgery (estrogen receptor negative patients)[48]	80% vs 71%	None	Mild	$6000
1989	Tamoxifen (estrogen receptor positive patients)[49]	83% vs 77%	None	Mild	$4750
1989	*Six 4-week cycles CMFP[50]	84% vs 69%	None	Moderate	$1830

*This was three-year data (the numbers could be closer at 4 years)
C=cyclophosphamide   M=methotrexate   F=5-fluorouracil
L=leukovorin   P=prednisone

Is there a better way to decide which negative axillary node patients will truly benefit from adjuvant systemic therapy? In June of 1990, the National Institutes of Health convened another consensus conference on "the treatment of early stage breast cancer."[52] One of the major purposes of the conference was to provide guidelines for the use of systemic adjuvant therapy for breast cancer patients with negative axillary nodes. The panel failed to issue any real statement about this matter and in fact dumped it back into the laps of the practicing physician and his or her patient with the following statement:

All patients with node negative breast cancer should be made aware of the benefits and risks of adjuvant systemic therapy, a thorough discussion of which should include the likely risk of recurrence without adjuvant therapy, the expected reduction in risk without adjuvant therapy, the toxic effects of therapy, and the impact of therapy on quality of life. Some degrees of improvement may be so small that the disadvantages of therapy outweigh them.[52]

The panel did conclude from a review of ten randomized trials that adjuvant systemic therapy reduced the rate of recurrence by approximately one-third but had no effect on improving overall survival.

Certain prognostic factors can predict a patient's overall risk for recurrence, and/or a shortened survival. These well-described prognostic factors should help guide us in determining which patients with negative axillary lymph nodes be offered adjuvant systemic therapy.

Table 22.2 indicates the prognostic factors that define low risk and high risk for breast cancer patients with negative axillary lymph nodes. The low-risk and high-risk categories have been determined by five-year recurrence rates for each prognostic factor[53,54] and other information.

Prognostic factors are assigned to either the low-risk category or the high-risk category based on their individual five-year recurrence rates, which are depicted in Table 22.3. For instance, the five-year recurrence rate for simply having ductal carcinoma *in situ* is only 1 or 2 percent, which means only 1 or 2 percent of the people with this

Table 22.2 Prognostic Factors That Define Low-Risk and High-Risk for Breast Cancer Patients With Negative Axillary Lymph Nodes

Low-Risk	High-Risk
Tumor diameter <1 cm	Tumor diameter >3 cm
Tumor diameter 1–3 cm but no high-risk factors	
Ductal carcinoma *in situ*	
Pure tubular, mucinous, papillary, adenoid, invasive lobular (all <2 cm)	
Typical medullary (may be <3 cm and/or high S-phase)	
Grade I	Grade III
Low S-phase	High S-phase (>7%)
Diploid	Aneuploid*
Age >50	High Cathepsin D (50 units)
Healthy lifestyle**	Negative estrogen receptor
	Cancer-promoting lifestyle factors
	High-fat, low-fiber diet
	Obesity
	No antioxidant nutrients or
	B vitamins
	Smoker or inhales others' smoke
	Alcohol: 3+ drinks per week
	Sedentary lifestyle
	Use of hormones
	Stress—uncontrollable

*Aneuploid with low S-phase is not high risk.
**Lifestyle factors as outlined in the ten-point plan on pages 317–333.

**Table 22.3   Five-Year Recurrence Rates With or Without Adjuvant
Systemic Treatment for Prognostic Risk Factors
in Breast Cancer Patients With Negative Axillary Lymph Nodes**

Prognostic Factors	Five-Year Recurrence Rates	
	No Treatment	Treatment
Ductal carcinoma *in situ*	1%	0.75%
Tumor <1.0 cm	6%	4.5%
Grade I	6%	4.5%
Low S-phase	10%	7.5%
Diploid	12%	9%
Tumor 1–3 cm	12%	9%
Grade II	25%	18.75%
Positive estrogen receptor	26%	19.5%
Aneuploid	27%	20.25%
Grade III	28%	21%
High S-phase	30%	22.5%
Negative estrogen receptor	35%	26.25%
High Cathespin D	50%	37.5%
Aneuploid + high Cathespin D	60%	45%

diagnosis will have a recurrence of their tumor in the first five years.
If a patient has a tumor less than 1 cm in size, the five-year recurrence
rate for that prognostic factor is only 6 percent, which is the same rate
for having a nuclear grade I.

*Remember, the review of 133 randomized clinical trials demonstrated that
systemic adjuvant treatment reduced the odds of recurrence by 25 percent.* So
with regard to an individual person, the absolute reduction is greatest
when the patient is predicted to have a high recurrence rate. For example, let's refer to Table 22.3 and consider a woman with prognostic
factors consisting of aneuploid and high Cathespin D levels. Her five-
year recurrence rate is 60 percent, which means that if she receives no
treatment, she has a 60 percent chance of having a recurrence. If, however, she receives adjuvant systemic treatment, that 60 percent would
be reduced by one-quarter. Hence, her five-year recurrence rate after
having received systemic adjuvant treatment would be 45 percent, 15
percent less. If a woman has only ductal carcinoma *in situ*, her five-year
recurrence rate is 1 percent and if that were reduced by one-quarter, she
would have a five-year recurrence rate of about .75 percent. It would,
therefore, make no sense to treat that particular patient. It would, on the
other hand, make sense to treat the first patient with an aneuploid status
and a high Cathespin D level.

Now let's look at a group of one hundred patients each having a
favorable recurrence rate of 10 percent. That means only ten of those

one hundred people will have recurrent disease without any adjuvant systemic treatment. Of these ten, about three will benefit from adjuvant treatment. Hence, only three of the original one hundred patients treated with adjuvant systemic treatment will benefit.

About 25 percent of all patients with negative nodes have small tumors and favorable histological types and hence have a low rate of recurrence. This group should not be treated at all with adjuvant systemic treatment. At the other end of the spectrum is another 25 percent of all patients with negative nodes who have large tumors and other poor prognostic risk factors conferring a much higher rate of recurrence who would benefit from adjuvant systemic treatment. The other 50 percent of patients will have a recurrence rate of about 30 percent because of tumor size alone. It is in this group that all the other prognostic risk factors must be assessed. If people in this middle group have more high-risk prognostic factors than low-risk prognostic factors as in Table 22.2, they will probably benefit from adjuvant systemic treatment.

If the patient is postmenopausal, has positive estrogen receptors, and a tumor size greater than 1 but less than 3 cm, tamoxifen has been shown to reduce the recurrence rate.[49] If the patient is postmenopausal, has positive estrogen receptors, but a tumor greater than or equal to 3 cm, tamoxifen or chemotherapy has been shown to reduce the recurrence rate.[48,49] And if the patient is postmenopausal with negative estrogen receptors, chemotherapy has been shown to reduce the recurrence rate. In all of these examples, there has been no change in survival rates at all.

Since there seems to be no difference in survival or recurrence rates in premenopausal women treated with ovarian ablation or combination chemotherapy, ovarian ablation should probably be offered to the patient if adjuvant systemic therapy is indicated. Chemotherapy can be used when there is rapidly growing tumor, liver metastases, or poor performance status, all of which heralds a poorer prognosis.

Can adjuvant chemotherapy given to breast cancer patients with negative axillary lymph nodes improve their quality of life? One study investigated two groups of women. The 45-year-old-woman's group was found to have an average lifetime benefit from chemotherapy of 5.1 quality-months at a cost of $15,400 per quality-year. The 60-year-old women gained only 4 quality-months at a cost of $18,800 per quality-year. Under the best scenarios, the benefit of chemotherapy varied from 1.4 to 14.0 quality-months for each group. The benefit of chemotherapy markedly diminished if the life span was deemed to be shortened (rapidly growing tumor, liver metastases, or poor performance status). The study concludes that the benefit from chemotherapy may be too small for many women to choose it as the adjuvant form of systemic treatment.[55] Similar results and high costs have been demonstrated in other studies.[56]

Are alternative therapies effective for breast cancer patients? There was no significant difference in survival or disease-free survival between patients receiving alternative therapies in a cancer hospital in England versus their controls. This particular study also reviewed cases from other studies using alternative therapies.[57]

TREATMENT OF LOCALLY ADVANCED BREAST CANCER

Patients who have very large breast masses (those measuring greater than 5 cm) have a very high rate of local recurrence and distant metastases.[58,59] Most of these locally advanced cancers are also inoperable and modalities other than surgery must be considered. Sometimes, these breast cancers extend directly to the chest wall and become immobile, or they grow through the skin so that you can visibly see tumor. These patients also have multiple positive axillary nodes.

Radiation therapy can be used initially with a dose of 60 Gy followed by a boost dose of more radiation to the large tumor mass. This can lead to good control of the local breast region, but side effects occur in about 20 percent of the patients. Combination chemotherapy may produce responses in over 70 percent of patients. After a good response to chemotherapy has been obtained, a limited surgical procedure may be done followed by radiation therapy. Good local control is achieved in many patients, but survival is unaffected.

Patients who have bleeding and fungating masses through the skin may be treated with large doses of radiation over a course of only two or three or four days. The radiation will stop the bleeding and start killing the cancer cells quickly so that the mass is no longer weeping, and the foul smell will subside.

Patients who have inflammatory breast cancer should have systemic therapy and radiation therapy as discussed on page 264.

SIMULTANEOUS BREAST CANCERS IN EACH BREAST

The same thought processes must be applied to patients with cancer in each breast and those with single-breast cancer. If there is no evidence of disease elsewhere in the body (normal bone scan, chest X-ray, and liver function tests) and the patient is deemed to have early stage breast cancers in each breast, each breast is then independently treated. For instance, if a woman is a candidate for lumpectomy, axillary node dissection followed by radiation therapy, then the same procedure can be applied to both breasts at the same time. Or if she elects to have mastectomies, they can be done simultaneously as well. In one particular patient, mastectomy may be required on one side and yet a breast-conserving procedure may be an option for the opposite side. But each breast should be considered independently with appropriate options given.

AUTOLOGOUS BONE MARROW TRANSPLANTATION

In the past, patients with acute leukemia, testicular carcinoma, advanced Hodgkin's disease, or aggressive lymphoma usually died of their disease until the proper combination of chemotherapeutic agents, doses, and schedules was empirically found. This thinking became the rationale for the use of more intensive chemotherapeutic regimens in breast cancer patients—to find that magic dose or scheduling of agents that will lead to better survival results.

The major side effect of most chemotherapeutic agents is their destruction of white and red blood cells and their precursors, all of which are formed and manufactured in the bone marrow. If one receives very high doses of chemotherapeutic agents, high enough to get rid of "all possible tumor cells," the majority of cells in the bone marrow will be destroyed; therefore, bone marrow cells will have to be replaced. In an autologous bone marrow transplant, bone marrow cells are given back to the patient after intensive chemotherapy. Prior to this intensive chemotherapy, the patient donated and had stored her own marrow cells. The technology of autologous bone marrow transplantation has been mastered. In many cases, bone marrow transplantation is merely a technique that allows the administration of a higher dose of chemotherapy. Drug dosages are typically escalated until toxicity occurs and with it congestive heart failure, thrombophlebitis, pulmonary fibrosis, interstitial pneumonitis, renal dysfunction, and/or hepatitis. High doses of chemotherapy produce higher response rates in patients with metastatic breast cancer than conventional doses.[60-68] The complete response rate (the percentage of people who had all their disease disappear with treatment) ranges from 0–55 percent. The partial response rate (the percentage of people who had 50 percent or more of their disease disappear with treatment) ranges from 6–60 percent. The median survival ranges from eight to twenty-three months. The toxicity is relatively high. In fact, treatment-related deaths ranged from 0–23 percent of the people involved in these studies. All these studies were conducted and reported in the early 90s so the technology was relatively sophisticated.

Several of these studies demonstrated that patients did better if they had not had chemotherapy prior to the high-dose chemotherapy needed before marrow transplantation. Drug resistance limits the success of high-dose therapy. But, curiously, autologous bone marrow transplantation is unlikely to give a patient long-term benefit if the initial tumors did not respond to conventional doses of chemotherapy.[69]

Even though the technology for performing bone marrow transplantation has improved and the selection of patients has improved, the median survival after transplant is only eighteen to twenty-three months. So it was thought that intensive treatment should begin early in the course of metastatic disease to possibly improve results. In one study, high-dose chemotherapy was followed by autologous bone marrow transplantation, yielding almost the same complete response of around 50 percent, but the median survival dropped down to nine months.

Adjuvant Autologous Bone Marrow Transplant

Having gained experience with performing transplantation on women with metastatic disease, oncologists turned their attention to women with stage II disease at high risk of recurrence. As you remember, women who have stage II disease had cancer in breast and axillary nodes. With standard adjuvant systemic chemotherapy, the recurrence rate at five years ranges between 55–90 percent in patients with ten or more positive axillary nodes. However, when high-dose chemotherapy and autologous bone marrow transplantation were used in women with stage II disease (ten or more positive lymph nodes), the disease-free survival rate was 72 percent at two and one-half years in one study,[70] and 93 percent at twenty-one months in another.[71] Some investigators believe that these numbers look very good. But compare them to the numbers for conventional standard doses of adjuvant combination chemotherapy, which give similar or better results. In any event, two high-priority randomized national trials have begun to evaluate high-dose therapy as an adjuvant. It is not known when these studies will finish.

One of the stumbling blocks in bone marrow transplantation is getting rid of possible malignant cancer cells in the marrow harvested from the patient who has breast cancer. If there are even a few cancer cells in the harvest, they will be injected back into the patient after she has been "cleaned" with high-dose chemotherapy. And although this technique has improved, it still has a way to go.

The use of growth factors have undoubtedly been beneficial for bone marrow transplantation because they do reduce morbidity and mortality. Growth factors promote the growth of white and red blood cells, thereby reducing the incidence of infection and mouth ulcerations.

Cost of Autologous Bone Marrow Transplantation

A breast cancer patient who has complications with an autologous bone marrow transplantation can incur a total cost of $175,000–$200,000. Without complications, the cost can range between $65,000–$140,000. Costs can be further reduced with more outpatient follow-up as opposed to hospitalizations. Patients should, therefore, receive transplants only if they are participating in a clinical trial designed to aid our understanding of newer techniques. Some consider this still experimental, others do not. Numerous law suits have been levied by breast cancer patients against their health insurance carriers in attempts to receive autologous bone marrow transplants. One case was settled in 1993 for close to $80 million.

Look at the numbers for yourself and decide if the survival is better with autologous bone marrow transplantation versus so-called "conventional" treatment. The early data reviewed above show that bone marrow transplantation may not be as effective as "conventional" treatment. The answer is simply not in yet, and it may not be in until the year 2000 or 2005. Until then, the anxieties and emotional outcries from patients who have been told by the media, organizations, and physicians that their only hope is bone marrow transplantation will continue. This subject is well reviewed in a recent study.[72]

PERIPHERAL BLOOD STEM CELL TRANSPLANTATION

Breast cancer was one of the first cancers to be treated with peripheral blood stem cell transplantation. Peripheral blood stem cells are cells that circulate in the bloodstream and have the ability to restore normal bone marrow and blood cell production. These stem cells are rare in the bloodstream and are relatively difficult to separate from the rest of the blood cells. Once they are separated, there is only one way to know if they are of good quality—put them back into the same person ("transplantation") and await the response.

Who is a candidate for peripheral blood stem cell transplantation?

- Patients who have breast cancer that has already spread to the bone marrow.
- Patients who have already had radiation therapy to their pelvic bones.
- Patients who are medically unable to undergo general anesthesia.

Peripheral blood stem cell transplantation was studied and employed because results with autologous bone marrow transplantation were modest at best: (1) two-year disease-free survival was only 10 percent to 20 percent; (2) transplant related mortality ranged from 3 percent to 23 percent; (3) there were only a few five-year survivors; (4) short-term costs are high; and finally, (5) long-term costs and toxicities are unknown.

The results of peripheral blood stem cell transplantation[73,74] compared to autologous bone marrow transplantation are: (1) No significant difference in response rates and long-term disease free survival; (2) Decreased toxicity and cost.

Hence, a lot more work and investigation must be done before either of these transplantation techniques are used routinely, if at all.

IMMUNOLOGICAL METHODS

At present there seems to be no convincing evidence that immunological treatments or biological response modifiers have a significant role to play in the treatment of breast cancer.

TREATMENT OF OLDER BREAST CANCER PATIENTS

Does age have anything to do with survival in breast cancer patients? A number of reports have shown that premenopausal women have a less favorable prognosis than postmenopausal women.[75,76] Another study shows that the oldest women, those older than 75, fared less favorably than any other age group.[77]

Should older (>65) breast cancer patients be treated any differently than younger breast cancer patients? The incidence of breast cancer has increased by almost 10 percent in women above age 50. And almost half of all breast cancers occur in women over the age of 65. Generally, breast cancers in older patients tend to be less aggressive biologically. Older patients generally have more favorable low-risk prognostic factors including positive estrogen-progesterone receptors in about 60–70 percent of the patients, lower S-phase fraction, and more diploid than aneuploid conditions.

Most clinically detected breast masses in older women tend to be malignant. And, in most cases, breast-conserving surgery as well as radiation therapy is an option for older patients with breast cancer. At present, once treatment is initiated, there is no convincing evidence that close follow-up improves survival.

Older patients with early stage breast cancer can be treated with tamoxifen instead of lumpectomy or mastectomy, and this therapy reduces the tumor in 50–75 percent of the patients. There is no difference in overall survival benefit between a group treated with tamoxifen and one treated with lumpectomy or mastectomy.[78]

However, over half the patients treated with tamoxifen alone had disease progression after four or five years. At that time, radiation therapy or surgery can be used if disease is present in the breast alone and has not spread to other distant organs. Using tamoxifen as an initial therapy may be the best option for patients who have poor health or abundant local-regional disease confined to the breast, axilla, and supraclavicular region, or metastatic disease at time of initial diagnosis.

When it was deemed necessary to use adjuvant systemic therapy in postmenopausal patients, tamoxifen significantly decreased the recurrence rate and prolonged survival slightly, especially in patients aged 70 or more.[79] Estrogen receptor status was important in determining the benefit derived from tamoxifen. All this information has been reviewed and noted in the investigation involving 133 randomized trials (see page 265).

In a trial that specifically looked at women aged 65–84 with positive axillary nodes, tamoxifen improved disease-free survival but not end-point life span survival.

If chemotherapy is to be used, the patient's kidney, liver, and cardiac function must be assessed. The use of low-dose chemotherapy is probably of little or no benefit; therefore, if chemotherapy is to be used at all, full doses should be administered whenever possible. Patients older than 65 experience the same toxicities to chemotherapy as patients aged 50–69. Probably the only indication for using chemotherapy in older patients is when the tumor is progressing extremely rapidly and/or there is liver metastases. Generally, tamoxifen or another hormonal manipulation should be used as initial therapy.

Once breast cancer has become metastatic, it is deemed incurable and all treatment is therefore palliative (soothing). In this setting, unless there is life-threatening disease, women should receive a hormonal therapy regardless of the estrogen or progesterone receptor status. Hormonal manipulation produces good responses in patients with soft tissue or bony metastases, and liver and pulmonary metastases may also respond. About 15–20 percent of breast cancer patients have negative estrogen receptor cancers but can still have a complete or partial response to hormonal manipulation.

When combination chemotherapy CMF was compared to tamoxifen or when cyclophosphamide + adriamycin was compared to tamoxifen, survival was identical in all treatment groups. Disease-free survival also was similar, but response rates were slightly different.

Generally, a response to a hormonal manipulation lasts an average of a year, at which time another hormonal manipulation may be administered. A person who responds to one initial hormonal manipulation is likely to respond to a second or third.

Summary Recommendations for Older Breast Cancer Patients

1. Early staged breast cancer patients can be treated with breast-conserving surgery and radiation therapy or mastectomy depending upon the indications as already defined.
2. All older breast cancer patients should receive tamoxifen as adjuvant systemic therapy or for treating metastatic disease.
3. Since survival and disease-free survival are the same with combination chemotherapy or tamoxifen, there is little or no indication for using combination chemotherapy in older patients[78] especially those who have compromised liver, kidney, or cardiac status.

MENOPAUSAL SYMPTOMS AND ESTROGEN USE IN BREAST CANCER PATIENTS

Almost half of all breast cancer patients are menopausal, and the premenopausal patients who receive some adjuvant systemic therapy generally are rendered menopausal secondary to the therapy. Hence, all these patients undergo hot flashes, accelerated bone loss, and osteoporosis, and will be susceptible to the risk of cardiovascular disease—all of which were prevented by estrogen.

In an earlier section in this chapter (see page 260), we learned that high doses of estrogen were used in the 1950s to actually treat breast cancer. But, theoretically, low-dose estrogens may actually stimulate breast cancer cells in the body.

To my knowledge, although there are no prospective randomized trials to address the risk of estrogen replacement in breast cancer patients, one report does describe seventy-seven breast cancer patients who desired estrogen replacement after breast cancer therapy.[79] This report shows minimal risk to these patients. However, this study was not randomized, and the only criteria for selection of patients was that they desired to have the estrogen replacement; therefore, it does not ensure absolute safety for estrogen replacement.

TREATMENT OF METASTATIC DISEASE

Breast cancer may metastasize to various organs including liver, bone, brain, the eye, soft tissues like the skin, and many other sites. Treatment is directed to the symptoms that are produced by these metastatic lesions. For instance, if the patient can identify one area of bone pain, radiation therapy is most appropriate for treating this problem. And radiation can be given over a course of one to three weeks or even four weeks depending on the site, the total dose desired to be delivered, and the complications that may ensue.

When breast cancer metastasizes to the brain and produces symptoms, radiation is generally given to the whole brain over a course of two weeks, five days a week. And if liver metastases cause pain that is not well controlled by properly administered analgesics, radiation therapy can be directed to the liver over a course of one, two, or three days in small doses. Blood counts must be closely monitored before each successive delivery of radiation. About 5–10 percent of the patients with breast cancer can have a metastatic lesion to the eye. Eye metastasis is generally a late manifestation of metastatic breast cancer, and radiation therapy is the preferred treatment.

Hormonal manipulation may be administered for any site that has metastatic disease. It works less well if liver or brain is involved with metastases.

Combination chemotherapy can be considered for patients who have liver metastases or disease that is unresponsive to hormonal manipulations. Realize that survival is unchanged in all cases.

FOLLOW-UP FOR BREAST CANCER PATIENTS

The conventional wisdom for breast cancer patients' follow-up is:

Physical examination by a physician:

- First two years, every three months; if a cancer is going to recur, it generally does so within the first two years.
- Years two to four, every four months.
- Years five to six, every six months.
- Seven years and after, annually.

Laboratory tests:

- Mammogram, chest X-ray, and liver function tests are done annually on the anniversary of the diagnosis.
- Bone scans should rarely be done. Studies demonstrate that unless a patient has a specific and persistent pain in one region of the skeletal system, the bone scan is rarely positive in routine follow-up.

Let us now look at the real value of the above follow-up procedures. About 70 percent of all recurrences are detected by patients themselves.[83] About 15 percent of abnormalities are detected by physicians in otherwise asymptomatic patients during routine follow-up visits. Hence, routine physical exams and symptoms from the patient lead to detection of recurrences in 85 percent of all cases.

With regard to bone scan use, only 0.06 percent of all the bone scans done in close to 8,000 patients detected bone metastases in asymptomatic patients in the National Surgical Adjuvant Breast Project. And all other studies done, totaling about nine, have demonstrated that patients who are symptomatic with bone pain will have a positive bone scan, otherwise the bone scans are invariably negative.

With regard to annual routine chest X-rays, two good studies were done. Less than 2 percent of all asymptomatic breast cancer patients have an abnormality on a routine annual chest X-ray.

And with regard to blood chemistry studies for liver testing, less than 2 percent of asymptomatic patients on routine follow-up were found to have abnormal liver chemistries. Another enzyme called alkaline phosphatase, which had been thought helpful in detecting bony metastases, was likewise useless in asymptomatic patients.

What are the costs involved in surveillance? "Routine" follow-up as has been done includes a physical examination ($60–$70), complete blood count ($40), blood chemistry studies ($80), annual mammography ($50–$100), chest X-ray ($100), and bone scan ($500). Sufficient follow-up testing need include only the review of the patient's history, examination by a physician, and an annual mammogram in certain age groups. Now in stage I and II patients, about one-third will receive six months of adjuvant systemic chemotherapy. The cost for five years of "routine" follow-up for asymptomatic patients is about $5,735 in 1990 dollars. About 18 percent of that amount or $1,025 is for physical examinations and mammography. Thus, the savings per patient is $4,710 if a minimal but sufficient amount of follow-up is done. This minimal follow-up results in the same survival rates and the same detection rates of recurrent disease.

About 90 percent of all breast cancer patients are stage I or stage II at initial detection and will need follow-up for a minimum of five years. If the minimal but sufficient follow-up is done on 171,000 patients (90 percent times 190,000 new breast cancer patients in 1994), the savings at $4,710 per person is over $800 million a year.

Once patients with breast cancer develop metastases, they are incurable.[84–87] Complete remissions are rarely seen whether the tumor burden at the time of recurrence is large or small.[85] And, curiously, the interval of time between initial management of the early breast cancer and the diagnosis of metastases is just about the same whether the patient is undergoing follow-up or not.[88,89] Therefore, follow-up after surgery and primary treatment does not lead to earlier detection of metastases nor does it affect the overall survival.[90,91]

Remember that recurrences are detected 86 percent of the time by the patient or by the physician during physical examination.

A belief system again, and not hard facts, has dictated our follow-up times and studies. We constantly hear from the media and various organizations that early detection is best. The driving force behind intensive follow-ups may be the threat of malpractice suits. A malpractice case is composed of two issues: deviation from the standard of care and "proximate cause." Based on the hard scientific data outlined above, it should be agreed by physicians that a minimal surveillance per follow-up is reasonable, cost effective, and, importantly, does not jeopardize survival at all. This should be the standard of care. Proximate cause, the second part of a malpractice case, also would not be applicable because a patient is essentially incurable once a recurrence is detected. Remember, also, routine surveillance does not affect the interval of time until the discovery of metastases. Proximate cause simply asks the question: Does a potential delay in a diagnosis of metastases make any difference in the ultimate outcome or survival?

Because of the scientific data presented, I advocate a minimal amount of follow-up testing: a good physical examination and surveillance by the patient and physician with an annual mammogram.

TOXICITY OF SYSTEMIC THERAPY

In this section, we will review only the chemotherapeutic drugs used most frequently in the treatment of breast cancer, even though there are many more as was initially stated in this chapter. Table 22.4 lists chemotherapeutic drugs and their toxicities.

Individual Chemotherapeutic Agents

Cyclophosphamide

Cyclophosphamide is given either intravenously or orally. Acute toxic signs include nausea and vomiting. Moderate doses will depress peripheral blood counts, and excessive doses lead to bone marrow depression. It may take two to three weeks for maximal toxicity to be seen after the last dose. Hair loss and bleeding from the urinary bladder can occur. It is very important to drink eight to ten large glasses of water a day to prevent bladder bleeding and decrease the risk of bladder cancer. If cyclophosphamide lies in the bladder for long periods of time, chemical breakdown produces a substance that can cause bladder cancer.

Table 22.4 Chemotherapy Toxicities

Drug	Organ Likely to Have a Toxic Reaction							
	Eye	Lung	Heart	Liver	Bone Marrow	Nerves	Brain	Skin (With Radiation)
Cyclophos-phamide	Yes	Yes	Yes*	Yes	Yes			
Methotrexate	Yes	Yes			Yes			Yes
5-FU	Yes		Yes**	Yes	Yes		Yes	
Adriamycin	Yes	Yes	Yes***		Yes			Yes
Taxol		Yes			Yes	Yes		

*Only with very high doses not commonly used in breast cancer care.
**With high-dose continuous infusion, generally not used in breast cancer care.
***Dose related.

Methotrexate

Methotrexate can be given orally, intravenously, or intramuscularly. Ulcerations occur in the mouth and the rest of the gastrointestinal tract. Bone marrow depression occurs, and all toxicities are worsened with poor kidney function. Do not drink alcohol, which can further compromise the liver. Avoid sunlight because methotrexate can sensitize your skin to sunlight. Aspirin should not be taken unless you check with your doctor first.

5-Fluorouracil

5-Fluorouracil (5-FU) is generally given intravenously and produces oral (mouth) ulceration, bone marrow depression, hair loss, and gastrointestinal injury.

Doxorubicin (Adriamycin)

Adriamycin is given intravenously and causes mouth ulcerations as well as gastrointestinal injury, hair loss, and bone marrow depression. At cumulative doses over 500 mg per meter square of patient body surface area, cardiac dysfunction is produced. This medicine is red in color and oftentimes turns the urine reddish in color so don't be alarmed by that. If some of the medicine leaks from the vein into the surrounding tissues, it may cause damage to the tissues and your physician should be notified. The patient experiencing leaking will have immediate pain and burning.

Tamoxifen

Tamoxifen is usually given orally, and some people experience nausea, vomiting, hot flashes, blurred vision, confusion, leg swelling, and weight gain. Intense bone pain may occur in the first two weeks if a patient has bony metastases from her breast cancer. A small number of patients (1 to 2 in 1,000) who use tamoxifen run the risk of developing endometrial cancer,[92,93] liver dysfunction, and ocular problems.

The longer you are on tamoxifen, the higher the risks. Some investigators think no routine surveillance is needed and check symptoms (e.g., vaginal bleeding) only when they arise.[94] Others think that routine transvaginal ultrasound of the uterus is indicated,[95] with uterine biopsy if endometrial thickening exceeds 8 mm.[96,97] There is no consensus.

Taxol

Taxol is administered intravenously, generally in a twenty-four-hour infusion, together with steroids and antihistamines to suppress any allergic reaction that may be triggered by the base in which taxol is delivered.[98] Taxol can suppress white blood cell count, cause hair loss, oral ulcerations, some vomiting, and diarrhea. Peripheral neurotoxicity such as numbness and burning in the hands and feet may occur. Cardiac abnormalities, which include slowing of the rhythm in about 30 percent of the patients, other electrical cardiac problems, and also fatal heart attack, and atypical chest pains have been reported. Early results of studies with taxol do indicate a minimal response in breast cancer patients.

Long-Term Toxicities

In addition to the long-term toxicity reported to lung, heart, liver, brain, and bone marrow, 5 of 10,000 women treated with combination chemotherapy for breast cancer have a real risk of developing a particular leukemia. This particular leukemia does not respond to any other future treatment.[99,100] The risk of developing this leukemia in the breast cancer group of almost 83,000 women after having radiation therapy alone was 2.4, the risk of developing a leukemia after receiving chemotherapeutic agents alone was 10.0, and when radiation was combined with chemotherapy, the risk was 17.4 times higher than in people who received no treatment at all. In other studies with combined chemotherapy and radiation therapy, radiation did not contribute to an increased risk; only combination chemotherapy of CMF or cyclophosphamide alone increased the risk of new cancers by a factor of 1.1 to 1.7.[101,102] In another study involving only 1,100 patients, there seemed to be no difference in relative risk of chemotherapy versus primary radiation therapy.[103] For additional information, you may refer to "Chemotherapy and You," NIH Publication No. 91-1136 (call 301-496-4000).

DECISION-MAKING: BREAST MASS TO TREATMENT

The following flow diagram, Figure 22.1, outlines decision-making for a person who finds a breast mass and needs to go through all the steps necessary for detection, diagnosis, and ultimately treatment of breast cancer.

BREAST CANCER TREATMENT BY STAGE

Ductal carcinoma *in situ*. Ductal carcinoma *in situ* can be handled in one of two ways. If microcalcifications are seen on a mammogram that led to a biopsy, this patient with a small amount of disease can be followed with no further therapy. If, on the other hand, there is a large amount of gross disease per the pathologist's review, then lumpectomy, axillary lymph node dissection, or radiation therapy is an option.

Lobular carcinoma *in situ*. Whereas ductal carcinoma *in situ* is an early stage of a malignant process, lobular carcinoma *in situ* is considered a pre-malignant process. You have a higher risk of developing an invasive cancer in one or both breasts. An excisional biopsy alone is probably adequate with no further therapy; however, close follow-up examinations must be provided for this patient. Some surgeons, however, may perform a modified radical mastectomy and some may remove both breasts, since there is a high risk in both breasts. There is no evidence that prophylactic mastectomies (see page 254) are beneficial.

Stage I Breast Cancer is defined as:
- Cancer less than 2 cm with negative lymph nodes.
  1. Breast local-regional treatment is mandatory. Choice of:
        either
     Surgical removal of the breast *mass* and lymph node dissection followed by radiation therapy,
        or
     Modified radical mastectomy.
        and
  2. Adjuvant systemic treatment.
     If you are in the high-risk category of prognostic factors—high S-phase, aneuploid, grade 3, high Cathepsin D level, negative estrogen receptor—you may be considered for adjuvant systemic therapy: either hormonal manipulation (ovarian castration) or

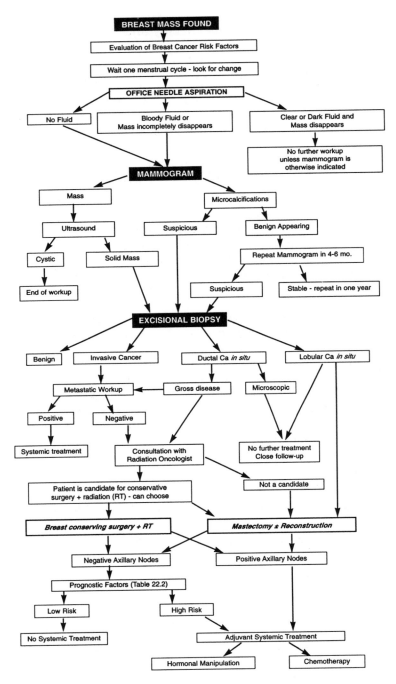

Figure 22.1 Decision Making: Breast Mass to Treatment

combination chemotherapy. If systemic adjuvant therapy is to be used, hormonal manipulation is best for patients who are estrogen receptor positive. Disease-free interval and overall survival seem to be similar whether hormonal therapy or chemotherapy has been used.

There is no need for systemic treatment if the tumor size is less than 1 cm in diameter and you have other low-risk prognostic factors per Table 22.2.

Stage II Breast Cancer is defined as:
- Breast cancer is 2 cm or less with positive lymph nodes.
- Cancer diameter is between 2 and 5 cm and the lymph nodes may be positive or negative, or
- Cancer is larger than 5 cm but lymph nodes are negative.

 1. Breast local-regional treatment is mandatory. Choice of:
      either
    Breast-conserving surgery with radiation therapy
        or
    Modified radical mastectomy.
        and
 2. Adjuvant Systemic Treatment:
    If you have Stage II with positive lymph nodes
    Postmenopausal women—should receive tamoxifen for at least two years and probably five. Disease-free survival is improved and a slight increase in survival is obtained.

    Premenopausal patients—hormonal manipulation (ovarian ablation) and chemotherapy produce identical results.

    If you have Stage II with negative lymph nodes
    Postmenopausal women may benefit from tamoxifen if they are estrogen receptor positive or estrogen receptor negative. Tamoxifen has been shown to decrease the rate of cardiovascular disease and decrease the risk of a new cancer's forming in the opposite breast. Adjuvant systemic treatment may be indicated for estrogen receptor negative patients if there are multiple high-risk prognostic factors (see Table 22.2).

Stage III Breast Cancer is divided into two groups.
  Stage IIIA is defined as:
- Cancer smaller than 5 cm with positive axillary nodes that have grown onto each other or onto other structures, or
- Cancer is larger than 5 cm with positive axillary lymph nodes.

 1. Breast local-regional treatment for Stage IIIA is mandatory.

Choice of:
> *either*

Modified radical or radical mastectomy,
> *or*

Radiation therapy either pre-operatively to shrink the mass down, or post-operatively delivered to the chest wall.
> *and*

2. Adjuvant Systemic Treatment is mandatory. Choice of:
> *either*

Hormonal manipulation
> *or*

Combination chemotherapy.

Stage IIIB, which is initially inoperable, is defined as:
- The cancer has spread from the breast to nearby tissues including chest wall, or,
- The cancer has spread to lymph nodes near the collar bone (supraclavicular nodes), or,
- Inflammatory breast carcinoma.

1. Systemic chemotherapy with radiation therapy is important to control local and regional disease as well as metastatic disease. Surgery may be used after radiation therapy and chemotherapy if it is judged to be helpful. If combination chemotherapy is contraindicated, systemic hormonal therapy may be used in patients who have positive estrogen receptors. Those therapies may include ovarian ablation in premenopausal patients, tamoxifen use for postmenopausal patients, or other hormonal agents as previously described.

Stage IV Breast Cancer is defined as:
- The breast cancer has already spread from the breast to other organs of the body especially bones, lungs, liver, or brain, or other sites. A biopsy must be done to determine that it is breast cancer and to obtain estrogen receptor status.

1. Because the cancer has spread from the breast to other organ(s), the objective is to use systemic treatment. There is no need to treat the local-regional area of the breast unless an ulcerating mass is causing problems.
2. If estrogen receptor and progesterone receptor are positive, hormonal therapy should be instituted first. This can include tamoxifen or ovarian ablation for premenopausal patients, tamoxifen for postmenopausal patients, and other hormonal agents that we have already described.

3. If, however, there is rapidly progressive disease or disease involving the liver and estrogen receptor status is negative, combination chemotherapy may be instituted as well as tamoxifen.
4. Radiation can be used to palliate symptoms of localized origin like pain in the bone.

Table 22.5 presents the percent of survival for breast cancer patients based on stage, tumor size, and axillary nodal status. As you can see, as the tumor size increases with positive lymph nodes, survival decreases.

FACTORS THAT IMPROVE SURVIVAL

Immune system parameters and lifestyle factors have never been adequately evaluated for overall survival benefit in any breast cancer study using hormonal therapy or chemotherapy. A patient's defense factors may be as important as other breast cancer prognostic factors (Table 22.2) and can actually be independent of them, which would separate a person from the normal statistics presented.[104] There have only been a few studies that demonstrate the importance of the patient's immune system and its competence in relation to survival in the first several years *after* chemotherapy for Stage I and II breast cancer patients.[105,106]

Rabbits that accidentally get cut in their cages while producing antibodies for experiments, produce higher levels of antibodies with

Table 22.5 Percent Survival for Breast Cancer Patients Based on Stage, Tumor Size, and Axillary Lymph Node Status

Stage	Tumor Size (cm)	Lymph Nodes	Percent Survival		
			5 Year	10 Year	20 Year
Non-invasive Stage I	0	Negative		95	
	<1 & special cell types (Table 22.2)	Negative			95
	<1	Negative		90	86
Stage II	1–2	Negative		80	70
	<2	Positive		70	
	2–5	Negative		65	
	2–5	Positive		50	
	>5	Negative		40	
Stage IIIA	<5	Pos. & Fixed	13		
	>5	Positive		35	
Stage IIIB	Cancer fixed to chest wall	Positive	5		

stronger affinity to their targets. Likewise, patients with breast or ovarian cancer have had unexpected longer survival if they have had a previous infection with tuberculosis and a positive tuberculin test.[107] In a few controlled studies, repeated injections of Bacilli Calmette-guerin (BCG) were given to breast cancer patients during but not after chemotherapy for stage II or advanced diseases to see if their survival could be increased.[108] Chemotherapy, however, is immunosuppressive and no benefit was demonstrated for patients who received BCG during this period of time. However, no studies have used BCG months or years after chemotherapy when the immune system would not be under the suppressive effects of chemotherapy drugs. This is only one example of factors that have not been studied in patients.

We know from the Japanese data that older women with breast cancer in Japan live longer than American women because 1) they are less obese and 2) they eat a low-fat, high-fiber diet with nutrients and other lifestyle factors that are healthy. Healthy lifestyle factors are presented in the Ten-Point Plan on page 317.[109]

Are survival and quality of life the same for patients receiving "unproven" or "conventional" cancer therapy? The Select Subcommittee on Quackery estimated that more than $10 billion are spent annually on unproven methods of treating cancer.[110] Large numbers of patients are using "unproven" treatments for their cancer, those that have not been sent through the rigors of randomized controlled trials. Among the many reasons people seek unproven treatments are their disillusionment with results of "conventional" treatment, and the low or nonexistent toxicity with "unproven" treatments. Better educated patients generally seek unproven therapies because they have become increasingly dissatisfied with conventional care due to toxicity, the lack of real benefit in cancer survival rates, and poor quality of life as well.

A recent study compared the length of overall survival and quality of life in patients who received both "conventional" and "unorthodox" treatment at an "unorthodox" cancer clinic in California, with matched control patients from a traditional academic cancer center in Philadelphia, Pennsylvania, who received only "conventional" treatment. The investigators were from the traditional cancer center in Philadelphia. All patients had documented histologically proven cancers with a predictable survival of less than one year. The investigators "hypothesized that survival time would not differ between the two groups, on the basis of the assumption that the unproved remedy would be no more effective in patients with end-stage disease than conventional care, itself largely ineffective. A second hypothesis was that the quality of life of the patients receiving unproved therapy would be superior to that of the patients receiving conventional care."[111]

There was no difference between the two patient groups in overall length of survival, about fifteen months. It was reported that quality of life scores were somewhat better among the conventionally treated patients.

Many of the agencies and/or "benevolent" charities in the United States have developed a "hit list" of unproven therapies and their proponents. More often than not, these therapies and their proponents are put on the hit list without the agency or charity having the therapy investigated—the therapy is guilty of quackery until proven otherwise. I am convinced that *all* therapies, unproven or otherwise, should be put through the same rigors of science to the degree that they can, and then people should evaluate the findings.

Rather than classify treatment as "conventional," or "unproven," or "alternative," treatments should have only two broad classifications: *effective* or *noneffective* therapy. The one basic question that should be asked in every study is whether that treatment is effective or not in terms of the patient's survival and quality of life. To use one simple example, breast-conserving surgery with radiation therapy is as effective as a modified radical mastectomy with respect to overall survival, and these procedures are more effective than the severe and more mutilating surgeries done for over one hundred years. The same question of whether systemic therapies are effective or not must be applied to hormonal therapy and chemotherapy. We have learned that chemotherapy does not increase survival but does produce a poor quality of life. Hormonal therapy likewise does not appreciably increase survival, as shown in Figure 22.2, but does produce a better quality of life compared to chemotherapy.

This is the question that must be asked when doing a study: Is the treatment effective, does it work? And at the same time, does the treatment do little or no harm? We needn't ask whether a treatment is unproven or conventional because we have already learned that conventional surgical methods done for hundreds of years are not effective.

This does not mean that unproven treatments are better. If there were a cure for cancer somewhere, in someone's hideaway clinic, it would not remain secret or unproven, and all the fuss about the correct cancer treatment would be over. A cure for cancer could never be kept a secret.

Patients considering unproven treatments must always ask, "What are the risks and what are the benefits?" If the risks are minimal and

Figure 22.2   Survival (Lifespan) for Breast Cancer Patients

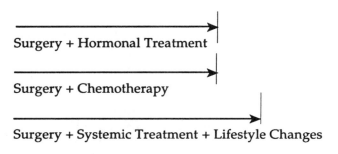

Surgery + Hormonal Treatment

Surgery + Chemotherapy

Surgery + Systemic Treatment + Lifestyle Changes

the benefit is great, then there is no question that the treatment should be entertained. However, if the risks are great and the benefit is minimal, you should reject that treatment.

CONCLUSION

Systemic hormonal therapy disrupts growth factor loops and combination chemotherapy kills dividing cells. The average duration of response, disease-free interval, and survival are approximately the same for both systemic therapies. **Conventional combination chemotherapy is no more curative for patients with advanced breast cancer than is hormonal therapy.** Generally, combination chemotherapy will produce its successes in the first few weeks or months (an average of six to nine months). Some patients do respond to subsequent different chemotherapy, but almost all patients die of their disease. Patients who had a response with CAF (cancers shrunk), had the same life span whether they continued receiving the same chemotherapeutic agents or were simply followed with no further treatment until their disease progressed and was detected. This group of patients, however, did have a greater disease-free interval if they received continuous chemotherapy, but the overall life span, survival, did not increase at all.[112]

Other reviews also state, "Currently available drugs, while active against breast cancer, have had modest clinical impact."[113] The *Lancet* editorial staff wrote on February 6, 1993, "Breast cancer: have we lost our way?"[114] In this editorial, it was stated, ". . . we acknowledge the failures of primary therapy and secondary prevention" and a convention was called for to review new issues that would help breast cancer patients and acknowledge the failure of existing treatment. The *Lancet* staff concluded: "This house believes that chemotherapy in the management of breast cancer has a dim future."[115]

With traditional treatment of breast cancer patients, survival figures have changed little since 1930. However, I am convinced, based on the Japanese and other data already reviewed, that women who follow an optimal lifestyle coupled to effective treatment using non-immunosuppressing agents when possible, will fare better. They will be more competent immunologically, and their tumors will not be fed by lifestyle factors that we know perpetuate tumor growth. (An outline of a complete plan like this begins on page 319.)

23
Male Breast Cancer

Every year in the United States, about 1,400 men develop breast cancer. And every year in the United States, about 350 men die of the disease. Male breast cancer was first recorded in 3000 B.C., and in the past century—especially in recent years—information about large numbers of cases has been accumulated for review.[1]

There are many similarities between male breast cancer and breast cancer developed by postmenopausal women. The incidence of breast cancer in men increases dramatically at around age 85 and above with 11 men in every 100,000 developing breast cancer. It is extremely rare in men below the age of 30.

RISK FACTORS

As with female breast cancer, the incidence for male breast cancer is low in Japan and Finland and higher in North America and England. A high-fat, low-fiber diet and lack of vitamins and minerals are the nutritional factors associated with male breast cancer as well.

About one-third of the men who develop breast cancer have a family member who has breast cancer.[2] Many of the family members who have breast cancer are females; however, many cases have been reported where father and son or grandfather and grandson or other close male family members have had breast cancer. There is no information concerning the incidence of breast cancer among female descendants of men who have breast cancer. Some true genetic linkages are found for men who develop breast cancer. For instance, men who have Klinefelter's syndrome (men who have an extra X chromosome) are obese and develop gynecomastia. About 3 percent of this group develop breast cancer.

RADIATION

Women who had exposure to ionizing radiation from either chest X-rays or X-ray treatment before the age of 20 have a very high risk of developing breast cancer. The same is true for men. Men have had radiation for a variety of conditions including gynecomastia (increase in breast tissue), enlarged thymus, eczema of the chest, chest burns, tuberculosis, lymphomas, etc. Men below the age of 20 who had radiation have a very high rate of developing breast cancer thereafter.[3]

HORMONES

Exogenous estrogens administered in large amounts have been associated with breast cancer in male transsexuals,[4,5,6] as well as in male heart and ulcer patients.[4,6] The incidence of breast cancer in men is very high in certain areas of Africa where infection of the liver, cirrhosis, or chronic malnutrition exists. These conditions raise the level of estrogens in the blood because those hormones are no longer broken down by the liver. Male breast cancers account for 15 percent of all the cancers of the breast in Zambia, 6.4 percent in Egypt, and 4.6 percent in India but only 0.8 percent in the United States.[7]

Gynecomastia is an excess of breast tissue in men. High levels of estrogen are evident in men with gynecomastia. With the larger amount of breast tissue, there is a larger risk for developing breast cancer. Gynecomastia is associated with male breast cancer in up to 40 percent of all the cases. However, other studies show that men who had a history of injury to their testicles, inguinal hernias, history of gynecomastia, history of head trauma, use of drugs that increase a hormone called prolactin, previous radiation, family history of breast cancer, and the use of soaps or perfumes containing estrogen, all had a higher risk for developing breast cancer.[8,9]

The following risk factors are also important for developing male breast cancer: being a Jewish male (Jewish women also are at high risk for breast cancer); a history of mumps orchitis (testicular inflammation) or mumps as an adult; testicular injury, undescended testes, late marriage with no children; and obesity.[10]

DETECTION

When a mass is palpated and detected, it must be differentiated from benign gynecomastia. The physician must take a history of drug use, hormone use, excess alcohol consumption, and all the other risk factors already mentioned. When a physician examines the axilla, there is about a 75 percent correlation between what is palpable or not and what is truly evident as seen under the microscope. The mammogram is useful and with today's techniques can be done rather efficiently and effectively. There is usually a spiculated mass (one with many jagged edges) seen beneath the nipple region and microcalcifications are rather unusual. No routine screening in the male population is recommended, however.

If the mass is large and firm, a needle aspiration may be helpful for initial diagnosis. However, as with any other mass in the breast, it must be removed for pathological examination as well as estrogen and progesterone receptor status. In addition, the other prognostic factors like S-phase, ploidy status, DNA analysis, etc. must be assayed.

DIAGNOSIS

The average age for developing breast cancer in men is 60. It has occurred in men as young as 5 years old and as old as 93 years old. Since men and many physicians tend to ignore symptoms or masses in the breast, men with breast cancer often come to see a physician at a very late stage in the disease as compared to women. Generally, there is between eighteen to twenty-four months delay in seeing a physician from the onset of symptoms.

Because the majority of the breast tissue in men as compared to women is centrally located around the nipple, men with breast cancer often initially report a painless mass in the center of the breast region. It is usually only on one side. The second most common presentation is in the upper outer quadrant. If a mass is detected peripheral to the breast, the physician should think of possibilities other than primary breast cancer. A bloody nipple discharge, with or without nipple inversion, is commonly seen in about 80 percent of all male breast cancers. Paget's disease of the nipple is rare in men.

PATHOLOGY

The pathological types of both male and female breast cancers are almost identical. Infiltrating ductal carcinomas represent the majority of male breast cancers as they do in female breast cancers. Since there is no routine screening of male breasts with mammograms, an early diagnosis of a lesionlike ductal carcinoma *in situ* is rare but still found. Paget's disease of the nipple as well as inflammatory breast carcinoma has also been seen in men.

STAGING

The staging procedure is identical to that described on pages 243 through 244: the size of the lesion in the breast, axillary lymph node status, and the other laboratory and X-ray studies that define whether the disease has spread from the breast region into other parts of the body.

Because of the small size of the male breast, it is not uncommon for the breast cancer to be fixed to the chest wall. The breast cancer usually has a diameter of about 4 centimeters or so, and in over half of the cases of male breast cancer, the axillary nodes are positive. As the primary breast cancer increases in diameter, so does the rate of involvement of the axillary lymph nodes, as is the case for women. And as with women, prognosis and survival correlates well with the size of the primary breast cancer and the presence or absence of axillary lymph node metastases. The nuclear grade is equally important but there are not enough data to determine how important are the other prognostic factors like S-phase, ploidy status, DNA content, etc.

Breast cancer in men was always thought to be more deadly than compared to women of the same stage. However, we now realize the prognosis is similar to that for women for the exact same stage and other factors. Remember: men usually come to the doctor at more advanced stages than women; if a breast mass is palpated by a man, he generally ignores it; the physician generally does not routinely examine male breasts for breast masses, and older men generally have a higher mortality from other causes.

"CONVENTIONAL" LOCAL TREATMENT

Until recently, the standard approach for men with breast cancer has been a radical mastectomy. Recently, modified radical mastectomies have been performed more routinely and dominate surgical procedures for men with breast cancer. A radical mastectomy and a modified radical mastectomy produce the same survival rate.

Primary radiation therapy with breast-conserving surgery has also been used and is equal in terms of both survival and local tumor control compared to modified radical mastectomy.[11,12] Men also have a true choice between modified radical mastectomy and the more conserving procedure. Although it has been said that men don't need "to have their breasts conserved," more and more of them, in fact, are conscious of the appearance and desire the more conserving surgery. In fact, the overriding concern for the men I have treated has been to conserve their breasts so they chose the primary radiation therapy/breast-conserving surgical approach.

Radiation therapy directed to the chest wall and lymph node draining sites after a radical or modified radical mastectomy does not increase survival but can reduce the frequency of recurrent disease to that site.

"CONVENTIONAL" SYSTEMIC TREATMENT

Here again, treatment is similar to that for women. Since the total number of men with breast cancer is so small, there have been no randomized trials and every trial that has been done involved a small number of patients.

In 1987, the National Cancer Institute reported the first prospective trial involving adjuvant systemic chemotherapy for men with breast cancer. The same indications apply to men and to women concerning prognostic factors and positive axillary nodes for the use of systemic adjuvant therapy (see page 264).

Estrogen receptors are usually high for male breast cancer patients. These patients are in the same age group as postmenopausal women who also have higher estrogen receptors compared to women who are premenopausal. Hence, tamoxifen has also been used in the adjuvant systemic setting for men with breast cancer.

Management of recurrences or metastatic disease is handled in an identical manner as for women. Almost half of the patients who receive tamoxifen for treatment of metastatic disease have a complete or partial response. When diethylstilbestrol (DES) is used, a response rate of about 40 percent is obtained. And, curiously, earlier reports show that about 50 percent of the patients respond also to orchiectomy (removal of the testicles). If tamoxifen was used first and disease progressed, orchiectomy was effective thereafter.

About 80 percent of men with breast cancer have estrogen receptor positive tumors. In this group, orchiectomy, tamoxifen, or other hormonal maneuvers have produced tumor regressions in about 80–85 percent of the men.[13-15]

Psychological and cultural issues limit the routine performance of orchiectomy in these patients. Tamoxifen and DES are usually employed and progesterone and megestrol also can produce tumor regressions. And as we have seen in women using high doses of estrogen to treat female breast cancer, high doses of testosterone have been effective in causing tumor regression in as many as 60 percent

Table 23.1 Five-Year Survival by Stage for Male Breast Cancer

Stage	Range of Five-Year Survival
Stage I	75%–85%
Stage II	44%–75%
Stage III	16%–43%
Stage IV	0%– 8%

of cases.[16-18] And even cortisone has been beneficial in about 40 percent of the cases.

Antiandrogens like cyproterone acetate (CPA) and flutamide can block androgen receptors. And although these agents have been used, there has not been a lot of experience with male breast cancer.

The main objective in hormonal therapy is simply to alter the current hormonal milieu that is feeding the tumor. So if estrogens feed the tumor, take it away; if testosterone feeds the tumor, take it away. If a person, male or female, responds to one hormonal manipulation, that person can respond to a different one and a third one and perhaps even a fourth change in hormonal manipulation.

Combination chemotherapy or even single-agent chemotherapy is less effective than hormonal manipulation and is usually considered a secondary treatment in male breast cancer. All the usual agents or combinations we have discussed already can produce regressions. But they are less durable than a hormonal manipulation.

Because the number of patients in various studies is so small, there is a wide range of survival statistics for each stage. Table 23.1 demonstrates the range for five-year survival by stage for men with breast cancer.[19,20]

CONCLUSION

It seems that male breast cancer behaves similarly to female breast cancer including risk factors for developing the cancer; natural history; response rates to various treatment modalities such as surgery, radiation, and systemic therapies; as well as prognosis. Although lifestyle factors have not been discussed for men, we know from the Japanese experience for women that if these are modified, survival is much improved compared to survival with the existing American lifestyle and conventional treatment. It behoves all people with breast cancer, regardless of sex, to modify lifestyle factors in an attempt to improve their survival and quality of life as well as general well-being.

24

Quality of Life and Ethics

Since 1930, overall survival (life span) has not changed for patients with breast cancer. In the ensuing years, treatments have become increasingly toxic. Issues concerning quality of life and ethics have, therefore, become quite important.

QUALITY OF LIFE

Disease-free survival and overall survival should no longer be considered the only appropriate end points to evaluate a treatment for breast cancer. The patient's quality of life is also very important and should be evaluated for any treatment given to a breast cancer patient. Quality of life should measure physical symptoms, psychological well-being, social functioning, daily activity levels, cognitive abilities, sexual dysfunction, and overall general life satisfaction. Quality of life assessments have been used for many illnesses including cardiovascular disease, strokes, and now cancer.

Since 1990, the National Cancer Institute has recommended that clinical trials include quality of life assessments whenever possible and appropriate. The U.S. Food and Drug Administration recognizes the benefit to quality of life as a basis for approval of new anticancer drugs.[1] NCI's recommendation came about because attempts to increase survival required more toxic chemotherapeutic agents. This produced no gain in survival and deteriorated quality of life proportionately to the number of drugs and their side effects.

Quality of life assessments in clinical cancer trials are important. When two treatment arms yield similar disease-free survival and/or survival, the treatment that affords a better quality of life should be recommended. Conversely, if one treatment is very effective but diminishes the quality of life so much that its use is unacceptable, that treatment is not worth undertaking. And finally, if a treatment doesn't yield a significant medical advantage regarding disease-free survival and/or overall survival but does, in fact, ameliorate symptoms from the illness thereby improving the quality of life, that treatment regimen also should be chosen.

A number of studies have been done to determine effects of treatment on quality of life. In fifty consecutive breast cancer patients with early stage infiltrating ductal carcinoma who were treated with lumpectomy, axillary node dissection, and radiation therapy, and/or chemotherapy, I demonstrated substantial reductions of side effects from radiation therapy and/or chemotherapy if the patient followed the pertinent aspects of the Ten-Point Plan that included nutrients as has been already reviewed in Chapter 6. The overall quality of life was much improved for the majority of women. The qualities of life investigated in the study included physical symptoms (skin reaction, fatigue, mouth sores, nausea, vomiting, dizziness, vertigo, light headedness, muscle cramps), performance, general well-being, cognitive abilities, sexual dysfunction, and life satisfaction. The majority of patients in this study were convinced that their qualities of life were improved when they took the nutrients and followed the proper lifestyle during radiation therapy or concomitant radiation and chemotherapy.

In another study, six or seven months of adjuvant chemotherapy or chemoendocrine therapy improved the quality of life for patients with node positive breast cancer compared with a single short course of perioperative combination chemotherapy.[2] The investigators argued that this is so because the disease-free interval is better in those patients treated with six or seven courses of combination chemotherapy than in the patients treated with a single dose of perioperative chemotherapy.

An international study showed substantial differences in quality of life scores between national groups. English-speaking patients in Europe were best able to cope with their cancer. German and Swedish patients, however, coped moderately well with their cancers. And the Italians were least able to cope.[3] This pattern fits with the conception that Northern people in Europe are more reserved and complain less about symptoms than Southern Europeans. Another study reports no difference in survival or quality of life for patients treated with conventional or unproven therapies.[4]

Studies of quality of life for patients receiving bone marrow transplants have not had clear-cut results. Some patients have an excellent quality of life following bone marrow transplant, but others do not fare as well. Physical difficulties, sexual dysfunction, and mood disturbances are among many of the problems that patients face. Some patients go back to work in a matter of weeks whereas others are permanently disabled. Many of the studies, including routine medical studies, indicate that patients who undergo bone marrow transplantation do quite well, however, the "survivors" don't indicate that.[5]

Some of the physical and psychological problems that negatively affect quality of life for bone marrow transplants include:

- low-grade rejection of the transplant
- chronic fatigue
- sterility
- cataracts
- pulmonary problems
- relapse of disease treated by bone marrow
- development of secondary malignancies

A significant minority of survivors suffer psychological and social affects that include:

- cognitive dysfunction
- sexual dysfunction
- occupational disability
- discrimination
- financial and insurance problems
- problems of personal identity and meaning in life[6]

However, many patients do not have these social and psychological affects and seem to do well.

Sexuality and Body Image

Any illness brings about changes in feelings of well-being, in sexual functioning, and in overall function. Although rarely dealt with by the physician, sexual function is an integral part of an individual's well-being.[7,8] Sexuality is an important issue for older as well as younger cancer patients. Many patients with breast cancer desire sexual health information. One large study demonstrated that 60 percent of the individuals wanted more information on the impact of cancer on sexuality, and 55 percent wanted to discuss the topic of sexuality openly with their physicians. Unfortunately, this rarely occurs.

Psychosexual dysfunction in breast cancer patients ranges from 20 to 50 percent.[9-11] Many investigators reporting on sexuality in breast cancer have commented that the breast is a symbol of womanhood and sexuality, and mastectomies usually devastate a woman's feelings of attractiveness and sexual desire. Women whose self-esteem or body image is connected to their breast as a source of attractiveness may be at particular risk after mastectomy or other alterations of the breast. There is a high correlation between increasing sexual dysfunction and the degree of surgical intervention. But a woman's overall psychological health, satisfaction with the relationship to her partner, and current sexual life are important predictors of sexual satisfaction after a diagnosis of breast cancer—perhaps more important than is the extent of damage to her breast. It appears that women who have problems with sexuality and body image in a relationship, generally have these problems long before a diagnosis of cancer is made. And although the diagnosis of cancer heightens these anxieties, breast cancer per se has a minimal impact on the sexuality of a small number of patients.

Although most studies simply ask about satisfaction with sex and maybe frequency of intercourse, specific questions with regard to sexuality are rarely asked. One investigator, however, is convinced that the following questions should be made part of any breast cancer questionnaire to determine the woman's quality of life with regard to sexuality.[12]

- How often does the woman have sex with her partner?
- How often does she feel desire for sex?
- How often does she masturbate?
- In a sexual situation, does she experience subjective excitement and pleasurable genital sensations?
- Is there enough vaginal lubrication for comfortable sexual activity?
- Has systemic cancer treatment created problems of vaginal dryness or pain with sex?
- What kinds of stimulation help her reach orgasm, and with what consistency?
- What range of sexual practices is comfortable for her?
- Have her breast cancer diagnosis and treatment changed her sexual frequency, function, or the types of touch used?
- Has she had a loss of pleasure from breast caressing?

Altered social-sexual function is attributed to change in partner relations, depression and anxiety, loss of energy and libido, loss of control, altered body image, isolation and fear, and treatment effects. It is thought that the most common cause of sexual dysfunction in breast cancer patients may be the premature or severe menopausal symptoms caused by systemic treatment and not necessarily surgical changes of the breast. Only about 25 percent of women have significant anxiety, depression, and sexual problems after having had modified radical mastectomy. When women with mastectomies were compared to women who underwent breast biopsies for benign disease or to other women who underwent gall bladder removal, no increased rate of psychological or sexual dysfunction was found in any of these groups.[13,14]

Another study compared postmastectomy women who received chemotherapy with women who had treatment for gynecological cancer and found breast cancer patients had sex less often but orgasm and sexual practices were not affected.

Women who had lumpectomy and radiation therapy had less sexual dysfunction than women who underwent mastectomy.[15-17] In a review of twelve studies comparing mastectomy and breast conservation and its effect on quality of life, the following conclusions were made:

- There seems to be no significant difference between the two groups with regard to marital satisfaction, psychological adjustment, frequency of intercourse, or sexual dysfunction.
- Patients who underwent breast conservation and radiation therapy had less fear of cancer recurrence than patients who underwent mastectomy.
- Importantly, women whose breasts were conserved had more positive feelings about their bodies, particularly their appearance in the nude than women who had mastectomy.

Breast reconstruction improves body image as is seen among women who have breast conservation surgery and radiation therapy.[18-20] Women who undergo reconstruction feel "whole again." They can wear a variety of clothing and feel comfortable with all the styles. There seems to be equal satisfaction for women who have immediate reconstruction versus women who have reconstruction at a later time.

Systemic therapy has been shown to have a negative impact on sexuality. Side effects like fatigue, nausea, vomiting, low white blood count, infections, etc., all lower libido. Postmenopausal symptoms rapidly develop in young women undergoing chemotherapy, particularly in those between the ages of 35 and 40. Body image also changes in women undergoing chemotherapy due to the loss of their hair, change in skin texture, and weight changes. Even when hair does grow back after chemotherapy is stopped, it does not regrow identically to what it was. The use of tamoxifen or bilateral ovarian ablation will bring on postmenopausal symptoms or slightly intensify those already existing. Tamoxifen, however, may add slightly to the health of the vaginal mucosa because it does have a mild estrogenlike effect. Hence, there may be enough vaginal lubrication for women taking tamoxifen so that there is little or no pain during intercourse.

Table 24.1 reviews the female sexual response cycle for women as described in Masters and Johnson.[21] Among women who receive systemic treatment for breast cancer, there are definite differences in the response cycle for older women compared to younger women. When you add chemotherapy or hormonal manipulation to these respective age groups, some aspects of each stage will be decreased somewhat. In fact, the probable culprit in causing sexual dysfunction in breast cancer patients is related to the premature or severe menopausal symptoms induced or promoted by systemic therapy. Alteration of the breast, except for body image, may have litle to do with sexuality.

Table 24.1 Female Sexual Response Cycle

	Young Women	Older Women
Excitement	Vaginal lubrication Expansion of inner ⅔ of vagina Elevation of cervix/uterus Clitoral, labial swelling Mild increase in breast size	Slowed response Reduced lubrication No increase in breast size Reduced vaginal expansion
Plateau	Outer ⅓ of vagina swells called "orgasmic platform" Increased uterine elevation leading to "tenting" and clitoral retraction Increased labial color Areolar swelling, nipple erection Sex flush	Reduced uterine elevation Reduced vaginal elasticity Reduced sex flush Less muscle tension
Orgasm	Uterine contractions Contractions of outer ⅓ of vagina and anal sphincters Increased sex flush	Shorter duration Weaker/spastic contraction
Resolution	Orgasmic platform disappears Labial color fades Breasts, clitoris decrease in size Uterus moves back to resting position Multi-orgasmic capacity	Multi-orgasmic capacity retained Faster return to prearousal state

Home Care and Quality of Life

The home should be the principal setting for care of the breast cancer patient in the terminal stages. Oftentimes, the terminal cancer patient will feel less anxious and more at ease in the home setting than in a hospital or nursing-home setting. The older patient has more concerns regarding transportation, finances, and symptoms from other chronic illnesses in addition to the cancer. All the creature comforts that the patient is used to are there at hand. And truly the ideal setting for such a patient is in the home because a hospital setting can offer little that home care can't offer. Family members, thus, must assume responsibility for physical and psychosocial demands of the patient with cancer. Everyone in the family has a new set of physical and psychosocial demands as care-givers. The quality of life for both the patient and the family is a major issue and concern.

The needs of the patient and care-giver are different and yet similar. A patient needs physical comforts and information. A care-giver needs household management skills first and information second. When both groups are considered, the priority need is psychological. But there are four major areas that must be addressed when caring for the terminal breast cancer patient at home:

1. Pain control
2. Self-care difficulties
3. Managing side-effects of treatment
4. Caring for patients at home who still require extensive treatment like chemotherapy or blood transfusions

According to one study,[23] the terminal cancer patient and the family desire the following from nurses giving home care:

1. Teach the care-giver to recognize signs that death is approaching.
2. Stay with the patient during difficult times.
3. Stay with the care-giver during difficult times.
4. Answer all questions honestly, openly, and willingly.
5. Inform the care-giver about changes in the patient's condition.
6. Reduce the patient's fears.
7. Show the care-giver how to keep the patient comfortable physically.
8. Listen to the patient.
9. Allow the patient to do as much for herself as possible.

In summary, quality of life issues are extremely important for any patient and particularly the breast cancer patient. Each of the qualities of life must be addressed: physical symptoms, performance, general well-being, cognitive abilities, sexual dysfunction, and overall life satisfaction. And the quality of life may be the determining factor for the breast cancer patient with regard to choice of treatment. Quality of life issues are now on equal footing with efficacy when a new drug is being considered for approval by the Food and Drug Administration.

ETHICS

In my experience, all cancer patients who receive treatment, and, hence, interact with physicians and other patients in treatment areas, know their situation. Even very young people know. A six-year-old boy who I was treating for leukemia at the National Cancer Institute, asked me what it was like in heaven.

A national survey conducted on noncancer patients in 1982 found that 96 percent of Americans wanted to be told if they had a cancer, and 85 percent wanted a realistic estimate of how long they would live if their cancer usually led to death in less than a year.[24] Half of the physicians said they give one of the following two answers:

1. Straight statistical prognosis (13 percent) or
2. Say they cannot tell how long the patient might live, but stress that in most cases people live no longer than a year (28 percent).

Do patients with cancer really want to know the exact day they are going to die? And if a doctor does give them a range of time for life, how many patients then go home, mark the calendar, and proceed to die on that day? The practice of medicine is an art as well as a science. It involves compassion and honesty. A good physician will always give a ray of hope as well as discuss the implications of a grave situation. Most people who grow up in an industrialized society with multimedia communications are aware that patients who have cancer generally will die of it. This is not a revelation. But some in the legal community have taken issue with this.

A case involving ethical informed consent (*Arato* v. *Avedon*[25]) asked whether the law should force physicians to report statistical life expectancy information to their patients in cases of terminal illnesses. In 1980, Mr. Arato was found to have a tumor in the tail of his pancreas, surrounding lymph nodes and tissues, which were removed during a surgical procedure. The surgeon told the patient and his wife that he thought he had removed all the tumor and then referred them to an oncologist. At that time, the surgeon did not tell

the patient and his wife that only 5 percent of the patients with
pancreatic cancer survive for five years. Nor did the surgeon give the
patient a prognosis or reasonable estimate of his life expectancy. I
wonder how many cancer patients really are concerned about prognosis or life expectancy when they first hear the diagnosis of cancer?
Not only does the fear of death immediately come upon people who
hear that they have cancer, but the next several thoughts are what can
they do about this problem.

To go on with the story, however, the oncologist did tell the patient
that there is a high chance of recurrence and that a recurrence would
mean that the disease was incurable. Because there is no good treatment for this illness, the oncologist recommended experimental chemotherapy and radiation therapy and told the patient that this might
produce no beneficial effect at all. The oncologist did not volunteer a
prognosis nor was he asked for it by the patient or his wife. During
treatment, a recurrence was detected. The physicians realized that the
life expectancy for this patient would be measured in months, but
they did not tell him that. The patient died one year after his cancer
had been diagnosed. Soon thereafter, the patient's wife and two adult
children sued the surgeon and oncologist. They claimed the doctors
had been obligated under California's informed consent law to tell
the patient, before asking him to consent to chemotherapy, that about
95 percent of the people with pancreas cancer die within five years.

At trial, it was decided that Mr. Arato should have been informed
that he had a serious illness. The surgeon, in response, thought it
medically inappropriate to talk about a specific mortality rate given
the patient's great anxiety. The oncologist's answer was that patients
like Mr. Arato "wanted to be told, but did not want a cold shower."
He thought that if the high mortality rate for pancreas cancer was
given to the patient, the patient would be deprived of any hope. And
during the seventy visits with his physicians over a year, the patient
had avoided asking specifics about his own life expectancy, and this
indicated to the doctors that he did not want to know. Also, all the
physicians testified that the life expectancy of a group of patients had
little predictive value when applied to a particular patient.

The patient's wife thought that if the patient had known the facts,
he would not have undergone experimental chemotherapy but would
have chosen to live at home with no treatment, taking care of his
business affairs. And since the patient did not arrange his financial
affairs properly before death, there were substantial tax losses. My
question is: How many people with cancer really need to be told to
"get their affairs in order"? Anyone with a chronic illness—heart
disease, stroke, cancer, kidney disease, pulmonary disease, etc.—

should get their affairs in order because there are no cures for chronic illnesses. In fact, anyone, young or old, should have a will.

The lower court returned a verdict in favor of the physicians. The family appealed and the decision was reversed, stating that the physicians were obligated to disclose statistics of life expectancy. The physicians appealed to the California Supreme Court, which upheld the appeals court decision in favor of the family. The California Supreme Court said that the doctrine of informed consent is based on four tenets:

1. Patients are generally ignorant of medicine.
2. Patients have a right to control their own bodies and thus to decide about medical treatment.
3. To be effective, consent to treatment must be informed.
4. Patients are dependent upon their physicians for truthful information and must trust them (making the doctor-patient relationship a "fiduciary" or trust relationship rather than an arm's-length business relationship).

The court concluded:

Rather than mandate the disclosure of specific information as a matter of law, the better rule is to instruct the jury that a physician is under a legal duty to disclose to the patient all material information—that is, information which would be regarded as significant by a reasonable person in the person's position when deciding to accept or reject a recommended medical procedure—needed to make an informed decision regarding a proposed treatment.[25]

Perhaps the good of this particular case is that physicians will be required to tell the patient about the probability that a proposed treatment will be successful and specifically define what the word "successful- means. A reasonable person should know the probability of success from a particular treatment and then decide whether to accept that treatment or not. The poor results with conventional medicine are, of course, the whole basis for the ground swell concerning alternative medicine in the United States. Our culture emphasizes life and youth and vitality. We tend to shy away from talking about death and dying. When it does come to cancer treatment, hope can always be given while, at the same time, informing the patient of studies regarding particular treatments and life expectancy and/or benefits from those treatments. Sometimes there are financial conflicts that arise when one treatment is considered over another treatment.

It has been said that the chief beneficiaries of cancer treatments that don't change survival and cause harm are often the appointment books of the oncologist, and pharmaceutical companies and their stockholders.[26] We really need to start thinking in terms of *effective or noneffective* treatment and tell patients about treatments in those terms. For instance, chemotherapy is noneffective for pancreas cancer. And perhaps, as I have said in the past, aggressive treatment to keep a person alive in the last several weeks of his or her life would stop if the patient and the family were truly informed about the futility of such efforts. The costs of health care provided to a patient in terminal stages in a hospital are enormous and consume anywhere from 20 to 30 percent of all the health-care dollars. The patient and the family may be responsible for this because they "want everything done." The physician is partly responsible because "our technology should help these people." And the legal profession may, in part, be responsible as well; if everything is not done, will the family sue the physician?

25
Untreated Breast Cancer: Its Natural History

The natural history of a disease is defined as that which happens to a person who has that disease and is unable or unwilling to receive any treatment for it. In many instances, there were no treatments for a particular disease in the 1800s. In other cases, patients may not accept treatments for religious or other beliefs, or may have another medical condition that precludes the use of certain treatments. Hence, these patients can be studied and followed. Treatment results may then be compared to the results in patients who have had no treatment.

One of the first studies of the natural history of breast cancer was published in 1962.[1] In a hospital cancer ward in England between the years 1805 and 1933, 250 patients were seen. Most of these patients had advanced breast cancer, the only stage at which patients in those days would have been admitted. Patients with stage III and IV comprised about 97 percent of the entire group in the study. There were only 2 percent who had stage II breast cancer. Close to 70 percent of these patients had ulcerations when first seen and not one of these patients was treated with surgery, radiation therapy, hormone therapy, or any other systemic intervention. These patients were admitted only for terminal care and, in every instance, a postmortem examination was performed. Only about 35 percent of the cases had histological documentation, but the records at the hospital were meticulous and well documented. Quite interestingly, 20 percent of this group was still alive after five years and 5 percent survived ten years. These figures are relatively comparable to those seen in other studies. Hence, the survival of breast cancer patients who are untreated can be quite long and approaches the numbers already seen in Chapter 22 for patients who have been treated with various modalities.

When these results are compared to results of modern "conventional" treatment, there are tremendous similarities. A study conducted by the End Results Section of the Biometry Branch of the National Cancer Institute of patients treated with modern conventional treatment showed there are two groups of patient outcomes almost identical to the untreated English study outcomes. About 40 percent of all breast cancer patients make up one group and these patients die at the same rate as in the English study—about 25 percent per year. The second group, consisting of 60 percent of all breast cancer patients treated with conventional treatment, dies at a rate of 2.5 percent per year, which is again similar to the rate for the second group in the English study, which is proportionate in size. Therefore, the results of these analyses show that breast cancer patients make up approximately two groups: one group that dies at a rate of about 25 percent per year and another group that dies at 2.5 percent per year. This indicates that breast cancer has a protracted course in about 60 percent of the population and in the other 40 percent of breast cancer patients (who die at a rate of 25 percent per year), it doesn't matter whether they are treated or not, they die at that rate.

This has obvious implications. For instance, based on these data it doesn't matter whether a patient is treated or not in 40 percent of the cases. Secondly, when the survival rates of the totally untreated English group are compared with the patients who had the benefit of "conventional treatment," the numbers are similar at five years and ten years for people who were treated or for people who were not treated. Secondly, as was stated before, because of the long natural course of breast cancer, mammogram screening may only detect the disease earlier in the natural course without altering its outcome, regardless of treatment. Breast cancer is probably a fifteen- to twenty-year disease. Older mammographic techniques and equipment could detect a breast cancer when the patient had only three or four years left to live. Now, with better mammographic techniques, we simply detect it earlier but the course of the disease is the same. This is called "lead-time bias." Mammographic screening can detect slow-growing or less aggressive tumors rather than fast-growing tumors. So even though mammographic screening may appear to improve survival, it simply does not, and probably only identifies patients with either favorable tumors or those early in the course of the disease, without really altering the long-term overall survival.

Analysis of what is called tumor doubling times provides another piece of evidence regarding the natural history of breast cancer. Most cancers are detected when the diameter is about 1 cm; this size contains about 1 billion cells, or 1×10^9 cells. To accumulate that number of cells, and assuming no other factors are involved in the process of cellular division (but there are many), it takes about 20 divisions from the initial single cancer cell. One study states an average doubling time is about 109 days, and if one assumes that no other factors are involved it would take about 8 to 9 years to reach 1 billion cells.[2] Many cancers at this size have already metastasized.[3] It has been estimated that 90 percent of tumors have already metastasized by the time the tumor has reached a diameter of 6 cm.[4] If a cancer is discovered between annual mammogram screening, the doubling time is about 30 to 70 days.[5] About 75 percent of all breast cancers grow fast enough to be detected on a mammogram 1 year after nothing had been detectable with mammography.[6] On the other hand, the long survival of some breast cancer patients, whether treated or untreated, shows that there is a slow growth of some breast cancers as well. The slowest doubling time recorded is 944 days[2] by one investigator, and as long as 5 years by another investigator.[7]

The natural history data are also supplemented by reviewing autopsy findings. About 6 percent of all women dying of other causes have breast carcinoma *in situ*, and 20 percent have dysplasia (abnormally developed tissues, organs, or cells).[8] About 25 percent of women had invasive breast carcinoma or premalignant lesions.[9]

IS BREAST CANCER CURABLE?

The data suggest that breast cancer is not curable the way it is treated today. However, that is a difficult issue to resolve given that breast cancer has a late age of onset, generally, and a long natural history, which means death occurs long after the initial diagnosis is made. Hence, claims of "cure" in studies having only a short follow-up time—less than twenty to forty years—are unjustified.[10-14] Long survival of a particular breast cancer patient who has had "conventional treatment" may actually be due to the natural history of the disease and have nothing to do with the treatment.

Papers and textbooks often define "cure" in different ways. The most common way is to make the numbers in a particular report look very good. For instance, if the majority of patients survive at least 5 years, that paper will discuss a 5-year cure. If a patient lives 5 years and 1 day, that person is counted as a cure. However, that patient is nonetheless dead. If, on the other hand, a patient lived 4 years and 364 days, that patient is not cured and will be entered into the statistics as such. The word "cure" should only be applied when a patient is given a treatment (e.g., antibiotics for a sore throat) and the patient then lives an uninterrupted life having the same life expectancy as a person who never got that sore throat. The same concept of cure should be applied for cancers in general and breast cancer specifically.

Some papers report a "personal cure," which is defined as having no events referable to breast cancer during the rest of the patient's life, and the patient dies of another illness.[12,15] In each of these reports, about 25 percent of the patients are sufficiently old that they have no further events from their breast cancer and die from other causes.

The controversy of whether breast cancer is curable or not stems back for over one hundred years. The "belief system" has been operational for this period of time and longer. The majority of surgeons have believed for a long time that the more disease removed, the better the chance to effect a cure. Even today, the great majority of breast cancer patients are treated with modified radical mastectomies, although the data clearly show the same survival rates for lumpectomy, axillary node dissection, and radiation therapy.

Even in the late 1800s, it was known that less was as effective as more. A surgeon in 1888 said there was no evidence to suggest that a simple mastectomy was inferior to the very radical operations that were being done in his time, which included removal of all axillary lymph nodes, clearance of the entire axilla, removal of the lymph nodes above the collar bone, total mastectomy, or even removal of the entire upper limb at the shoulder joint.[16] Jackson commented that these radical operations were unscientific and needlessly "cruel" to many women. And he said that clinicians should not ignore the clinical experience that had shown radical surgery did not decrease recurrence: "I hope we shall not, ignoring the opinion of Sir James Paget as to the constitutional nature of the disease . . . wander on the strength of a delusion as to the local nature of the disease."[16] Even now, over one hundred years later, the same "non-sense" wishful thinking abounds, justifying more surgery versus less surgery.[17-19] Lewison, in his textbook for breast cancer, stated "we must now be born again believers and anticipate the golden age of cancer surgery, complemented by radiotherapy, hormone therapy, chemotherapy, and immunotherapy."[20] If we cannot conquer cancer, at least let us give it the full works.[21]

Breast cancer is a systemic disease. It metastasizes early before it is detectable by current screening methods.[22,23] Time of diagnosis will have little effect on the development of metastases; therefore, delay in diagnosis does not unfavorably influence survival for those with breast cancer.[23]

Fashions in conventional treatment change rapidly and don't allow too much time for reasonable assessment of those therapies. "One must be astonished at the sudden plethora of therapeutic talent, though not without fear of the coming day of reckoning."[24]

We know scientifically that lesser amounts of surgery are as good as very radical forms of surgery. We know that added radiation therapy will help achieve a better rate of local control. But we don't know if patients would survive as long if the breast were not removed and only irradiated. Survival rates, on the other hand, are not affected by any methods currently used, whether radical or simple mastectomy, with or without radiation therapy, with or without hormonal or chemotherapeutic methods. Removal of lymph nodes or radiation of those nodes with or without metastases does not improve survival either.[25-27] Hence, survival is more closely related to the actual biology of the breast cancer than to early detection, diagnosis, and treatment.

From the data for mammographic screening techniques, we learned that early detection does not mean increased survival. In fact, by the time we can detect it by whatever technology we have, breast cancer is already disseminated from the breast to other parts of the body. Because of our limited technology, we are unable to detect cancer masses less than 1 cm in diameter. So if there is 1/2 cm of disease in a particular organ, we will never see it. If there are 100,000 cells or 1,000,000 cells or 10 million cells in an organ or site other than the breast, we cannot find it with our current technology. Generally, cancers less than 1 cm in diameter will be demonstrated clinically after about 10 years.[28] And many studies show that early treatment intervention after a breast cancer has been "detected early" has not changed survival curves probably because these early cases had cancers of either very low or nonlethal potential. For instance, cancers less than 1 cm in diameter that had been removed surgically from the breast should not have been treated at all. Patients with these lesions will do quite well. We are simply detecting breast cancer earlier along its natural history of growth than we would without our current mammogram technology. Many of the cancers that we are detecting earlier as per our mammographic techniques are *in situ* carcinomas.

When people are desperate, they often perform aggressively. And the belief system in medicine is no different. In 1977, about 50 percent of all breast cancer surgeries in the United States were radical mastectomies, and in 1981, about 77 percent of all breast surgical operations were modified radical mastectomies. Today, little has changed. Modified radical mastectomies are still performed even though we know that conservative surgical procedure (i.e., lumpectomy and axillary node dissection) with radiation therapy yields identical survival rates.

Our zeal also to find the right combination of chemotherapeutic agents, the right high dose, and to subject breast cancer patients to more and more aggressive treatment in hopes of finding the "cure" is no different.

The truth is that if we employ only current conventional techniques, we will obtain the same survival figures for patients with breast cancer that were obtained over one hundred years ago. If we apply the same current conventional techniques, we will obtain the same survival curves as obtained for women who never had treatment at all. We must rethink what we are doing, what we are administering, and shift to a brand new paradigm.

We must recommend that patients with breast cancer radically change their lifestyles. Per the Japanese data, which have shown lifestyle factors have a pronounced effect on overall survival, we must add lifestyle modification to the *judicious* use of conventional techniques and treatments. A proper lifestyle as described in the following Ten-Point Plan cannot hurt anyone; with regard to breast cancer and perhaps other dietary related tumors, it may, in fact, actually add years to the survival curve.

PART FIVE

Simone Ten-Point Plan for Adjunctive Breast Care

26

The Simone
Ten-Point Plan
for Adjunctive
Breast Care

You can do many things to control the destiny of your life and the lives of your loved ones. Eighty percent of women experience benign breast disease; the breast pain and other symptoms simply do not have to be. You can decrease the severity of these symptoms and the risk of developing breast cancer from benign breast disease.

Cancer, the most dread of all diseases, will affect one of every three Americans now and by the year 2000, two in five. Breast cancer affects one in eight women now, and those odds are getting worse. Eighty to ninety percent of all cancers are related to nutritional factors (a high-animal-fat, high-cholesterol, low-fiber diet), lifestyle (tobacco smoking, excessive alcohol consumption), the environment (chemical carcinogens, ozone, air pollution, industrial exposure), and some hormones and drugs. As we have learned, many of these cancer risk factors also put you at risk for developing and worsening cardiovascular diseases. Since we can now identify many of these factors, we should modify them accordingly to lessen our risks.

The likelihood of drastically increasing the number of cancer cures by conventional cancer therapies in the foreseeable future is not great, even though some of the very best American minds and technologies are involved in cancer research. Cancer is the most complex group of diseases known, and there are many different causes. We must all do

our part to try to *prevent* cancer in order to substantially reduce the
number of new cancer cases. Americans need to know the risk factors
for cancer and cardiovascular diseases. Adults who become aware of
these risk factors and then modify their diets and lifestyles accordingly will reduce their risk of developing the diseases. Table 26.1
provides a check list of the risk factors for cancer and heart disease
that you can control and those you cannot control. As you now know,
you have direct control over the majority of them.

Children will benefit the most from properly modified nutritional
factors and daily habits. Information on nutrition should be part
of a child's education throughout the school years, because nutritional practices and habits are easily modified in youth. The main risk
factors for the development of cancer and cardiovascular disease are
poor nutrition and tobacco smoking. If parents and teachers set the
example of correct nutritional practices, no smoking, and very modest
alcohol consumption, the children will continue these practices
throughout their own lives. There will be a consequent decrease in
the incidence of cancer and cardiovascular disease.

What can you do to help yourself? My recommendations to modify
your risk factors for benign breast disease as well as breast cancer
(and also cancer generally and cardiovascular disease) will increase
the possibility of breast health. The Ten-Point Plan is not anything
like the popular fad diets or the crash schemes for weight reduction,
longevity, or reversal of diseases. Primary prevention is the major
goal of my plan for risk factor modification—no fads.

Simply, I have presented the current body of scientific information
concerning benign breast disease, breast cancer, and the factors that
promote an existing breast cancer. I now will discuss how those risk
factors can be modified. Whether you have a benign breast problem
or breast cancer, you will be better off when you closely adhere to my
recommendations. As you have read, survival—lifespan—is positively affected mainly by proper lifestyle and not by existing "conventional" treatments. The preponderance of scientific information
suggests that breast health can be achieved by following the Ten-
Point Plan. This plan can help to prevent breast disease and increase
the possibility of survival for those who have breast cancer.

POINT 1: NUTRITION

Maintain an ideal weight. Remember, repeated fluctuations in your
weight, per se, can increase your risk for heart disease and death. You
will find several medically sound weight-reduction diets in *Cancer
and Nutrition*, along with a table of foods and their compositions.

Table 26.1   Risk Factors for Cancer and Heart Disease

Risk Factors	Controllable
• Nutritional	Yes
Fat Intake	Yes
Fiber Intake	Yes
Vitamin/Mineral Intake	Yes
Food Additives/Contaminants	Yes
Caffeine Intake	Yes
• Obesity	Yes
• Tobacco Use	Yes
• Alcohol Use	Yes
• Drug Use	Yes
• Pesticides	Yes
• Environmental Factors	
Air Pollution (Outdoor, Ozone Depletion, Acid Rain)	Yes
Indoor Pollution	Yes
Water Treatment and Pollution	Yes
Electromagnetic Fields	Yes
• Radiation	
Sun Exposure	Yes
Suntanning Booths	Yes
Multiple Unnecessary X-Rays	Yes
• Sexual-Social	
Female Promiscuity	Yes
Male Promiscuity	Yes
AIDS Spread	Yes
• Hormonal Factors	
Menstrual History	Yes/No*
First Pregnancies	Yes
Abortion First Trimester, First Pregnancy	Yes
Benign Breast Disease	Yes
Failure to repair Undescended Testicle	Yes
DES	Yes
Oral Contraception	Yes
Estrogen Use	Yes
Androgen Use	Yes
• Sedentary Lifestyle	Yes
• Stress	Yes
• Silicon Breast Implants	Yes
• Occupational Factors	Yes
• High Blood Pressure	Yes
• Age	No
• Lack of Physical Examination	Yes

*A high-fat diet triggers early menarche.

Reduce your cholesterol intake. No matter what your cholesterol level, but especially if it is over 200, eliminate:

- Red meats (beef, lamb, luncheon and processed meats, pork, veal)
- Whole, 2 percent, and 1 percent dairy products (butter, cheese, eggs, ice cream, milk, yogurt). Skim (nonfat) products are okay.
- Shellfish

When you avoid these foods, your cholesterol will begin to decrease in four to six *months*.

If your triglycerides are over 150, eliminate:

- Alcohol
- Fruit and fruit juices
- Cookies, cakes, candies, ice cream, sweet rolls, etc.

When you eliminate these foods, your triglycerides will decrease in four to six *weeks*.

Remember, there are no cholesterol or triglyceride fairies who come at night and sprinkle these evils into your body while you are sleeping!

Consume a low-animal-fat, low-cholesterol diet. Following the rec-ommendations under this heading will provide you with more than enough fats necessary for all bodily functions and, at the same time, modify disease risks. If your total dietary fats are less than 20 percent of your total calories, you will attain breast health and decrease your risk of cancer and other health risks. It is also virtually impossible to gain weight on such a low-fat diet.

- *Eat poultry*. White meat is best. Remove all skin before cooking. Chicken, turkey, Cornish hen, and game birds are good. Do not eat any fatty poultry like goose or duck.
- *Eat fish*. All fish are recommended except shellfish, sardines, mack-erel, and fish canned in oil, all of which are high in fat or cholesterol.
- *Eliminate red meat* or eat only lean red meat, and limit consumption to about once every ten days. Eliminate all fatty meats like bacon, fatty hamburger, spareribs, sausage, luncheon meats, sweetbreads, hot dogs, kidney, brains, liver, etc. Do not eat smoked or salt-cured foods. Limit the amount of barbecued and charcoal-broiled foods.
- *Limit dairy products*. Only nonfat products should be eaten: skim milk, skim powdered milk, evaporated skim milk, nonfat yogurt and but-termilk, and cheeses made only with skim milk. Eliminate whole and low-fat milk and the products made from them: cream, half and half, all cheeses containing greater than 0 percent fat, whipped cream, etc. Do not eat whole eggs. Eat only a few egg whites per week or a cholesterol-free egg substitute a couple of times a week.

Simone Ten-Point Plan for Breast Health

POINT 1: NUTRITION.

- Maintain an ideal weight. Lose weight even if it is just 5 or 7 pounds.
- Decrease the number of daily calories.
- Eat a low-fat, low-cholesterol diet: fish, especially those rich in omega-3 fatty acids; poultry without the skin; and if you must consume dairy products, not whole, 1 percent, or 2 percent. No red meat, lunch meat, or oils.
- Consume both *soluble* and *insoluble* fiber (25 to 30 grams per day). Fruits, vegetables, cereals are mainly *insoluble* fibers. Pectins, gums, and mucilages have *soluble* fibers which can decrease cholesterol, triglycerides, sugars, and carcinogens. Use a supplement of soluble fiber to insure a consistent amount of fiber each day.
- Supplement your diet with certain nutrients in the proper doses, form, and combination based on your lifestyle. Take high doses of all antioxidants (beta-carotene, vitamins E and C, selenium, cysteine, flavonoids, copper, zinc), and the B vitamins. Calcium and its enhancing agents should be taken at bedtime.
- Eliminate salt, food additives, smoked, and pickled foods. Limit barbecues.
- Take one aspirin every day if you are able.

POINT 2: TOBACCO.   Do not smoke, chew, snuff, or inhale other people's smoke.

POINT 3: ALCOHOL and CAFFEINE.   Avoid all alcohol, or have one drink or less per week. Avoid caffeine (coffee, tea, chocolate).

POINT 4: SEXUAL-SOCIAL FACTORS, HORMONES, DRUGS.   Avoid promiscuity, hormones, and any unnecessary drugs.

POINT 5: ENVIRONMENTAL EXPOSURE.   Keep air, water, and work place clean by using filters.

POINT 6: RADIATION.   Have X-rays taken only when needed. Avoid electromagnetic fields from home appliances, office equipment, and outside electric fields. Use #15 sunscreen, wear sunglasses.

POINT 7: LEARN THE SEVEN EARLY WARNING SIGNS.

- Lump in breast.
- Change in wart or mole.
- Nonhealing sore.
- Change in bowel or bladder habits.
- Persistent cough or hoarseness.
- Indigestion or trouble swallowing.
- Unusual bleeding.

POINT 8: EXERCISE.

POINT 9: STRESS MODIFICATION, SPIRITUALITY, AND SEXUALITY.

POINT 10: GET EXECUTIVE PHYSICAL EXAM YEARLY.   Prevention is the key to wellness.

You will feel better and stay well by following this Simone Ten-Point Plan.

- *Eliminate all oils and fats* including butter, margarine, meat fat, lard, and all oils. Both saturated and polyunsaturated fats are detrimental.
- *Limit garnishes and sauces.* Use products that do not have fats, oils, or egg yolks. Dry white wine may be used in cooking, and you can also use ketchup and vinegar. Do not use salad dressings, prepared gravies and sauces, mayonnaise, sandwich spreads, or other products containing fats, oils, or egg yolks.

It is important to know how to read a nutritional label and then determine the percentage of fat calories from it. You need to know two numbers from the label: the total number of calories per ounce, second, the number of fat grams per ounce, then add an imaginary zero to that number. Let's look at specific examples:

"Light" Potato Chips
Total calories: 120 calories per serving
Total fat: 6 grams per ounce—add that zero—60 fat calories/serving

$$\% \text{ Fat} = \frac{\text{Fat calories/serving}}{\text{Total calories/serving}}$$

$$\% \text{ Fat} = \frac{60 \text{ Fat calories/serving}}{120 \text{ Calories/serving}}$$

% Fat for "light potato chips" = 50%

Eating these "light potato chips" you will:
Gain weight
Decrease your breast health
Increase your risk for disease
Promote an existing disease

Non-salted Pretzel
Total calories: 100 calories/serving
Total fat: 1 gram per serving—add that zero—10 fat calories/serving

$$\% \text{ Fat} = \frac{\text{Fat calories/serving}}{\text{Total calories/serving}}$$

$$\% \text{ Fat} = \frac{10 \text{ Fat calories/serving}}{100 \text{ Calories/serving}}$$

% Fat for this pretzel = 10%

Eating these pretzels you will:
Not gain weight
Increase your breast health
Decrease your risk for disease
Not promote an existing disease

What if there is no food label to read? Then you simply must remember the information here or refer to the information in Table 26.2.

Eat a high-fiber diet. The typical American eats about 3–8 grams of fiber each day. I recommend that you consume 25 to 35 grams per day, which studies suggest can protect you from diseases.

Low-fiber diets correlate with: breast cancer, benign breast disease, colorectal cancer, other cancers, cardiovascular disease, diabetes, obesity, elevated cholesterol, elevated triglycerides, irritable bowel syndrome, constipation, diverticular disease, hemorrhoids, appendicitis, gall bladder disease, and hiatal hernia.

There are two types of fiber: *soluble* and *insoluble*. Both increase fecal bulk and bowel movement frequency, slow an irritable bowel, or speed up a constipated bowel. Insoluble fiber occurs in most fruits, vegetables, and cereals. Soluble fiber, however, is more important and available only in pectin, gum (guar and oat gums), and mucilages (kelp and psyllium). These are foods we ordinarily don't eat. Soluble fiber:

- Entraps harmful bile acids, bile estrogens, and carcinogens.
- Lowers cholesterol, LDL-cholesterol, triglycerides, and blood sugar level.
- Taken with water, makes you feel full due to longer time in stomach and, hence, can be used effectively to decrease your appetite so that you lose weight.
- Provides stool "lubricant."

Vegetables of the Brassicaceae family provide fiber and induce enzymes to destroy certain carcinogens. These include Brussels

Table 26.2 Percent Fat Calories in Foods

Food	% Fat Calories
Vegetables/Fruit	<10%
Breads	10–20%
Fish	10–20%
Pasta, grains, cereals	10–20%
Poultry (no skin)	20–35%
Beef and Lamb	50–80%
Pork ("the other white meat")	80%
Dairy (nonskim)	60–90%
Eggs	70%
Nuts, seeds, peanut butter	80%
Olive, avocado, coconut	85%
Cookie, cake, muffin	90%
Diet margarine/Vegetable oil	100%

sprouts, broccoli, and cabbage. You can eat whole or lightly milled grains like rice, barley, and buckwheat. Whole-wheat bread and whole-wheat pasta, cereals, crackers, and other grain products can also be eaten as can unsweetened fruit juices and unsweetened cooked, canned, or frozen fruit.

Do not eat cooked, canned, or frozen fruit with added sugar, fruit syrups with added sugar, fruit juices with added sugar, or bleached white flour, and grain products made with added fats, oils, or egg yolks. Avoid butter rolls, commercial biscuits, muffins, doughnuts, sweet rolls, cakes, egg bread, cheese bread, and commercial mixes containing dried eggs and whole milk.

Add food supplements to your diet. You should supplement your diet with vitamins, minerals, and fibers in the proper dosages and combinations. Some people today are taking supplements that contain the right buzz-word nutrients. These, generally, are in a less effective or less stable chemical form like the gelcap oil-based capsule form of vitamin E, beta-carotene, or any other nutrient. Sometimes, the nutrients are in the wrong ratios relative to other nutrients, or are in very low amounts but just enough to be listed on the label and advertised, "with beta-carotene," for instance.

Most nutrients should be taken with food. However, calcium and nutrients that enhance its metabolism should be taken at bedtime or on an empty stomach because most foods (fiber) will bind calcium and render it useless. Here again, most supplements have calcium in the same tablet with the other nutrients—and, in effect, you get little or none of it when taken this way.

Also, beware of supplements that contain iron because iron is associated with cancer promotion. There are many causes of anemia so unless you have a *true iron deficiency anemia,* there is no reason to take any supplemental iron, and this applies to menstruating women, too. If you do have a documented iron deficiency anemia, then you should be treated by a physician with therapeutic doses of iron in a thirty-day period. Patients who have a cancer and/or receive chemotherapy or radiation therapy usually have an anemia related to chronic disease and/or to therapy. No amount of iron will correct this anemia because it is not due to an iron deficiency.

The supplement doses I recommend are outlined in Chapter 5. They contain effective doses of all nutrients, especially antioxidants, and fibers as discussed above.

Eliminate table salt. Add only a minimal amount of salt while cooking. Most condiments, pickles, dressings, prepared sauces, canned vegetables, bouillon cubes, pot pies, popcorn, sauerkraut, and caviar have high amounts of salt in them.

Avoid food additives. Avoid all foods containing nitrates, nitrites, or other harmful additives, or that were processed using a harmful technique (see Chapter 10). Do not eat pickle relish.

Watch your snacks and desserts. Acceptable snacks or desserts include fresh fruit and canned fruit without added sugar, water ices, gelatin, and (sparingly) puddings made with skim milk. Do not eat commercially prepared cakes, pies, cookies, doughnuts, and mixes; coconut or coconut oil; frozen cream pies; potato chips and other deep-fried snacks; whole-milk puddings; ice cream; candy; chocolate; or gum with sugar.

Watch your beverages. Acceptable beverages are skim milk or nonfat buttermilk, mineral water, unsweetened fruit juices, and vegetable juices. Avoid caffeine-containing beverages—coffee, tea, cola, etc.

Remember good nutrition when dining out. Call the restaurant to see if your needs as outlined here can be accommodated. Airlines and ocean liners will also help you. Request that your food be prepared without any salt products (Chinese food is high in sodium). Use lemon juice or vinegar on your salad.

POINT 2: TOBACCO

Do not smoke! Do not chew or snuff tobacco. If you are smoking, quit now. There is no easy, painless way to quit. The best way is simply to go "cold turkey" without tapering off or using any expensive smoke-ending courses.

The American Lung Association can help you. Call this organization. Remember, tobacco smoke also endangers the health of nonsmokers.

As a nonsmoker, demand that smokers not smoke in your presence, especially in public or work-related areas.

POINT 3: ALCOHOL AND CAFFEINE

Abstain from alcohol consumption or reduce to a minimum (less than one drink per week). Remember, consumption of even modest amounts of alcohol in a week is a risk factor for benign breast problems, breast cancer and other cancers, and can perpetuate an existing breast cancer. Avoid caffeine from all sources, including chocolate.

POINT 4: SEXUAL-SOCIAL FACTORS, HORMONES, AND DRUGS

Female promiscuity. The earlier the age of starting sexual intercourse and the more male sexual partners a female has (particularly uncir-cumcised partners), the higher is her risk of developing cancer of the cervix.

Benign breast disease is, in part, influenced by hormonal changes (Chapter 2). Take steps to minimize your risk by following this Ten-Point Plan.

Birth control pills. Birth control pills should not be used. Other means of birth control should be sought. Do not use estrogens to treat other conditions.

DES exposure. Tell your physician if you have been exposed to DES, or if you are the daughter or son of a DES-exposed mother.

Drugs. Avoid all unnecessary drugs. Take drugs only when they are prescribed by your physician. Check to see if the drug interferes with vitamin function.

POINT 5: ENVIRONMENTAL EXPOSURE

Environmental protection standards for air, water, and the work place should be rigorously observed. Several specific industries, such as the manufacturing of boots, shoes, furniture, and cabinets, are risk factors for the development of cancer of the nasal sinuses. Other indus-tries that use certain chemicals (see Table 3.1 on page 32) pose an increased risk for persons working with those chemicals. All these industries have safety standards that should be strictly observed. For instance, a person working with asbestos (insulation, brake lining, etc.) should wear a mask to protect the respiratory and gastrointestinal systems. Frequently, workers find a mask to be a nuisance and will not wear one, especially on hot days. This simply increases their risk of developing cancer. Firefighters are indirectly exposed to many hazard-ous chemicals when objects made from them burn.

Avoid prolonged exposure to household cleaning fluids, solvents, and paint thinners. Some may be hazardous if inhaled in high con-centrations. Pesticides, fungicides, and other home garden and lawn chemicals are also dangerous.

POINT 6: RADIATION

X-ray exposure (ionizing). X-ray pictures are certainly needed in many circumstances and should be taken on a physician's recommen-dation. The equipment is getting better and less radiation is now delivered to a person per film. However, there are hypochondriacs who want X-ray studies, and some people involved in motor-vehicle accidents also want X-rays done for possible legal purposes. These people receive unnecessary radiation exposure.

Inform your physician if you had radiation to your head and neck as a child.

Electromagnetic Fields. Avoid all unnecessary exposure to electromagnetic fields from home appliances, office equipment, and outside electric fields. "Safe distance" codes should be established for housing, offices, hotels, etc.

Sunlight. Sunscreens should be used when you sunbathe. Remember, sunlight causes skin cancer and ages skin rapidly. Avoid suntanning booths. Wear sunglasses.

POINT 7: LEARN THE SEVEN WARNING SIGNS OF CANCER

- A lump or thickening in the breast.
- A change in a wart or mole.
- A sore that does not heal.
- A change in bowel or bladder habits.
- A persistent cough or hoarseness.
- Constant indigestion or trouble swallowing.
- Unusual bleeding or discharge.

If any of these signs appear, contact your physician immediately.

POINT 8: EXERCISE

Everyone should start a program of exercise, but see a physician before doing so if you are at risk for cardiovascular disease. Initially the exercising should start out slowly, then increase to a comfortable level. Fast walking is a good form of exercise and should be part of your program. Two miles is a satisfactory distance to briskly walk four out of seven days. I stress fast walking because it is easier to do than other forms of exercise—no equipment to buy, no change of clothing, no one to rely on except yourself. You can walk in a shopping mall in inclement weather. Calisthenics should also be done to firm up abdominal-wall muscles and decrease that "spare tire." Five to ten sit-ups, with knees bent, can readily be done at home every day. Lower back pain is one of the most common pains in America. Simple stretching and flexing exercises will prevent and treat lower back pain.

Remember, the data show that some amount of exercise is better than none. Just a little exercise every day will benefit you enormously. Choose an exercise program that you are likely to follow, and stick with your exercise routine.

POINT 9: STRESS MODIFICATION, SPIRITUALITY, AND SEXUALITY

Stress is a risk factor for the development and promotion of breast disease. To promote breast health, you must modify your stress. Control stress by whatever means you can: meditation, self-hypnosis, intimacy, or self-love, biofeedback, music, hot-water showers, or other methods you find relaxing. Stress is a killer! So find out what will help you relax.

Spirituality, or the Life Force, is what gives people hope and produces a calming and peaceful effect. Spirituality is often ignored by many people until they get into trouble with an illness or other aspects of life. Spirituality is comprised of many components.

The scientific connection between the mind and body is inescapable. The mind has great control over the body and the immune system. So your attitude in dealing with any crisis is critical. Good spiritual attitude is important for good health and the proper functioning of the immune system. Having a good spiritual life is important for wellness and health. Lack of spirituality is a risk factor for illness. Remember the words of the Bible:

"Pleasant words are like a honeycomb, sweetness to the soul and health to the body."—Book of Proverbs (16:24)

"A man's spirit will endure sickness; but a broken spirit who can bear?"—Book of Proverbs (18:14)

Seek the psychological and emotional comfort of other people as well. Avoid loneliness.

Sexuality is also important. Re-read the section in Chapter 24 on Sexuality and Body Image. Do what makes you feel good; this will further relieve stress.

POINT 10: EXECUTIVE PHYSICAL EXAMINATION

It is well known that people with localized cancer will live longer than those who present with widespread cancer. All women who have lumpy breasts should have a comprehensive executive type physical examination (combines a thorough history and a scalp-to-toe examination) with appropriate counseling and laboratory studies in order to prevent or detect early cancer or heart disease. If a physician is looking for early cancer and it is present, it then can probably be found. A thorough history should include questions about all the risk factors for cancer that are listed in Chapter 3, as well the questions at the end of this plan.

The physical examination is important and should be complete, starting at the scalp and finishing at the toes. One capable, highly trained specialist should perform the entire examination, rather than your gynecologist doing the Pap smear and breast exam, your cardiologist checking the heart, your dentist looking in your mouth, and so on. The examining physician must be thorough in examining your breasts. All the examination techniques outlined in Chapter 19 should be followed for a complete breast examination.

Laboratory tests are another part of an asymptomatic noncancerous person's work-up. Little more than one ounce of blood and urine is taken and assayed. Table 26.2 lists the laboratory tests, the normal range of the tests, and the functions tested.

Since breast cancer patients have a higher incidence of colon cancer, testing the stool for trace amounts of blood is another important laboratory examination. Trace amounts of blood in the stool can result from some lesion(s) in the gastrointestinal tract, which can be a gastrointestinal cancer. Prior to and during the collection of the stool specimens, it is important to completely avoid red meat for three entire days, because red meat contains animal blood that will produce a positive result in the test. All other instructions must also be followed.

Certain fiberoptic procedures should be done when indicated. By using a fiberoptic laryngoscope, we have found many lesions of the nasopharynx and larynx when examining patients who have been exposed to passive smoke for several hours a day, patients who have been hoarse for two weeks or more, or other high-risk patients.

A colonoscopy is used to examine the colon with a fiberoptic flexible instrument, looking for abnormalities like lesions that may bleed. Indications for doing a fiberoptic colonoscopy are:

1 To evaluate the colon when an abnormality was found with a barium enema.

2. To discover and excise polyps.

3. To evaluate unexplained bleeding:
    • A positive occult blood stool test (detection of blood in the stool that could not be seen by the eye).
    • Bleeding from the rectum.

4. To investigate an unexplained iron deficiency anemia.

5. To survey for colon cancer:
    • A strong family history of colon cancer.
    • To check the entire colon in a patient with a treatable cancer or polyp.
    • A follow-up after resection of polyp or cancer at eighteen- to thirty-six-month intervals, depending on the clinical circumstances.
    • In a patient with ulcerative colitis.

Table 26.2 Laboratory Tests for the Executive Physical

Laboratory Test	Normal Range
Stool for occult blood	Negative
Blood count	
Hemoglobin	Male: 12.5–17; Female: 11.5–15
Hematocrit	Male: 36–50 Female: 34–44
White blood cells	3,700–10,500
Platelet count	155,000–385,000
Blood lipids	
Cholesterol	130–200
HDL cholesterol	30–90
Triglycerides	30–150
Blood proteins	
Total protein	6.0–8.5
Albumin	3.5–5.5
Fasting blood sugar	
Glucose	65–115
Electrical function of cells	
Calcium	8.5–10.8
Phosphate	2.4–4.5
Magnesium	1.3–2.1
Sodium	135–147
Chloride	96–109
Potassium	3.5–5.3
CO_2	23–33
Uric acid	3.0–9.0
Kidney function	
Blood urea nitrogen	5–25
Creatinine	.6–1.5
Liver function and enzymes	
Alkaline phosphatase	25–140
SGPT	0–45
SGOT	0–40
LDH	0–240
Total bilirubin	0.1–1.2

6. To investigate chronic inflammatory bowel disease.

7. To control bleeding.

An annual chest X-ray should be done in high-risk asymptomatic patients. If a cancer mass is found in the periphery of the lung, it can be surgically removed thereby affording the patient an excellent chance for cure. A person's lung function can be readily assessed by pulmonary function testing—a series of tests that determine the quantity and speed of the air moving in and out of the lungs, the volumes of the lungs, etc.

Breast Surveillance: Asymptomatic Women. In the order of importance, the following should be done:

1. Physical Examination by Physician—all women starting at age 35.
2. Annual Mammogram—women aged 50–65.
3. Self-Breast Exam—all women, all ages.

Surveillance Follow-Up: Asymptomatic Breast Cancer Patients (looking for recurrence or metastases)

Current Convention	Sufficient

Physical exam by physician
  First 2 years: every 3 months
  Years 2 to 4: every 4 months
  Years 5 to 6: every 6 months
  6+ years: annually
	Physical exam by physician
	  First 2 years: every 3 months
	  Years 2 to 4: every 4 months
	  Years 4 to 6: every 6 months
	  6+ years: annually

Laboratory tests
  Mammogram, chest X-ray,
  liver function tests
	Laboratory tests—not indicated*

*With these "routine" tests, an abnormality is found in less than 2 percent of all asymptomatic breast cancer patients.

The Cancer Questionnaire that begins on the next page will help you to work with your physician. If, after answering the questions, you find you have three or more of the possible "yes" answers in any one category, consult your physician.

CANCER QUESTIONNAIRE*

	No	Yes

General
1. Have you ever been told by a physician that you had cancer? ___ ___
   If yes, cancer of what?_____

2. Have any of your blood relatives had cancer? ___ ___
   If yes, cancer of what?_____
3. Have you lost 10 to 15 pounds over the past 6 months without knowing why? ___ ___

Lungs
4. Have you coughed up blood in the past several weeks? ___ ___
5. Have you had a chronic daily cough? ___ ___
6. Have you been told that you have emphysema? ___ ___
7. Have you had pneumonia twice or more in the past year? ___ ___
8. Have you ever smoked? ___ ___
9. Did you quit smoking less than 15 years ago? ___ ___
10. Do you smoke now? ___ ___
    Cigarettes: Number of packs/day ___.
                 Number of years ___.
    Cigars: Number of cigars/day ___.
    Pipe: Number of bowls/day ___.
11. Do you inhale others' smoke for one or more hours/day? ___ ___

Larynx (voice box)
12. Have you had persistent hoarseness? ___ ___

Mouth and Throat
13. Have you had any of the following symptoms lasting more than a month?
    Pain or difficulty swallowing ___ ___
    Pain or tenderness in the mouth ___ ___
    A sore or white spot in your mouth ___ ___
14. Do you drink more than 4 oz. of wine, 12 oz. of beer, or 1 ½ oz. of whiskey every day? ___ ___

Stomach
15. Have you vomited blood in the past month? ___ ___
16. Have you had black stools in the past 6 months? ___ ___
    Does this happen when you are not taking pills with iron in them? ___ ___
17. Have you had stomach pains several times a week? ___ ___

*Adopted from Cancer Prevention and Detection Screening Program.

	No	Yes
Stomach (continued)		
18. Has a physician told you that you an ulcer or stomach growths called polyps?	___	___
Large Intestine and Rectum		
19. Have you had a change in your usual bowel habits?	___	___
20. Has your stool been becoming more narrow in diameter?	___	___
21. Does this happen with every bowel movement?	___	___
22. Have you had bleeding from the rectum, either with bowel movements or at other times?	___	___
23. Have you had mucus in your stool every time you had a bowel movement?	___	___
24. Have you been told that you had a polyp in the large intestine?	___	___
25. Have you had ulcerative colitis?	___	___
Breasts		
26. Have you failed to self-examine your breasts each month?	___	___
27. Do you have a lump in either breast?	___	___
28. Have you had breast pain recently? If yes, does the pain occur when you are not menstruating?	___	___
29. Has there been discharge or bleeding from your nipples, or have they begun to pull in (retract)?	___	___
30. Are there any changes in the skin of your breasts?	___	___
31. Have you ever had a breast biopsy?	___	___
Cervix, Uterus, and Vagina		
32. Do you have vaginal bleeding or spotting? If yes:	___	___
Is it between periods?	___	___
Is it after sexual intercourse?	___	___
Is it after menopause?	___	___
33. Have you stopped having your periods? At what age? _____	___	___
Since then, have you ever had hormone therapy?	___	___
Have you had a hysterectomy?	___	___
34. Have you ever had sexual intercourse?	___	___
Did you first have intercourse before age 16?	___	___
35. Did your mother use the hormone DES when she was pregnant with you?	___	___
Skin		
36. Has there been bleeding or a change in a mole on your body?	___	___

	No	Yes

Skin (continued)

37. Do you have a mole on your body where it may be irritated by underwear, a belt, etc.?

38. Do you have a sore that does not heal?

39. Do you have a severe scar from a burn?

40. Do you have fair skin and sunburn easily?

41. Do you sunbathe for long hours or use a suntanning booth?

Thyroid

42. Can you see or feel a lump in the lower front of your neck?

43. Have you had X-ray treatment to your face for acne, tonsil enlargement, or other reasons?

Kidney and Urinary Bladder

44. Have you had blood in your urine?

CONCLUSION

The Cancer Questionnaire is only good if you take the time to answer the questions. Similarly, the points in my plan are only good if *you* follow them. The ball is in your court.

If you've read the book, you, hopefully, already understand some of the ways in which you can reduce your risk of cancer. Now, take the test. Find out where you stand. You'll gain a better understanding of your odds, and you will be better prepared to do something. Start by following the Ten-Point Plan presented here. And turn the page to find out what comes next.

27
Now What?

This may be the ending of my book, but it should be just a beginning for you. I hope the book has given you the information you need to understand what breast health is all about. Armed with this information, there are things you can and *should* do.

The responsibility for breast health does not lie with other people. It falls directly in your hands. It's up to you to do something. Start by taking care of yourself. Modify your lifestyle with your optimum health in mind. And if you should feel a lump, don't let fear immobilize you. See your health-care paractitioner.

Next, take care of those close to you. Tell them to do something. You can also take care of them by following my suggestions for protecting the environment.

If you want to take it one step further, join an organization or group. Work with others in support groups that aid and educate cancer patients and their families. Join with others to lobby against such cancer risks as second-hand smoke, air pollution, and toxic wastes. Anything can be accomplished if we work together.

Afterword

You have read quite a bit of information. But you should come away with a single important thought: You have almost total control over the destiny of your health. Work in the prevention of disease is exploding. More and more people realize that by controlling risk factors—especially the major ones like nutrition, tobacco use, and alcohol consumption—you can control your well-being.

You now have the knowledge and the tools to modify your lifestyle to optimize your health and the health of your loved ones. You have the chance for a rendezvous with your well-being. Determine your own health's destiny. Seize this opportunity! Do it now!

For more information, please write to:

Charles B. Simone, M.D.
Simone Protective Cancer Center
123 Franklin Corner Road
Lawrenceville, New Jersey 08648

Notes

Introduction

1. U.S. Department of Health and Human Services, Public Health Service. 1990. The Surgeon General's Report on Nutrition and Health. Washington, D.C., U.S. Government Printing Office.
2. Boring, et al. 1995. Cancer statistics. *CA–A Cancer J for Clinicians* 45:8–30.
3. Bailar, J., and E. Smith. 1986. Progress against cancer? *NEJM* 314 (19):1226–32.
4. Boyd, J., ed. 1985. NCAB approves year 2000 report. *The Cancer Letter* 11(28):1–6.
5. Kolata, G. 1985. Is the war on cancer being won? *Science* 229:543–44.
6. Boffey, P. 1984. Cancer progress: Are the statistics telling the truth? *New York Times* (Sept 18): C1.
7. Bush, H. 1984. Cancer cure. *Science* 84:34–35.
8. Blonston, G. 1984. Cancer prevention. *Science* 84:36–39.
9. Marshall, E. 1990. Experts clash over cancer data. *Science* 250:900–902.
10. Simone, C.B. 1983. *Cancer and Nutrition*. McGraw-Hill: 1–237.
11. National Academy of Sciences, National Research Council, Food and Nutrition Board. 1989. *Diet and health: Implications for reducing chronic disease risk*. Washington, D.C.: National Academy Press.
12. The Surgeon General's Report on Nutrition and Health. 1988.
13. Butrum, et al. 1988. NCI dietary guidelines: Rationale. *Am J Clin Nutrition* 48:888–95.
14. U.S. Bureau of Vital Statistics from 1900 to present.
15. *Ca–A Cancer J for Clinicians*. 1962–present.
16. Perception of cancer risks. 1993. *JNCI* (Sept. 1).

Chapter 1
The Scope of Breast Disease

1. Boring, et al. 1995. Cancer statistics. *CA–A Cancer J for Clinicians* 45 (1):8–30.
2. Cohen, P., et al. 1983. Seasonality in the occurrence of breast cancer. *Canc Res* 43:892–893.
3. Parkin, D.N., et al. 1984. Estimates of the worldwide frequency of 12 major cancers. *Bull WHO* 62:163182.
4. Mittra, I., et al. 1989. Early detection of breast cancer in developing countries. *Lancet* (April 1):719–720.
5. Boyle, R., et al. 1993. Trends in diet related cancers in Japan: A conundrum? *Lancet* 342:752.

Chapter 2
Benign Breast Syndromes

1. Boyd, et al. 1988. Effects of a low fat, high carbohydrate diet on symptoms of cyclical mastopathy. *Lancet* ii:128–132.
2. Facchinetti, F., et al. 1991. Oral magnesium successfully relieves premenstrual mood changes. *Obstet Gynecol* 78:178–181.
3. Minton, et al. 1979. Response of fibrocystic disease to caffeine withdrawal and correlation of cyclic nucleotides with breast disease. *Am J Obstet Gynecol* 135:157–158.
4. Ernster, et al. 1982. Effects of caffeine free diet on benign breast disease: A randomized trial. *Surgery* 91 (3):263–267.
5. Dupont, W., et al. 1994. Longterm risk

of breast cancer in women with fibroadenoma. *NEJM* 331:10–15.

6. McBride, G. 1992. Revised Consensus on Benign Breast Conditions. *Oncology Times* (December), 22.

7. Bannayan, G.A., S.I. Hajdu. 1972 Gynecomastia: Clinicopathologic study of 351 cases. *Am J Clin Pathol* 57:431.

8. Kapdi, C.C., N.J. Parekh. 1983. The male breast. *Radiol Clin North Am* 21:137.

9. Nydick, M., J. Bustos, et al. 1961. Gynecomastia in adolescent boys. *JAMA* 178:449.

10. Nuttal, F.Q. 1979. Gynecomastia as a physical finding in normal men. *J Clin Endocrinol Metab* 48:338.

11. Carlson, H.E. 1980. Current concepts: Gynecomastia. *NEJM* 303:671.

12. Williams, M.J. 1963. Gynecomastia: Its incidence, recognition and host characterization in 447 autopsy cases. *Am J Med* 334:103.

13. Nutall, F.Q. 1979. Gynecomastia as a physical finding in normal men. *J Clin Endocrinol Metab* 48:338–340.

14. Fletcher, S., et al. 1985. Physician's abilities to detect lumps in silicone breast models. *JAMA* 253(15):2224–2228.

15. Gail, et al. 1989. Projecting individualized probabilities of developing breast cancer for white females who are being examined annually. *JNCI* 81:1879–1886.

16. National Surgical Adjuvant Breast and Bowel Project Protocol P-1, Aug. 31, 1991. Food and Drug Administration Oncologic Drugs Advisory Committee.

17. Nayfield, et al. 1991. Potential roll of tamoxifen in prevention of breast cancer. *JNCI* 83:1450–1459.

18. Fornander, et al. 1990. Long term adjuvant tamoxifen in early breast cancer. *JNCI* 83:1450–1459.

19. Love, et al. 1988. Bone mineral density in women with breast cancer treated with adjuvant tamoxifen for at least two years. *Breast Cancer Res Treat* 12:279–302.

20. Gotfredson, et al. 1984. The effect of tamoxifen on bone mineral content in premenopausal women with breast cancer. *Cancer* 53:853–857.

21. Fentiman, et al. 1989. Bone mineral content of women receiving tamoxifen for mastalgia. *Br J Cancer* 60:262–264.

22. Powles, et al. 1989. A pilot trial to evaluate the acute toxicity and feasibility of tamoxifen for prevention of breast cancer. *Br J Cancer* 60:126–131.

23. Rossner, et al. 1984. Serum lipoproteins and proteins after breast cancer surgery and effects of tamoxifen. *Atherosclerosis* 52:339–346.

24. Love, et al. 1991. The effects of tamoxifen on cardiovascular risk factors in postmenopausal women. *Ann Intern Med* 115:860–864.

25. Bruning, et al. 1988. Tamoxifen, serum lipoproteins and cardiovascular risk. *Br J Cancer* 58:497–499.

26. *FDA Adverse Reaction Reports.* 1987–1990.

27. Fentiman and Powles. 1987. Tamoxifen and benign breast problems. *Lancet i* (November 7): 1070–1071.

28. Cuzick, et al. 1986. The prevention of breast cancer. *Lancet* (January 11):83–86.

29. Powles. 1992. The case for clinical trials of tamoxifen for prevention of breast cancer. *Lancet* 340:1145–1145–1147.

30. Special report: Breast Cancer Prevention Trial. 1992. *Oncology Bulletin.* (June) 4–19.

31. Symposium on Early Lesions and the Development of Epithelial Cancer. 1976. *Cancer Research.* 36:2475–2706.

32. Sporn. 1993. Chemoprevention of cancer. *Lancet* (June) 342:1211–1213.

Chapter 3
An Overview of Risk Factors

1. The National Academy of Sciences. 1982. *Nutrition, diet, and cancer.*

2. Wynder, E.L., and G.B. Gori. 1977. Contribution of the environment to cancer incidence: An epidemiologic exercise. *J Natl Cancer Inst* 58:825.

3. Workshop on Fat and Cancer. September 1981. Supplement to *Cancer Res* 41(9):3677.

4. Mulvihill, J.J. 1977. Genetic repertory of human neoplasia. In *Genetics of human cancer*, ed. J.J. Mulvihill, R.W. Miller, and J.F. Fraumeni. New York: Raven Press, 137.

5. Armstrong, B., and R. Doll. 1975. Environmental factors and cancer incidence and mortality in different countries, with special reference to dietary practices. *Intl J Cancer* 15:617.

6. Bjarnason, O., N. Day, G. Snaedal, and H. Tilinuis. 1974. The effect of year of birth on the breast cancer age incidence curve in Iceland. *Intl J Cancer* 13:689.

7. Miller, A.B. 1980. Nutrition and cancer. *Prev Med* 9:189.

8. Eskin, B.A. 1978. Iodine and mammary cancer. In *Inorganic and nutrition aspects of cancer*, ed. G.H. Schrauzer. New York: Plenum Press, 293–304.

9. Upton, A.C. 1980. Future directions in cancer prevention. *Prev Med* 9:309.

10. Alpert, M.E., M.S.R. Hutt, G.N. Wogan, et al. 1971. Association between aflatoxin content of food and hepatoma frequency in Uganda. *Cancer* 28:253.

11. Shank, R.C., G.N. Wogan, J.B. Gibson, et al. 1972. Dietary aflatoxins and human liver cancer.II. Aflatoxins in market foods and foodstuffs of Thailand and Hong Kong. *Food Cosmet Toxicol* 10:61.

12. MacMahon, B., S. Yen, D. Trichopoulos, et al. 1981. Coffee and cancer of the pancreas. *NEJM* 304:630.

13. Feinstein, A.R., R.I. Horwitz, W.O. Spitzer, and R.N. Battista. 1981. Coffee and pancreatic cancer. *JAMA* 246:957.

14. Goldstein, H.R. 1982. No association found between coffee and cancer of the pancreas. *NEJM* 306:997.

15. Tomatis, L., C. Agthe, H. Bartsch, et al. Evaluation of the carcinogenicity of chemicals: A review of the monograph program of the International Agency for Research on Cancer. *Cancer Res* 38:877.

16. Wattenberg, L.W. 1978. Inhibitors of chemical carcinogenesis. *Adv Cancer Res* 26:197.

17. Pierce, R.C., and M. Katz. 1975. Dependency of polynuclear aromatic hydrocarbons on size distribution of atmospheric aerosols. *Environ Sci Technol* 9:347.

18. U.S. Environmental Protection Agency. 1975. Preliminary assessment of suspected carcinogens in drinking water. Report to Congress. Environmental Protection Agency, Washington, D.C.

19. Harris, R.H., T. Page, and N.A. Reiches. 1977. Carcinogenic hazards of organic chemicals in drinking water. In *Book A. Incidence of cancer in humans*, ed. H.H. Hiatt, et al. Cold Spring Harbor Lab.

20. Gardner, M.J., et al. 1990. Results of case-control study of leukemia and lymphoma among young people near Sellafield nuclear plant in West Cumbria. *BMJ* 300:423–29.

21. Wing, S., et al. 1991. Mortality among workers at Oak Ridge National Laboratory: Evidence of radiation effects in follow-up through 1984. *JAMA* 265:1397–1408.

22. Jablon, S., et al. 1991. Cancer in populations living near nuclear facilities. *JAMA* 265:1403–8.

23. International Agency for Research on Cancer. 1980. Annual Report. World Health Organization. Lyon, France.

24. Fox, A.J., E. Lynge, and H. Malker. 1982. Lung cancer in butchers. *Lancet* i:156.

25. Johnson, E.S., and H.R. Fischman. 1982. Cancer mortality among butchers and slaughterhouse workers. *Lancet* i:913.

26. Miller, D.G. 1980. On the nature of susceptibility to cancer. *Cancer* 46:1307.

27. Walford, R.L. 1969. *The immunological theory of aging*. Munksgaard, Copenhagen.

28. Kahn, H.A. 1966. The Dorn study of smoking and mortality among U.S. veterans: Report on eight and one-half years of observation. In *Epidemiological study of cancer and other chronic diseases*. Natl. Cancer Inst. Mono. 19. Washington, D.C. U.S. Government Printing Office. 1.

29. Benditt, E.P., and J.M. Benditt. 1973. Evidence for a monoclonal origin of human atherosclerotic plaques. *Proc Natl Acad Sci USA* 70:1753.
30. Shu, H.P., and A.V. Nichols. 1979. Benzo(a)pyrene uptake by human plasma lipoproteins *in vitro*. *Cancer Res* 39:1224.
31. Pero, R.W., C. Bryngelsson, F. Mitelman, et al. 1976. High blood pressure related to carcinogen induced unscheduled DNA synthesis, DNA carcinogen binding, and chromosomal aberrations in human lymphocytes. *Proc Natl Acad Sci USA* 73:2496.
32. de Waard, F., E.A. Banders-van Halewijn, and J. Huizinga. 1964. The bimodal age distribution of patients with mammary cancer. *Cancer* 17:141.
33. Dyer, A.R., J. Stamler, A.M. Berkson, et al. 1975. High blood pressure: A risk factor for cancer mortality. *Lancet* i:1051.
34. Paffenbarger, R.S., E. Fasal, M.E. Simmons, et al. 1977. Cancer risk as related to use of oral contraceptives during fertile years. *Cancer Res* 39:1887.
35. Pike, M.C., H.A. Edmondson, B. Benton, et al. 1977. Origins of human cancer. In *Book A. Incidence of cancer in humans*. Cold Spring Harbor Lab., 423–27.
36. Cotton, T., et al. 1993. Breast cancer in mothers prescribed DES in pregnancy. *JAMA* 269(16):2096–2100.
37. Wobbes, T., H.S. Koops, and J. Oldhoff. 1980. The relation between testicular tumors, undescended testes, and inguinal hernias. *J Surg Onc* 14:45.
38. IARC. 1994. Hepatitis viruses: IARC monographs on the evaluation of carcinogenic risks to humans (vol. 59). Geneva: WHO Publications, 286.
39. IARC. 1994. Schistosomes, liver flukes and *Helicobacter pylori*: IARC monographs on the evaluation of carcinogenic risks to humans (vol. 61). Geneva: WHO Publications, 270.
40. Sharp, D.W. 1993. Gastric cancer: A new role for *Helicobacter pylori*? *Science Watch* 4 (7):5.
41. Sharp, D.W. 1995. Worms, spirals, flukes as carcinogens. *Lancet* 345:403–404.

Chapter 4
Nutrition, Immunity, and Cancer

1. Cannon, P.R. 1942. Antibodies and protein reserves. *J Immunol* 44:107.
2. Chandra, R. 1989. *Nutrition and immunology*. New York: Alan R. Liss, Inc. Press.
3. Rous, P. 1914. The influence of diet on transplanted and spontaneous mouse tumors. *J Exp Med* 20:433.
4. Tannenbaum, A. 1940. The initiation and growth of tumors. Introduction I. Effects of underfeeding. *Am J Cancer* 38:335.
5. Simone, C.B., and P.A. Henkart. 1980. Permeability changes induced in erythrocyte ghost targets by antibody-dependent cytotoxic effector cells: Evidence for membrane pores. *J Immunol* 124:954.
6. Burnet, F.M. 1970. *Immunological surveillance*. Oxford: Pergamon Press.
7. Kersey, J.H., G.D. Spector, and R.A. Good. 1973. Primary immunodeficiency diseases and cancer: The immunodeficiency-cancer registry. *Intl J Cancer* 12:333.
8. Spector, G.D., G.S. Perry III, R.A. Good, and J.H. Kersey. 1978. Immunodeficiency diseases and malignancy. In *The immunopathology of lymphoreticular neoplasms*, ed. J.J. Twomey, and R.A. Good. New York: Plenum Publishing, 203.
9. Penn, I. 1970. *Malignant tumors in organ transplant recipients*. New York: Springer-Verlag.
10. Birkeland, S.A., E. Kemp, and M. Hauge. 1975. Renal transplantation and cancer. The Scandia transplant material. *Tissue Antigens* 6:28.
11. Chandra, R. *Nutrition and immunology*.
12. Dworsky, et al. 1983. *JNCI* 71:265.
13. Delafuente, et al. 1988. *J Am Geriat Soc* 36:733.
14. Lichenstein, et al. 1982. *J Am Geriat Soc* 30:447.
15. Rosenkoetter, et al. 1983. *Cell Immunol* 77:395.
16. Halgren, et al. 1983. *J Immunol* 131:191.

17. Delafuente, and Panush. 1990. Potential of drug-related immunoenhancement of the geriatric patient. *Geriatric Med* 9 (4):32–40.
18. Aschekenasy, A. 1975. Dietary protein and amino acids in leucopoiesis. *World Rev Nutri Diet* 21:152.
19. Jose, D.G., and R.A. Good. 1971. Absence of enhancing antibody in cell-mediated immunity to tumor homografts in protein deficient rats. *Nature* 231:807.
20. Passwell, J.H., M.W. Steward, and J.F. Soothill. 1974. The effects of protein malnutrition on macrophage function and the amount and affinity of antibody response. *Clin Exp Immunol* 17:491.
21. Van Oss, C.J. 1971. Influence of glucose levels on the *in vitro* phagocytosis of bacteria by human neutrophils. *Infect Immunol* 4:54.
22. Perille, P.E., J.P. Nolan, and S.C. Finch. 1972. Studies of the resistance to infection in diabetes mellitus: Local exudative cellular response. *J Lab Clin Med* 59:1008.
23. Bagdade, J.D., R.K. Root, and R.J. Bulger. 1974. Impaired leukocyte function in patients with poorly controlled diabetes. *Diabetes* 23:9.
24. Stuart, A.E., and A.E. Davidson. 1976. Effect of simple lipids on antibody formation after ingestion of foreign red cells. *J Pathol Bacteriol* 87:305.
25. Santiago-Delpin, E.A., and J. Szepsenwol. 1977. Prolonged survival of skin and tumor allografts in mice on high fat diets. *J Natl Cancer Inst* 59:459.
26. DiLuzio, N.R., and W.R. Wooles. 1964. Depression of phagocytic activity and immune response by methyl palmitate. *Am J Physiol* 206:939.
27. Jeevan, A., and M.L. Kripke. 1993. Ozone depletion and the immune system. *Lancet* 342:1159–1160.
28. Cooper, K.D., et al. 1992. UV exposure reduces immunization rate and promotes tolerance to epicutaneous antigens in humans. *Proc Natl Acad Sci USA* 89:8497–8501.
29. Vermeer, M., et al. 1991. Effects of ultraviolet B light on cutaneous immune responses of humans with deeply pigmented skin. *J Invest Dermatol* 97:729–734.
30. Yoshikawa, T., et al. 1990. Susceptibility to effects of UVB radiation on induction of contact hypersensitivity as a risk factor for skin cancer in man. *J Invest Dermatol* 95:530–536.
31. Peters, E., et al. 1993. Vitamin C supplementation reduces incidence of post-race symptoms of upper respiratory tract infection in ultramarathon runners. *Am J Clin Nutr* 57:170–171.
32. Heath, G.W. 1991. Exercise and incidence of upper respiratory tract infections. *Med Sci Sports Exerc* 23:152–157.

Chapter 5
Antioxidants and Other Cancer-Fighting Nutrients

1. Pietrzik, K. 1985. Concept of borderline vitamin deficiencies. *Int J Vit Nutr Res Suppl* 27:61–73.
2. Brin, M. 1972. Dilemma of marginal vitamin deficiency. *Proc 9th Int Cong Nutrition, Mexico* 4:102–115.
3. U.S. Department of HEW. 1974. HANES: Health and Nutrition Examination Survey, Publication No. 74-1219-1. Rockville, Maryland.
4. U.S. Department of HEW. 1970. Ten State Nutrition Survey, Publication No. 72-8130 to 8134. Washington, D.C.
5. Baker, H., and O. Frank. 1985. Sub-clinical vitamin deficits in various age groups. *Int J Vit Nutr Res Suppl* 27:47–59.
6. Christakis, G. 1980. *Socio-economic factors of nutrition in New York City Schools.* New York: Elsiever Publishing.
7. McGanity, W. 1980. *Teenage nutrition in Miami: Threat or threshold to a healthy adult life.* New York, New York.
8. Brin, M., M.V. Dibble, A. Peel, E. McMullen, A. Bourquin, and N. Chen. 1965. Some preliminary findings on the nutritional status of the aged in Onondaga County, NY. *Am J Clin Nutr* 17:240–58.
9. Brin, M., S.H. Schwartzberg, and D. Arthur-Davies. 1964. A vitamin evaluation program as applied to 10 elderly residents in a community home for the aged. *J Am Geriat So* 12:493,99.

10. Davis, T.R.A., S.N. Gershoff, and D.F. Gamble. 1969. Review of studies of vitamin and mineral nutrition in the United States (1950—1968). *J Nutr Edn* suppl. 1:410–57.

11. Dibble, M.V., M. Brin, E. McMullen, A. Peel, and N. Chen. 1965. Some preliminary findings on the nutritional status of Syracuse and Onondaga County, New York Junior High School children. *Am J Clin Nutr* 17:218–239.

12. Thiele, V.F., M. Brin, and M.V. Dibble. 1968. Preliminary biochemical findings in Negro migrant workers at King Ferry, New York. *Am J Clin Nutr* 21:1229–38.

13. Vitamins and Health, Man and Molecules. 1977. American Chemical Society, Script #852, Washington, D.C. (April).

14. Food and Nutrition Board. 1974. Proposed fortification policy for cereal-grain products. Divsn. of Biol. Sci. Ass. of Life Sci., Natl. Research Council, Nat'l. Acad. of Sci. Washington, D.C.

15. U.S. Dept. of Agriculture. 1980. USDA Household Food Consumption Survey. Family Economics Research Group. Science and Education Administration. Hyattsville, Maryland.

16. U.S. Dept. of Agriculture, Human Nutrition Information Service, 1985. Nationwide Food Consumption Survey, Continuing Survey of Food Intakes by Individuals. Women 19–50 Years and Their Children 1–5 Years, 4 Days. NFCS, CSFII Report No. 85-4.

17. Ten State Nutrition Survey, Publ. No. 72-8130 to 8134. 1970. Washington, D.C.: United States Dept. of Health, Education, and Welfare.

18. Brin, M. Marginal deficiency and immunocompetence. Presented at *American Chemical Society Symposium*, Las Vegas, NV (Aug. 1980).

19. Schumann, I. Preoperative measures to promote wound healing. *Nursing Cl. of N.A.* 14 (Dec. 1979):4.

20. Statistical Abstracts of the U.S., 1980. U.S. Dept. of Commerce, Bureau of the Census, Washington, D.C.

21. Sheils, M. 1983. Portrait of America. *Newsweek* Special Report (Jan 17).

22. U.S. Dept. of Agriculture. Nationwide Food Consumption Survey.

23. Pao, E.M., and S.M. Mickle. Nutrients from meals and snacks consumed by individuals. Family Economics Review, U.S. Dept. of Agriculture, Science and Education Administration, Beltsville, MD.

24. Sheils, M. Portrait of America.

25. Pao and Mickle. Nutrients from meals and snacks consumed by individuals.

26. Ideas for better eating. 1981. Menus and recipes to make use of the dietary guidelines. Science and Education Administration/Human Nutrition. U.S. Dept. of Agriculture (January).

27. Dietary intake source data. United States 1976-80. Data from the National Health Survey, Series 11, No. 231, DHHS Publication No. (PHS) 83-1681 (March 1983).

28. U.S. Dept. of Agriculture. Nationwide Food Consumption Survey.

29. Leevy, C.M., L. Cardi, O. Frank, et al. 1965. Incidence and significance of hypovitaminemia in a randomly selected municipal hospital population. *Am J Clin Nutr* 17:259.

30. Sheils, M. Portrait of America.

31. Pao, E. and S. Mickle. 1981. Problem nutrients in the United States. *Food Technology* (September).

32. Krehl, W.A. 1981. The role of nutrition in preventing disease. Presented at Davidson Conference Center for Continuing Education. Univ. of Southern California School of Dentistry. (Feb. 29).

33. Roe, D. 1976. *Drug-induced nutritional deficiencies*. Connecticut: The AVI Publishing Company, Inc.

34. Leevy, C.M., and H. Baker. 1968. Vitamins and alcoholism. *Am J Clin Nutr* 21:11.

35. Lieber, C.S. 1975. Alcohol and malnutrition in the pathogenesis of liver disease and nutrition. Veterans Administration Hospital and Department of Medicine. Mt. Sinai School of Medicine of the City University of New York, Bronx, NY. (Sept.).

36. Baker, H., O. Frank, R.K. Zetterman, K.S. Rajan, W. ten Hove, and C.M.

Leevy. 1975. Inability of chronic alcholics with liver disease to use food as a source of folates, thiamine and vitamin B6. *Amer J Clin Nutr* 28:1377–1380.

37. Payne, I.R., G.H.Y. Lu, and K. Meyer. 1974. Relationships of dietary tryptophan and niacin to tryptophan metabolism in alcoholics and nonalcoholics. *Am J Clin Nutr* 27:572–579.

38. Lumeng, L., and T.K. Li. 1974. Vitamin B6 metabolism in chronic alcohol abuse. *J Clin Investigation* 53:57–61.

39. Hines, J.D. and D.H. Cowan. 1970. Studies on the pathogenesis of alcohol-induced sideroblastic bone-marrow abnormalities. *NEJM* 238:9.

40. Leevy, C.M., H. Baker, W. ten Hove, O. Frank, and G.R. Cherrick. 1965. B-complex vitamins in liver disease of the alcoholic. *Amer J Clin Nutr* 16:4.

41. Lieber, C.S., E. Baraona, M.A. Leo, and A. Garro. 1987. Metabolism and metabolic effects of ethanol, including interaction with drugs, carcinogens and nutrition. *Mutat Res* 186:201–233.

42. Halsted, C.H., and C. Heise. 1987. Ethanol and vitamin metabolism. *Pharmac Ther* 34:453–464.

43. Aoki, K., Y. Ito, R. Sasaki, M. Ohtani, N. Hamajima, and A. Asano. 1987. Smoking, alcohol drinking and serum carotenoids levels. *Jpn J Cancer Res Gann* 78:1049–1056.

44. Fazio, V., D.M. Flint, and M.L. Wahlqvist. 1981. Acute effects of alcohol on plasma ascorbic acid in healthy subjects. *Am J Clin Nutr* 34:2394–2396.

45. Pelletier, O. 1975. Vitamin C and cigarette smokers. Second Conference on Vitamin C. *Ann NY Acad Sci* 258:156–166.

46. U.S. Department of Health, Education and Welfare. The health consequences of smoking. January 1973.

47. Hornig, D.H., and B.E. Glatthaar. 1985. Vitamin C and smoking: Increased requirement of smokers. *Int J Vit Nutr Res Suppl* 27:139–155.

48. Menkes, M.S., G.W. Constock, J.P. Vuilleumier, K.J. Helsing, A.A. Rider, and R. Brookmeyer. 1986. Vitamin C is lower in smokers. *NEJM* 315:1250–4.

49. Chow, C.K., R.R. Thacker, C. Changchit, R.B. Bridges, S.R. Rehm, J. Humble, and J. Turbek. 1986. Lower levels of vitamin C and carotenes in plasma of cigarette smokers. *J Am Coll Nutr* 5:305–312.

50. Witter, F.R., D.A. Blake, R. Baumgardner, E.D. Mellits and J.R. Niebyl. 1982. Folate, carotene, and smoking. *Am J Obstet Gynecol* 144:857.

51. Gerster, H. 1987. Beta-carotene and smoking. *J Nutr Growth Cancer* 4:45–49.

52. Pacht, E.R., H. Kaseki, J.R. Mohammed, D.G. Cornwell, and W.B. Davis. 1986. Deficiency of vitamin E in the alveolar fluid of cigarette smokers: Influence on alveolar macrophage cytotoxicity. *J Clin Invest* 77:789–796.

53. Serfontein, W.J., J. B. Ubbink, L.S. DeVilliers, and P.J. Becker. 1986. Depressed plasma pyridoxal-5'-phosphate levels in tobacco-smoking men. *Atherosclerosis* 59:341–346.

54. Who's dieting and why. 1978. A.C. Nielsen Co.

55. Welsh, S.O., and R.M. Marston. 1982. Review of trends in food used in the United States, 1909 to 1980. *J A Dietetic Assn* (August 1982).

56. Kasper H. 1964. Vitamins in prevention and therapy: Recent findings in vitamin research. Fortschritte der Medizin 82:22.

57. Horo, E.H., M. Brin, and W.W. Faloon. Fasting in obesity: Thiamine depletion as measured by erythrocyte activity changes. *The Archives of Internal Medicine* 117:175–81.

58. Fisher, M.C. and P.A. Lachance. 1985. Nutrition evaluation of published weight-reducing diets. *J Am Diet Assoc* 85:450–454.

59. Bristrian, Bruce, et al. 1976. Prevalence of malnutrition in general medical patients. *JAMA* 235 (April 12) 15–18.

60. Lemoine, et al. 1980. Vitamin B1, B2, B6 and status in hospital inpatients. *Am J Clin Nutr* (December): 33–37.

61. Leevy, et al. 1965. Incidence and significance of hypovitaminemia in a randomly selected municipal hospital population. *Amer J Clin Nutr* (Oct. 17).

62. Driezen, S. 1979. Nutrition and the

immune response–a review. *Internat J Vit Nur Res*, 49.

63. Beisel, et al. 1981. Single-nutrient effects on immunologic functions. *JAMA* (Jan. 2) 245 (1).

64. Leevy C.M. 1972. Vitamin therapy: It means more than simply giving vitamins. *Drug Therapy* (February).

65. Pollack, S.V. 1979. Nutritional factors affecting wound healing. *J Dermatol Surg Oncol* (August):5:8.

66. Kaminsky, M.V. and Allan Windborn. 1978. Nutritional assessment guide. Midwest Nutrition, Educational and Research Foundation, Inc.

67. Pao and Mickle. Problem nutrients in the United States.

68. Nationwide Food Consumption Survey, Spring 1980. U.S. Dept of Agriculture, Science and Education Administration, Beltsville, MD.

69. Dietary intake source data. United States 1976–80.

70. Kirsch, A. and W.R. Bidlack. 1987. Nutrition and the elderly: Vitamin status and efficacy of supplementation. *Nutr* 3:305–314.

71. Baker, H., S.P. Jaslow, and O. Frank. 1978. Severe impairment of dietary folate utilization in the elderly. *J Am Geriatrics Soc* 26:218–221.

72. Pao and Mickle. Problem nutrients in the United States.

73. U.S. Department of Agriculture Nationwide Food Consumption Survey.

74. First Health and Nutrition Examination Survey. 1971. U.S. Public Health Service. Health Resources Administration. U.S. Dept. of Health, 72.

75. Connelly, T.J., A. Becker, and J.W. McDonald. 1982. Bachelor scurvy. *Intl J Dermatol* 21:209–211.

76. Schorah, C.J. 1978. Inapproprate vitamin C reserves: Their frequency and significance in an urban population. In *The importance of vitamins to health*, ed. T.G. Taylor. Lancaster, England: MTP Press, 61–72.

77. Garry, P.J., J.S. Goodwin, W.C. Hunt, E.M. Hooper, and A.G. Leonard. 1982. Nutritional status in a healthy elderly population: Dietary and supplemental intakes. *Am J Clin Nutr* 36:319–331.

78. Pao and Mickle. Problem nutrients in the United States.

79. Clark, A.J., S. Mossholder, and R. Gates. 1987. Folacin status in adolescent females. *Am J Clin Nutr* 46:302–306.

80. Sumner, S.K., M. Liebman, and L.M. Wakefield. 1987. Vitamin A status of adolescent girls. *Nutr Rep Intl* 35:423–431.

81. Lee, C.J. 1978. Nutritional status of selected teenagers in Kentucky. *Am J Clin Nutr* 31:1453–1464.

82. Saito, N., M. Kimura, A. Kuchiba, and Y. Itokawa. 1987. Blood thiamine levels in outpatients with diabetes mellitus. *J Nutr Sci Vitaminol* 33:421–430.

83. Mooradian, A.D., and J.E. Morley. 1987. Micronutrient status in diabetes mellitus. *Am J Clin Nutr* 45:877–895.

84. Pao and Mickle. Problem nutrients in the United States.

85. Vobecky, J.S., and J. Vobecky. 1988. Vitamin status of women during pregnancy. In *Vitamins and minerals in pregnancy and lactation*, ed. H. Berger. Nestle Nutrition Workshop Series, Vol. 16. Nestle Ltd. New York: Vevey/Raven Press, Ltd., 109–111.

86. Shenai, J.P., F. Chytil, A. Jhaveri, and M.T. Stahlman. 1981. Plasma vitamin A and retinol-binding protein in premature and term neonates. *J Pediatr* 99:302–305.

87. Heinonen, K., I. Mononen, T. Mononen, M. Parviainen, I. Penttila, and K. Launiala. 1986. Plasma vitamin C levels are low in premature infants fed human milk. *Am J Clin Nutr* 43:923–924.

88. Vitamin E status of premature infants. 1986. *Nutr Rev* 44:166–167.

89. Dietary intake source data. United States 1976–80.

90. Pao and Mickle. Problem nutrients in the United States.

91. First Health and Nutrition Examination Survey. U.S. Public Health Service.

92. Pao and Mickle. Problem nutrients in the United States.

93. Peterkin, B.B., R.L. Kerr, and M.Y. Hama. Nutritional adequacy of diets

of low income households. *J Nut Ed* 14(3):102.

94. Roe, D.A. 1985. *Drug-Induced Nutritional Deficiencies*, 2nd ed. Westport, CT: AVI Publishing Company, Inc., 1–87.

95. Brin, M. 1978. Drugs and environmental chemicals in relation to vitamin needs. In *Nutrition and Drug Interrelations*, ed. J.N. Hathcock and J. Coon. New York: Academic Press, 131–150.

96. Driskell, J.A., J.M. Geders, and M.C. Urban. 1976. Vitamin B6 status of young men, women, and women using oral contraceptives. *J Lab Clin Med* 87:813–821.

97. Prasad, A.S., K.Y. Lei, D. Oberleas, K.S. Moghissi, and J.C. Stryker. 1975. Effect of oral contraceptive agents on nutrients: II. Vitamins. *Am J Clin Nutr* 28:385–391.

98. Rivers, J.M., and M.M. Devine. 1972. Plasma ascorbic acid concentrations and oral contraceptives. *Am J Clin Nutr* 25:684–689.

99. Truswell, A.S. 1985. Drugs affecting nutritional state. *Br Med J* 291:1333–1337.

100. Benton and Roberts. 1988. Effect of vitamin and mineral supplementation on intelligence of a sample of school children. *Lancet* (Jan. 23):140–144.

101. Campbell, et al. 1988. Vitamins, minerals, and I.Q. *Lancet* (Sept 24):744–745.

102. Letters to the Editor. 1988. Vitamin/mineral supplementation and non-verbal intelligence. *Lancet* (Feb. 20):407–409.

103. Grantham-McGregor, S.M., et al. 1991. Nutritional supplementation, psychosocial stimulation, and mental development of stunted children: The Jamaican study. *Lancet* 338:1–5.

104. Brown, et al. 1972. *J Pediatrics* 81:714.

105. Webb and Oski. 1973. Iron deficiency and IQ. *J Pediatr* 82:827–30.

106. Grantham-McGregor, et al. Nutritional supplementation, psychosocial stimulation, and mental development.

107. Brown, et al. 1972.

108. Benton, et al. 1987. Glucose improves attention and reaction. *Biol Psychol* 24:95–100.

109. Benton. 1981. Influence of vitamin C on psychological testing. *Psychopharmacology* 75:98–99.

110. Pfeiffer, C., and E. Braverman. 1982. Zinc, the brain and behavior. *Biol Psychiat* 17:513–31.

111. Brin. 1973. Behavioral effects of protein and energy deficits. DHEW (NIH) publication No.79:1966. Washington, D.C.

112. Godfrey, P., et al. 1990. Enhancement of recovery from psychiatric illness by methylfolate. *Lancet* 336:392–394.

113. Shibata, A., et al. 1992. Intake of vegetables, fruits, beta-carotene, vitamin C, and vitamin supplements and cancer incidence among the elderly: A prospective study. *Br J Cancer* 66(4):673–679.

114. Barone, J., et al. 1992. Vitamin supplement use and risk for oral and esophageal cancer. *Nutr Cancer* 18(1):31–41.

115. Chen, J., et al. 1992. Antioxidant status and cancer mortality in China. *Int J Epidemiol* 21(4):625–635.

116. Blot, W.J., et al. 1993. Nutrition intervention trials in Linxian, China: Supplementation with specific vitamin-mineral combinations, cancer incidence, and disease specific mortality in the general population. *J Natl Cancer Inst* 85(18):1483–1492.

117. Smigel, K. 1993. Dietary supplements reduce cancer deaths in China. *J Natl Cancer Inst* 85(18):1448–1450.

118. Knekt, P., et al. 1991. Dietary antioxidants and the risk of lung cancer. *Am J Epidemiol* 134(5):471–479.

119. Stahelin, H.B., et al. 1991. Plasma antioxidant vitamins and subsequent cancer mortality in the 12-year follow up of the prospective Basel Study. *Am J Epidemiol* 133(8):766–775.

120. LeMarchand, L., et al. 1993. Intake of specific carotenoids and lung cancer risk. *Cancer Epidemiol Biomarkers and Prevention* 2(3):183–187.

121. Punnonen, R., et al. 1993. Activities of antioxidant enzymes and lipid per-

oxidation in endometrial cancer. *Eur J Cancer* 29a(2):266–269.

122. Palan, P.R., et al. 1992. Beta-carotene levels in exfoliated cervical vaginal epithelial cells in cervical intra-epithelial neoplasia and cervical cancer. *Am J Obstet-Gynecol* 167(6):1899–1903.

123. Hunter, D.J., et al. 1993. A prospective study of the intake of vitamins C, E, and A and the risk of breast cancer. *NEJM* 329:234–240.

124. Ennever, F.K. and Pasket. 1993. Vitamins and breast cancer. *NEJM* 329:1579–1580.

125. Jaakkola, et al. 1992. Treatment with antioxidant and other nutrients in combination with chemotherapy and irradiation therapy in patients with small cell lung cancer. *Anticancer Research* 12(3):599–606.

126. Gridley, G., et al. 1992. Vitamin supplement use and reduced risk of oral and pharyngeal cancer. *Am J Epidemiol* 135:1083–1092.

127. Zheng, W., et al. 1993. Serum micronutrients and the subsequent risk of oral and pharyngeal cancer. *Cancer Res* 53:795–798.

128. Li, J.Y., et al. 1993. Nutrition intervention trials in Linxian, China: Multiple vitamin and mineral supplementation, cancer incidence, and disease-specific mortality among adults with esophageal dysplasia. *J Natl Cancer Inst* 85:1492–1498.

129. Li, J.Y., et al. 1993. Nutrition intervention trials in Linxian, China.

130. Lippman, S., et al. 1993. Comparison of low dose isotretinoin with beta-carotene to prevent oral carcinogenesis. *NEJM* 328:15–20.

131. Toma, S., et al. 1992. Treatment of oral leukoplakia with beta-carotene. *Oncology* 49:77–81.

132. Benner, S., et al. 1993. Regression of oral leukoplakia with alpha-tocopherol: A community clinical oncology program chemoprevention study. *JNCI* 85:44–47.

133. Benner, and Hong. 1993. Clinical chemoprevention: developing a cancer prevention strategy (Editorial). *JNCI* 85:1446–1447.

134. Paganelli, et al. 1992. Effect of vitamin A, C, and E supplementation on rectal cell proliferation in patients with colorectal adenomas. *JNCI* 84:47–51.

135. Stampher, M., et al. 1993. Vitamin E consumption and the risk of coronary disease in women. *NEJM* 328:1444–1449.

136. Rimm, E., et al. 1993. Vitamin E consumption and the risk of coronary heart disease in men. *NEJM* 328:1450–1456.

137. Steinberg, D. 1993 Antioxidant vitamins and coronary heart disease (Editorial). *NEJM* 328:1487–1489.

138. Dieber-Rotheneder, et al. 1991. Effect of oral supplementation with D-alpha-tocopherol on the vitamin E content of human low-density lipoproteins and its oxidation resistance. *J Lipid Res* 32:1325–1332.

139. Enstrom, et al. 1992. Vitamin C intake and mortality among a sample of the United States population. *Epidemiology* 3(3):194–202.

140. Graziano, et al. 1990. Beta-carotene therapy for chronic stable angina. *Circulation* 82 (Suppl III):201.

141. Gey, et al. 1987. Plasma levels of antioxidant vitamins in relation to ischemic heart disease and cancer. *Am J Clin Nutr* 45 (Suppl):1368–1377.

142. Gey, et al. 1991. Inverse correlation between plasma vitamin E and mortality from ischemic heart disease in cross-cultural epidemiology. *Am J Clin Nutr* 53 (Suppl 1):326S–334S.

143. Gey, et al. 1993. Poor plasma status of carotene and vitamin C is associated with higher mortality from ischemic heart disease and stroke: Basel Prospective Study. *Clin Investig* 71(1):3–6.

144. Jialal and Grundy. 1992. Effect of dietary supplementation with alpha-tocopherol on the oxidative modification of low density lipoprotein. *J Lipid Res* 33:899–906.

145. Kok, et al. 1987. Serum selenium, vitamin antioxidants, and cardiovascular mortality: A 9 year follow-up study in the Netherlands. *Am J Clin Nutr* 45:462–468.

146. Kardinal, et al. 1993. Antioxidants in adipose tissue and risk of myocardial infarction: the EURAMIC study. *Lancet* 342:1379–1382.

147. Hertog, et al. 1993. Dietary antioxidant flavonoids and risk of coronary heart disease: the Zutphen Elderly Study. *Lancet* 342:1007–1011.

148. Enstrom, et al. 1992. Vitamin C intake and mortality among a sample of the U.S. population. *Epidemiology* 3:194–202.

149. Block, G. 1992. Vitamin C and reduced mortality. *Epidemiology* 3:189–191.

150. Regnstrom, J., et al. 1992. Susceptibility to low-density lipoprotein oxidation and coronary atherosclerosis in man. *Lancet* 339:1183–1186.

151. Princen, et al. 1992. Supplementation with vitamin E but not beta-carotene *in vivo* protects low-density lipoprotein from lipid peroxidation *in vitro*. *Arteriosclerosis & Thrombosis* 12:554–562.

152. Reaven, et al. 1993. Effect of dietary antioxidant combinations in humans. Protection of LDL by vitamin E but not by beta-carotene. *Arteriosclerosis & Thrombosis* 13(4): 590–600.

153. Riemersma, et al. 1991. Risk of angina pectoris and plasma concentrations of vitamins A, C, and E and carotene. *Lancet* 337:1–5.

154. Salonen, et al. 1985. Serum fatty acids, apolipoproteins, selenium, and vitamin antioxidants and the risk of death from coronary artery disease. *Am J Cardiol* 56:226–231.

155. Steinberg, et al. 1989. Beyond cholesterol: modifications of low-density lipoprotein that increase its atherogenicity. *NEJM* 320:915–924.

156. Trout. 1991. Vitamin C and cardiovascular risk factors. *Am J Clin Nutr* 53:322S–325S.

157. Luc and Fruchart. 1991. Oxidation of lipoproteins and atherosclerosis. *Am J Clin Nutr* 53:206S–209S.

158. Salonen, et al. 1988. Relationship of serum selenium and antioxidants to plasma lipoproteins, platelet aggregability, and prevalent ischaemic heart disease in eastern Finnish men. *Atherosclerosis* 70:155–160.

159. Murphy, et al. 1992. Antioxidant depletion in aortic cross clamping ischemia. *Free Radical Biology and Medicine* 13:95–100.

160. Simone, C.B. 1992. *Cancer and Nutrition: A Ten-Point Plan to Reduce Your Risk of Getting Cancer*. Garden City Park, NY: Avery Publishing Group, 101–104.

161. Hemila. 1991. Vitamin C and lowering of blood pressure. *J Hypertension* 9:1076–1078.

162. Riemersma, et al. 1991. Risk of angina pectoris and concentrations of vitamins A, C, E, and carotene. *Lancet* 337:1–5.

163. Sperduto, R., et al. 1993. Linxian cataract studies. Two nutritional intervention trials. *Arch Ophthalmol* 111:1246–1253.

164. Hankinson, S., et al. 1992. Nutrient intake and cataract extraction in women: A prospective study. *BMJ* 305:335–339.

165. Taylor, A. 1993. Cataract: Relationships between nutrition and oxidation. *J Am Coll Nutr* 12:138–146.

166. Jacques and Chylack. 1991. Vitamin C plasma level inversely related to cataract incidence. *Am J Clin Nutr* 53:352S–355S.

167. Leske, et al. 1991. *Arch Ophthalmol* 109:244–251.

168. Seddon, J.M., et al. 1994. The use of vitamin supplements and the risk of cataract among U.S. male physicians. *Am J Public Health* 84:788–792.

169. Vitale S., et al. 1993. Plasma antioxidants and risk of cortical and nuclear cataract. *Epidemiology* 4:195–203.

170. Robertson, et al. 1989. *Ann NY Acad Sci* 570:372–382.

171. Knekt, et al. 1992. Serum antioxidant vitamins and risk of cataract. *BMJ* 305:1392–1394.

172. West, S., et al. 1994. Are antioxidants or supplements protective for age-related macular degeneration? *Arch Opthalmol* 112:222–227.

173. Seddon, J.M., et al. 1994. Vitamins, minerals, and macular degeneration. *Arch Opthalmol* 112:176–179.

174. Seddon, J.M., et al. 1994. Dietary carotenoids, vitamins A, C, and E, and advanced age-related macular degeneration. *JAMA* 272:1413–1420.

175. Shriqui, C., et al. 1992. Vitamin F in the treatment of Tardive Dyskinesia: A double blind placebo controlled study. *Am J Psychiatry* 149:391–393.

176. Bower, B. 1992. Vitamin E may ease movement disorder. *Science News* 141:351.

177. Adler, L., et al. 1994. Vitamin E treatment of Tardive Dyskinesia. *Am J Psychiatry.* (In press.)

178. Levy, S., et al. 1992. The anticonvulsant effects of vitamin E, a further evaluation. *Can J Neurol Sci* 19:201–203.

179. Evans, P., et al. 1992. Aluminosilicate induced free radical generation by murine brain glial cells *in vitro. Dementia* 3:1–6.

180. Behl, C., et al. 1992. Vitamin E protects nerve cells from amyloid protein toxicity. *Biochem Biophys Res Commun* 186:944–950.

181. Yapa, S. 1992. Detection of subclinical ascorbic deficiency in early Parkinson's disease. *Public Health* 106:393–395.

182. Fahn, S. 1992. A pilot trial of high dose alpha-Tocopherol and ascorbate in early Parkinson's disease. *Ann Neurol* 32:S128–S132.

183. The Parkinson's Study Group. 1993. Effects of Tocopherol and Deprenyl on the progression of disability in early Parkinson's Disease. *NEJM* 328:176–183.

184. Mutations in the copper-zinc containing superoxide dismutase gene are associated with Lou Gehrig's Disease. 1993. *Nutr Rev* 51:243–245.

185. Fairburn, K., et al. 1992. Alpha-Tocopherol, lipids, and lipoproteins in knee joint fluid and serum from patients with inflammatory joint disease. *Clinical Science* 83:657–664.

186. Bendich, A. 1989. *Antioxidant vitamins and their function in immune responses.* New York: Plenum Publishing Corp.

187. Bendich, A. 1988. Safety of beta-carotene. Review. *Nutr Cancer* 11:207–214.

188. Haber, S.L., and R.W. Wissler. 1962. Effect of vitamin E on carcinogenicity of methylcholanthrene. *Proc Soc Exp Biol Med* 111:774.

189. Pryor, W. 1991. Can vitamin E protect humans against the pathological effects of ozone in smog? *Am J Clin Nutr* 53:702–722.

190. London, R., G.S. Sundaram, M. Schultz, et al. 1981. Alpha-tocopherol, mammary dysplasia and steroid hormones. *Cancer Res* 4:249–253.

191. Ceriello, et al. 1991. Vitamin E reduction of protein glycosylation in diabetics. *Diabetes Care* 14:68–72.

192. Bendich and Machlin. 1988. Safety of oral intake of vitamin E: A Review. *Am J Clin Nutr* 48:612–9.

193. Vitamin E. 1989. Tenth Edition of Recommended Dietary Allowances. National Research Council. National Academy Press. Washington D.C.

194. Bendich and Machlin. Safety of oral intake of vitamin E.

195. Kamm, J.J., T. Dashman, A.H. Conney, and J.J. Burns. 1973. Protective effects of ascorbic acid on hepatotoxicity caused by sodium nitrite plus aminopyrine. *Proc Natl Acad Sci* 70:743.

196. Weisburger, J.H. 1979. Mechanism of action of diet as a carcinogen. *Cancer* 43:1987.

197. Pipkin, G.E., R. Nishimura, L. Banowsky, and J.U. Schlegel. 1967. Stabilization of urinary 3 hydroxyanthranilic acid by oral administration of L-ascorbic acid. *Proc Soc Exp Biol Med* 126:702.

198. Schlegel, J.U. 1975. Proposed uses of ascorbic acid in prevention of bladder carcinoma. *Ann NY Acad Sci* 258:423.

199. Gluttenplan, J.B. 1978. Mechanism of inhibition of ascorbate of microbial mutagenesis induced by N-nitroso compounds. *Cancer Res* 38:2018.

200. Henning, S., et al. 1991. Glutathione blood levels and other oxidant defense indices in men fed diets low in vitamin C. *J Nutr* 121:1969–1975.

201. Pauling, L. 1972. Preventive nutrition. *Medicine on the Midway* 27:15.

202. Cameron, E. 1966. In *Hyaluronidase and cancer.* New York: Pergamon Press.

203. Bendich. Antioxidant vitamins and their function in immune response.

204. Hoffer, A. 1971. Ascorbic acid and toxicity. *NEJM* 285:635.

205. Klenner, F.R. 1971. Vitamin C and toxicity. *J Appl Nutr* 23:61.

206. Shamberger, R.J., and C. Willis. 1971. Selenium distribution and human cancer mortality. *Clin Lab Sci* 2:211.

207. Shamberger and Willis. Selenium distribution and human cancer mortality.

208. Shamberger, R.J. 1966. Protection against cocarcinogenesis by antioxidants. *Experientia* 22:116.

209. Ip, C., D.K. Sinha. 1981. Enhancement of mammary tumorigenesis by dietary selenium deficiency in rats with a high polyunsaturated fat intake. *Cancer Res* 41:31.

210. Kurkela, P. 1977. The health of Finnish diet. 22nd Gen. Conf. Internat. Fed. of Agricultural Producers. Helsinki, Finland.

211. Chinese Academy of Medical Sciences. 1977. Keshan Disease Group. Beijing. Epidemiologic studies on the etiologic relationship of selenium and Keshan disease. *Chin Med J* 92:477.

212. Young, V.R., and D. Richardson. 1979. Nutrients, vitamins, and minerals in cancer prevention. Facts and fallacies. *Cancer* 43:2125.

213. Sakurai, H., and K. Tsuchiya. 1975. A tentative recommendation for the maximum daily intake of selenium. *Environ Physiol Biochem* 5:107.

214. McMahon, L.J., D.W. Montgomery, A. Guschewsky, et al. 1976. *In vitro* effects of $ZnCl_2$ on spontaneous sheep red blood cells (E) rosette formation by lymphocytes from cancer patients and normal subjects. *Immunol Commun* 5:53.

215. Frost, P., J.C. Chen, I. Rabbini, et al. 1977. The effects of zinc deficiency on the immune response. *Proc Clin Biol Res* 14:143.

216. Lotan, R. 1979. Different susceptibilities of human melanoma and breast carcinoma cell lines to retinoic acid-induced growth inhibition. *Cancer Res* 39:1014.

217. Micksche, M., C. Cerni, O. Kokron, et al. 1977. Stimulation of immune response in lung cancer patients by vitamin A therapy. *Oncology* 34:234.

218. Mettlin, C., S. Graham, and M. Swanson. 1979. Vitamin A and lung cancer. *J Nat Cancer Inst* 62:1435.

219. Krishnan, S., U.N. Bhuyan, et al. 1974. Effect of vitamin A and protein calories undernutrition on immune response. *Immunol* 27:383.

220. Genta, V.M., D.G. Kaufmann, C.C. Harris, et al. 1974. Vitamin A deficiency enhances binding of benzo(a)pyrene to tracheal epithelial DNA. *Nature* 247:48.

221. Lefebvre, P., et al. 1993. Retinoic acid stimulates regeneration of mammalian auditory hair cells. *Science* 260:692–695.

222. Rosenberg, H., and A.N. Felzman. 1974. In *The Book of Vitamin Therapy.* New York: Berkley Publishing Corp.

223. Goodman, L.S., and A. Gilman, eds. *A pharmacological basis of therapeutics.* 1977. 5th ed. New York: Macmillan.

224. Bendich and Langseth. 1989. Safety of vitamin A. *Am J Clin Nutr* 49:358-371.

225. Vitamin D: New perspective. 1987. *Lancet* (May 16):1122–1123.

226. Reitsma, et al. 1983. Regulation of myc gene expression. *Nature* 306:492–495.

227. Reichel, et al. 1989. Role of vitamin D in the endocrine system in health and disease. *NEJM* 320:980–991.

228. Garland, et al. 1989. Serum vitamin D and colon cancer—8 year prospective study. *Lancet* (Nov. 18):1176–1178.

229. Rosenberg and Felzman. In *Book of vitamin therapy.*

230. Guggenheim, K., and E. Buechler. 1946. Thiamine deficiency and susceptibility of rats and mice to infection with Salmonella typhimurium. *Proc Soc Exp Biol Med* 61:413.

231. Yunis, J. 1984. Fragile sites and predisposition to leukemia and lymphoma. *Cancer Genetics and Cytology* 12:85–88.

232. Yunis and Soreng. 1984. Constitutive fragile sites and cancer. *Science* 226:1199–1204.

233. Morgan, A.F., M. Groody, and H.E. Axelrod. 1946. Pyridoxine deficiency in dogs as affected by level of dietary protein. *Am J Physiol* 146:723.

234. National Heart, Lung, and Blood Institute: Report of the National Cholesterol Education Program: Expert panel on detection, evaluation, and treatment of high blood cholesterol levels in adults. 1988. *Arch Intern Med* 148:36–69.

235. Morgan, Groody, and Axelrod. Pyridoxine deficiency.

236. Robson, L.C., and M.R. Schwartz. 1975. Vitamin B6 deficiency and the lymphoid system. I. Effects on cellular immunity and *in vitro* incorporation of ^{3}H-uridine by small lymphocytes. *Cell Immunol* 16:145.

237. Newmark, H. 1993. Teens' low-calcium diets may increase breast cancer risk. *Oncology News Intl* 2(11):2.

238. McCarron, et al. 1985. Blood pressure response to oral calcium in persons with mild to moderate hypertension. *Ann Intern Med* 103:825.

239. Garland, et al. 1985. Dietary vitamin D and calcium and risk of colorectal cancer: A 19 year prospective study in men. *Lancet* i:307.

240. Rozen, et al. 1989. *Gut* 30:650–655.

241. Deary, et al. 1986. Calcium and Alzheimer's disease. *Lancet* (May 24):1219.

242. Curhan, G., et al. 1993. A prospective study of dietary calcium and other nutrients and the risk of symptomatic kidney stones. *NEJM* 328:833–838.

243. Dawson-Hughes, et al. 1990. A controlled trial of the effect of calcium supplementation on bone density in postmenopausal women. *NEJM* 323:878–883.

244. Prince, et al. 1991. Prevention of postmenopausal osteoporosis. *NEJM* 325:1189–1195.

245. Recommended Dietary Allowances. 1989. 10th Edition. National Research Council. National Academy Press. Washington, D.C.

246. Bigg, et al. 1981. Magnesium deficiency: Role in arrhythmias complicating acute myocardial infarction. *Med J Aust* i:346–48.

247. Heptinstall, et al. 1986. Letters to the Editor. *Lancet* (March 8):551–552.

248. Myers, Gianni, and Simone. 1982. Oxidative destruction of membranes by Doxorubicin-iron complex. *Biochemistry* 21:1707–1713.

249. Stevens, R., et al. 1988. Body iron stores and the risk of cancer. *NEJM* 319:1047–1052.

250. Nelson, R., et al. 1994. Body iron stores and risk of colonic neoplasia. *J Natl Cancer Institute*. 86:455–60.

251. Burkitt, D. Etiology and prevention of colorectal cancer.

252. Goldin, Adlercreutz, Gorbach, Warren, Dwyer, Swenson, and Woods. Estrogen excretion patterns and plasma levels.

253. *American Journal of Clinical Nutrition*. 1978. Supp No. 31 (Oct. 31).

254. Miller, J.A., and E. C. Miller. 1969. The metabolic activation of carcinogenic aromatic amines and amides. *Prog Exp Tumor Res* 11:273.

255. Haung, C., B.S. Gopalakrishna, and B.L. Nichols. 1978. Fiber, intestinal steroid, and colon cancer. *Am J Clin Nutr* 31:512.

256. Phillips, R.L. Role of life-style and dietary habits in risk of cancer.

257. Rosen, Hellerstein, and Horwitz. The low incidence of colorectal cancer in a "high-risk" population.

258. Lyon, Gardner, Klauber, and Smart. Low cancer incidence and mortality in Utah.

259. Wynder and Reddy. The epidemiology of cancer of the large bowel.

260. Goldin, Adlercreutz, Gorbach, Warren, Dwyer, Swenson, and Woods. Estrogen excretion patterns and plasma levels.

261. Burkitt, D.P. 1975. Large-bowel cancer: An epidemiological jigsaw puzzle. *Natl Cancer Inst* 54:3.

262. MacDonald, I.A., R. Webb, and D.E. Mahony. 1978. Fecal hydroxysteroid dehydrogenase activities in vegetarian Seventh-Day Adventists, control subjects, and bowel cancer patients. *Am J Clin Nutr* 31:S233.

263. Graham, S., and C. Mettlin. 1979. Diet and colon cancer. *Am J Epidemiol* 109:1.

264. Roth, H.P., and M. Hehlman. 1978. Role of dietary fiber in health. Symposium. *Am J Clin Nut* 31(Suppl):51–91.

265. Hirayama, T. 1979. Diet and cancer. *Nutrition and Cancer* 1(3):67.
266. Kritchevsky, D., and J. Story. 1974. Binding of bile salts in vitro by non-nutritive fiber. *J Nutr* 104:458.
267. MacLennan, M.B., O.M. Jensen, J. Mosbech, and H. Vuoris. 1978. Diet, transit time, stool weight, and colon cancer in two Scandinavian populations. *Am J Clin Nutr* 31:S239.
268. Jain, M., et al. 1980. A case control study of diet and colo-rectal cancer. *Int J Cancer* 26:757.
269. Basu, T.K. 1976. Significance of vitamins in cancer. *Oncology* 33:183.

Chapter 6
Nutritional and Lifestyle Modification in Oncology Care

1. Speyer, et al. 1988. Protective effect of ICRF-187 against doxorubicin-induced cardiac toxicity in women with breast cancer. *NEJM* 319:745–752.
2. Filppi and Enck. 1990. A review of ADR-529: A new cardioprotective agent. *Clin Oncology* 16–18.
3. Speyer, J., et al. 1992. Cumulative dose-related doxorubicin cardiotoxicity can be prevented by ICRF-187. *Cancer Investigation* 10(1):26.
4. Carlson, R. 1992. Reducing the cardiotoxicity of the anthracyclines. *Oncology* 6(6):95p108.
5. Taper, H., et al. 1989. Potentiation of chemotherapy *in vivo* in an ascitic mouse liver tumor, and growth inhibition *in vitro* in 3 lines of human tumors by combined vitamin C and K3 treatment. European Association for Cancer Research Tenth Biennial Meeting. Sept. Galway, Ireland. p. 72.
6. Shimpo, et al. 1991. Ascorbic acid and adriamycin toxicity. *Am J Clin Nutr* 54:1298S–1301S.
7. Ripoll, E.A., et al. 1986. Vitamin E enhances the chemotherapeutic effects of adriamycin on human prostatic carcinoma cells in vitro. *J Urol* 136(2):529–531.
8. Pieters, R., et al. 1991. Cytotoxic effects of vitamin A in combination with vincristine, daunorubicin and 6-thio-guanine upon cells from lymphoblastic leukemic patients. *Jap J Cancer Res* 82(9):1051–1055.
9. Van Vleet, et al. 1980. *Cancer Treat Reports* 64:315.
10. Singal, P.K., et al. 1988. *Molecular and Cellular Biology* 84:163.
11. Wang, Y.M., et al. 1980. Effect of vitamin E against adriamycin-induced toxicity in rabbits. *Cancer Res* 40:1022–1027.
12. Milei, J., et al. 1986. Amelioration of adriamycin-induced cardiotoxicity in rabbits by prenylamine and vitamins E and A. *Am Heart J* 111:95.
13. Svingen, B., et al. 1981. Protection against adriamycin-induced skin necrosis in the rat by dimethyl sulfoxide and alpha-tocopherol. *Cancer Research* 41:3395–3399.
14. Mills. 1982. Retinoids and cancer. *Soc R Radiotherap and Congress* (May 13).
15. Okunieff, P. 1991. Interactions between ascorbic acid and the radiation of bone marrow, skin, and tumor. *Am J Clin Nutr* 54:1281S–1283S.
16. Meadows, G., et al. 1991. Ascorbate in the treatment of experimental transplanted melanoma. *Am J Clin Nutr* 54:1284S–1291S.
17. Taper, H.S., et al. 1987. Non-toxic potentiation of cancer chemotherapy by combined C and K3 vitamin pre-treatment. *Int J Cancer* 40:575–579.
18. Crary, E.J., et al. 1984. *Medical Hypothesis* 13:77.
19. Sprince, H., et al. 1975. *Agents and Actions* 5(2):164.
20. Poydock, E. 1984. *IRCS Medical Science* 12:813.
21. Holm, et al. 1982. Tocopherol in tumor irradiation and chemotherapy—experimental studies in the rat. Feb 12 Linderstrom-Lang Conference. Selenium, Vitamin E and Glutathioperoxidase (June 25). Icelandic Biochemical Society, p. 118.
22. Kagerud, A., et al. 1980. Effect of tocopherol in irradiation of artificially hypoxic rat tumours. Second Rome International Symposium: Biological Bases and Clinical Implications. (Sept. 21): 3–9.

23. Kagerud, A., and Peterson. 1981. To-copherol in tumour irradiation. *Anticancer Res* 1:35–38.

24. Shen, et al. 1983. Antitumour activity of radiation and vitamin A used in combination on Lewis lung carcinoma. Thirty-first Annual Meeting of the Radiation Research Society. Feb. 27. San Antonio, p. 145.

25. Seifter, et al. 1983. C3HBA tumor therapy with radiation, beta-carotene and vitamin A. A two year follow-up. *Fed Proc* 42:768.

26. Williamson, J.M., et al. 1982. Intracellular cysteine delivery system that protects against toxicity by promoting glutathione synthesis. *Proc Natl Acad Sci* 79:6246–6249.

27. Ohkawa, K., et al. 1988. The effects of co-administration of selenium and cis-platin on cis-platin induced toxicity and antitumour activity. *Br J Cancer* 58:38–41.

28. Waxman, S., et al. 1982. The enhancement of 5-FU antimetabolic activity by leucovorin, menadione, and alpha-to-copherol. *Eur J Cancer Clin Oncol* 18(7):685–692.

29. Watrach, A.M., et al. 1984. Inhibition of human breast cancer cells. *Cancer Letters* 25:41–47.

30. DeLoecker, W., et al. 1993. Effects of vitamin C and vitamin K3 treatment on human tumor cell growth *in vitro*. Synergism with combined chemotherapy action. *Anticancer Res* 13(1):103–106.

31. Ferrero, D., et al. 1992. Self-renewal inhibition of acute myeloid leukemia clonogenic cells by biological inducers of differentiation. *Leukemia* 6(2):100–106.

32. Schwartz, J.L., et al. 1992. Beta-carotene and/or vitamin E as modulators of alkylating agents in SCC-25 human squamous carcinoma cells. *Canc Chemo and Pharma* 29(3):207–213.

33. Zhang, L., et al. Induction by bufalin on human leukemic cells HL60 . . . and synergistic effect in combination with other inducers. *Cancer Res* 52(17):4634–4641.

34. Hofsli and Waage. 1992. Effect of pyridoxine on tumor necrosis factor activities *in vitro*. *Biotherapy* 5(4):285–290.

35. Petrini, et al. 1991. Synergistic effects of interferon and D3. *Haematologica* 76(6):467–471.

36. Saunders, et al. 1992. Inhibition of ovarian carcinoma cells by taxol combined with vitamin D and adriamycin. Proc Ann Meet Am Assoc Cancer Res. 33:A2641.

37. Ermens, A.A., et al. 1987. Enhanced effect of MTX and 5FU on folate metabolism of leukemic cells by B12. Proc Ann Meet Am Assoc Cancer Res. 28:275.

38. Dimery, et al. 1992. Reduction in toxicity of high-dose 13-cis-retinoic acid with vitamin E. Proc Ann Meet Am Soc Clin Oncol. 11:A399.

39. Wood, L.A. 1985. *NEJM* (April 18).

40. Komiyama, et al. 1985. Synergistic combination of 5FU, vitamin A, and cobalt radiation for head and neck cancer. *Auris, Nasus, Larynx* 12 S2:S239–S243.

41. Israel, L., et al. 1985. Vitamin A augmentation of the effects of chemotherapy in metastatic breast cancers after menopause. Randomized trial in 100 patients. *Annales De Medecine Interne* 136(7):551–554.

42. Nagourney, et al. 1987. Menadiol with chemotherapies: feasibility for resistance modification. Proc Ann Meet Am Soc Clin Oncol. 6:A132.

43. Ladner, H.L., et al. 1986. In *Vitamins and Cancer*, ed. F.L. Meyskens. Clifton, NJ: Humana Press, 429.

44. Sakamoto, A., et al. 1983. In *Modulation and Mediation of Cancer by Vitamins*. Karger, Basel, 330.

45. Smyth, J., et al. 1995. Glutathione may prevent cisplatin toxicity, raise response rates in ovarian cancer. *Oncology News* 4(1):1–4.

46. Schein, P. 1992. Results of chemotherapy and radiation therapy protection trials with WR-2721. *Cancer Investigation* 10(1):24–26.

47. Santamaria, Benazzo, et al. First clinical case-report (1980–88) of cancer chemoprevention with beta-caro-

tene plus canthaxanthin supplemented to patients after radical treatment.

48. Jaakkola, et al. 1992. Treatment with antioxidant and other nutrients in combination with chemotherapy and irradiation in patients with small cell lung cancer. *Anticancer Res* (May–June) 12(3):599–606.

49. Henriksson, et al. 1991. Interaction between cytostatics and nutrients. *Med Oncol Tumor Pharmacother* 8(2):79–86.

50. Simone, C.B. 1992. Use of therapeutic levels of nutrients to augment oncology care. Adjuvant Nutrition in Cancer Treatment Symposium. Nov. 6–7. Tulsa, OK, p. 72.

51. Williams, G.H. 1987. Quality of life and its impact on hypertensive patients. *Am J Med* 82:98–105.

52. Selby, P.J., et al. 1984. The development of a method for assessing the quality of life of cancer patients. *Br J Cancer* 50:13–22.

53. Aaronson, N.K. 1988. Quality of Life: What is it? How should it be measured? *Oncology* 2(5):69–76.

54. Tchekmedyian, N.S., and D.F. Cella, editors. 1990. *Quality of Life in Current Oncology Practice and Research* 4(5):11–234.

55. Cassileth, B., et al. 1991. Survival and quality of life among patients receiving unproven as compared with conventional cancer therapy. *NEJM* 324(17): 1180–1185.

56. Hopwood, P. and N. Thatcher. 1991. Current status of quality of life measurement in lung cancer patients. *Oncology* 5(5):159–164.

57. Gelber, R.D., et al. 1991. Quality of life adjusted evaluation of adjuvant therapies for operable breast cancer. *Ann Int Med* 114:621–628.

58. Gotay, C.C., et al. 1992. Building quality of life assessment into cancer treatment studies. *Oncology* 6(6):25–37.

59. Tchekmedyian, N.S., D.F. Cella, and A.D. Mooradian, editors. 1992. Care of the older cancer patient: clinical and quality of life issues. *Oncology* 6(2) Suppl:1–160.

60. Sensky, T. 1988. Measurement of the quality of life in end-stage renal failure. *Lancet* 319(20):1353–1354.

61. Hoffer and Pauling, L. 1990. Hardin Jones biostatistical analysis of mortality data for cohorts of cancer patients with a large surviving fraction surviving at the termination of the study using vitamin C and other nutrients. *J Orthomolecular Medicine* 5(3):143.

62. Goodman, M.T., et al. 1992. *European J Cancer* 28(2):495.

63. Carter, J.P., et al. 1993. *J Am College Nutr* 12(3):209.

64. Foster, H.D. 1988. *Intl J Biosocial Research* 10(1):17.

65. Sakamoto, et al. 1983. In *Modulation and Mediation of Cancer by Vitamins*. Karger, Basel. p. 330.

66. Jaakkola, et al. 1992. Treatment with antioxidant and other nutrients in combination with chemotherapy and irradiation in patients with small cell lung cancer. *Anticancer Res* 12(3):599–606.

67. Henquin, N., et al. 1989. Nutritional monitoring and counselling for cancer patients during chemotherapy. *Oncology* 46(3):173–177.

68. Wynder, E., et al. 1963. A comparison of survival rates between American and Japanese patients with breast cancer. *Surg Gyn Obstet* (August):196–200.

69. Nemoto, et al. 1977. Differences in breast cancer between Japan and the U.S. *JNCI* 58:193–197.

70. Sakamoto, et al. 1979. Comparative clinicopathological study of breast cancer among Japanese and American females. *Jpn J Cancer Clin* 25:161–170.

71. Ward-Hinds, et al. 1982. Stage-specific breast cancer incidence rates by age among Japanese and Caucasian women in Hawaii. *Br J Cancer* 45:118–123.

72. Kolonel, et al. 1981. Nutrient intakes in relation to cancer incidence in Hawaii. *Br J Cancer* 44:332–339.

73. Armstrong and Doll. 1975. Environmental factors and cancer incidence and mortality in different countries with special reference to dietary practices. *Int J Cancer* 15:617–631.

74. Ward-Hinds, et al. 1982. Stage-specific breast cancer incidence rates by

age among Japanese and Caucasian women in Hawaii.

75. Donegan, et al. 1978. The association of body weight with recurrent cancer of the breast. *Cancer* 41:1590–1594.
76. Abe, et al. 1976. Biological characteristics of breast cancer in obesity. *Tohoku J Exp Med* 120:351–359.
77. Donegan, et al. 1978. The prognostic implications of obesity for surgical cure of breast cancer. *Breast* 4:14–17.
78. Sohrabi, et al. 1980. Recurrence of breast cancer. *JAMA* 244:264–265.
79. Boyd, et al. 1981. Body weight and prognosis in breast cancer. *JNCI* 67:785–789.
80. Tartter, et al. 1981. Cholesterol and obesity as prognostic factors in breast cancer. *Cancer* 47:2222–2227.
81. Buchwald, H. 1992. Cholesterol inhibition, cancer, and chemotherapy. *Lancet* 339:1154–1156.

Chapter 7
Free Radicals

1. Tam, B.K., and P.B. McKay. 1970. Reduced triphosphopyridine nucleotide oxidase-catalysed alterations of membrane phospholipids, III. Transient formation of phospholipid peroxides. *J Biol Che* 245:2295.
2. Reich, L., and S.S. Stivala. 1969. *Autoxidation of hydrocarbons and polyoletins*. New York: Dekker.
3. Lundberg, W.O. 1961. *Autoxidation and antioxidants*. Vol. I. New York: Wiley.
4. Wills, E.D. 1970. *Int J Rad Res* 17:229.
5. Norins, A.L. 1962. Free radical formation in skin following exposure to ultraviolet light. *J Invest Dermatol* 39:445.
6. Zelac, R.E., H.L. Cromroy, W.E. Bloch, et al. 1971. Inhaled ozone as a mutagen. I. Chromosome aberration induced in Chinese hamster lymphocytes. *Environ Res* 4:262.
7. Pryor, W.A. 1973. Free radical reactions and their importance in biochemical systems. *Fed Proc, Amer Soc Exp Biol* 32:1862.
8. Slater, T.F. 1972. *Free radical mechanism in tissue injury*. London: Pion, Ltd.
9. Recknagel, R.O. 1967. Carbon tetrachloride hepatoxicity. *Pharmacol Rev* 19:145.
10. Cross, et al. 1987. Oxygen radicals and human disease. *Ann Int Med* 107:526–45.
11. Southorn, P., and Powis. 1988. Free radicals in medicine, chemical nature and biological reactions. *Mayo Clin Proc* 63:381–389.
12. Aruoma Okezie, I., et al. 1991. Oxygen free radicals and human diseases. *J Roy Soc Health* 111(5):172–177.
13. Saul, et al. 1987. Free radicals, DNA damage, and aging. In *Annals: Modern biological theories of aging*. New York: Raven Press, 113–29.
14. Cerutti. 1985. Pro-oxidant states and tumor promotion. *Science* 227:375–82.
15. Vuillaume, M. 1987. Reduced oxygen species, mutation, induction and cancer initiation. *Mutat Res* 186:43–72.
16. Halliwell, et al. 1985. *Free oxygens in biology and medicine*. Oxford: Clarion Press.
17. Draper, et al. 1984. Anti-oxidants and cancer. *J Agri Food Chem* 32:433–35.
18. Rubanyi. 1988. Vascular effects of oxygen-derived free radicals. *Free Rad Bio Med* 4:107–20.
19. Hennig and Chow. 1988. Lipid peroxidation and endothelial cell injury: Implications in atherosclerosis. *Free Rad Bio Med* 4:99–106.
20. Re-profusion injury after thrombolytic therapy for acute myocardial infarction. 1989. *Lancet* (Sept 16):655–57.
21. McCord. 1985. Oxygen derived free radicals in post ischemic tissue injury. *NEJM* 312:159–63.
22. Fridovich, I. 1975. Superoxide dismutases. *Ann Rev Biochem* 44:147.
23. Ogura, Y. 1955. Catalase activity at high concentrations of hydrogen peroxide. *Arch Biophys* 57:228.
24. Christopherson, B.O. 1969. Reduction of linoleic acid hydroperoxide by a glutathione peroxidase. *Biochem Biophys Acta* 176:463.
25. Wattenberg, W.L., W.O. Loub, L.K. Lam, and J.L. Speier. 1976. Dietary constituents altering the response to

chemical carcinogens. *Fed Proc* 35:1327.

Chapter 8
Nutritional Factors

1. Wynder, E., and P. Gori. 1977. Contribution of the environment to cancer incidence: An epidemiologic exercise. *JNCI* 58:825.
2. The National Academy of Sciences. 1982. *Nutrition, Diet, and Cancer.*
3. Simone, C.B. 1983. *Cancer and Nutrition: A Ten-Point Plan to Reduce Your Chances of Getting Cancer.* New York: McGraw-Hill Book Co.
4. Moody. 1973. *Aboriginal Health.* Canberra, Australia: Australian National University Press, p. 92.
5. Truswell and Hansen. 1976. Medical research among the Kung. In *Hunter-Gatherers,* Lee and DeVore Ed S. Kalahari. Cambridge, Mass: Harvard University Press.
6. Eaton, Konner. 1985. Paleolithic nutrition. *NEJM* 312 (5):283–289.
7. Tannenbaum, A. 1942. The genesis and growth of tumors. III. Effects of a high-fat diet. *Cancer Res* 2:468.
8. Rosen, P., S.M. Hellerstein, and C. Horwitz. 1981. The low incidence of colorectal cancer in a "high-risk" population. *Cancer* 48:2692.
9. Wydner, E.L., et al. 1969. Environmental factors of cancer of the colon and rectum. II. Japanese epidemiological data. *Cancer* 32:1210.
10. Phillips, R.L. 1975. Role of life-style and dietary habits in risk of cancer among Seventh-Day Adventists. *Cancer Res* 35:3513.
11. Lyon, J.L., J.W. Gardner, M.R. Klauber, and C.R. Smart. 1977. Low cancer incidence and mortality in Utah. *Cancer* 39:2608.
12. Baptista, J., W.R. Bruce, I. Gupta, J. Krepinsky, R. Van Tassell, T.D. Wilkins. 1984. On distribution of different fecapentaenes, the fecal mutagens, in the human population. *Cancer Letters* 22:299.
13. Bruce, W.R., A.J. Varghese, and R. Farrer. 1977. A mutagen in the feces of

normal humans. In *Origins of Human Cancer,* ed. H.H. Hiatt, J.D. Watson, and J.A. Winsten, Cold Spring Harbor Laboratory, Cold Spring Harbor, NY, pps. 1641–44.
14. Prentice, R.L., L. Sheppard. 1990. Dietary fat and cancer: consistency of the epidemiology data, and disease prevention that may follow from a practical reduction in fat consumption. *Cancer Causes Control* 1:81–97.
15. Boyle, P., et al. 1993. Trends in diet related cancers in Japan: A conundrum? *Lancet* 342:752.
16. Golden, B.R., et al. 1982. Estrogen excretion patterns and plasma levels in vegetarian and omnivorous women. *NEJM* 307(25):1542–1547.
17. Howe, G.R., et al. 1990. Dietary factors and risk of breast cancer; combined analysis of 12 case-control studies. *J Natl Cancer Institute* 82:561–569.
18. Graham, S., et al. 1982. Diet in the epidemiology of breast cancer. *Am J Epidemiol* 116:68–75.
19. Ewertz, M., G. Caroline. 1990 Dietary factors and breast cancer risk in Denmark. *Inst J Epidemiol* 46:779–784.
20. Van't Veer, P., et al. 1990. Dietary fat and the risk of breast cancer. *Int J Epidemiol* 19:12–18.
21. Graham, S., et al. 1991. Nutritional epidemiology of postmenopausal breast cancer in Western New York. *Am J Epidemiol* 34:552–566.
22. Frisch, R. 1987. Dietary fat and the risk of breast cancer. *NEJM* 317(3):165.
23. Lee, H.P., et al. 1991. Dietary effects on breast cancer risk in Singapore. *Lancet* 337:1197–1200.
24. Kritchevsky, D. 1991. Diet and cancer. *CA-A Cancer J for Clinicians* 41(6):328–333.
25. Weinhouse, S., et al. 1991. American Cancer Society Guidelines on diet, nutrition, and cancer. *CA-A Cancer J for Clinicians* 41(6):334–338.
26. Schatzkin, A., et al. 1989. The dietary fat-breast cancer hypothesis is alive. *JAMA* 261(22):3284–3287.
27. Willett, W.C., D.J. Hunter, et al. 1992. Dietary fat and fiber in relation to risk

of breast cancer. *JAMA* 268(15):2037–2044.

28. Giovannucci, E., et al. 1991. A comparison of prospective and retrospective assessments of diet in the study of breast cancer. *Am J Epidemiol* 134:714.

29. Friedenreich, C.M., G.R. Howe, A.B. Miller. 1991. The effect of recall bias on the association of calorie-providing nutrients and breast cancer. *Epidemiology* 2:424–429.

30. Marshall, E. 1993. Search for a killer: focus shifts from fat to hormones. *Science* 259:618–621.

31. Jones, D.Y., et al. 1987. Dietary fat and breast cancer in the National Health and Nutrition Examination Survey I: epidemiologic follow-up study. *J Nat Cancer Inst* 79:465–471.

32. Knekt, P., et al. 1990. Dietary fat and risk of breast cancer. *Am J Clin Nutr* 52:903–908.

33. Howe, G.R., et al. 1991. A cohort study of fat intake and risk of breast cancer. *J Natl Cancer Inst* 83: 336–340.

34. Kushi, L.H., et al. 1991. Dietary fat, breast cancer, adjustment for energy intake and categorization of risk. *Am J Epidemiol* 134:714.

35. Ganz, P., and A. Schag. 1993. Nutrition and breast cancer. *Oncology* 7(12):71–76.

36. Report of the Council on Scientific Affairs. 1993. Diet and Cancer: Where do matters stand? *Arch Intern Med* 153:50–56.

37. Toniolo, P., et al. 1989. Calorie providing nutrients and risk of breast cancer. *JNCI* 81:278.

38. LaVeccia, C., et al. 1988. Comparative cancer epidemiology in the U.S. and Italy. *Cancer Res* (Dec 15): 1202–1207.

39. Gaskill, S.P., et al. 1979. Breast cancer mortality and diet in the United States. *Cancer Res* 39:3628.

40. Reddy, B.S., Mastromarino A., and E. Wynder. 1977. Diet and metabolism: Large bowel cancer. *Cancer* 39:1815.

41. Reddy, B.S., and E. Wynder. 1977. Metabolic epidemiology of colon cancer. *Cancer* 39:2533.

42. Paptestas, A.E., et al. 1982. Fecal ster-

oid metabolites and breast cancer risk. *Cancer* 49:1201.

43. Brammer, S.H. and R.L. DeFelice. 1980. Dietary advice in regard to risk for colon and breast cancer. *Prev Med* 9:544.

44. Chan, P.C., J.F. Head, L.A. Cohen, et al. 1977. Effect of high fat diet on serum prolactin levels and mammary cancer development in ovariectomized rats. *Proc Am Assoc Cancer Res* 18:189.

45. Brammer and DeFelice. Dietary advice.

46. Petrakis, N.L., L.D. Gruenke, and J.C. Craig. 1981. Cholesterol and cholesterol epoxide in nipple aspirate of human breast fluid. *Cancer Res* 41:2563.

47. Aries, V.C., J.S. Growther, B.S. Drasar, M.J. Hill, and F.R. Ellis. 1971. The effect of a strict vegetarian diet on the fecal flora and fecal steroid concentration. *J Pathol* 103:54.

48. Burkitt, D. 1984. Etiology and prevention of colorectal cancer. *Hospital Practice* 67(Feb.):67–77.

49. *Nutrition and Cancer*, ed. DeWys, W.D. 1983. Seminars in Oncology. 10 (3):255–364.

50. Maier, B., M.A. Flynn, G.C. Burton, R.K. Tsutakawa, and D.J. Hentges. 1974. Effect of high-beef diet on bowel flora: A preliminary report. *Am J Clin Nutr* 27:1470.

51. Jacobs, L. 1987. Effect of dietary fiber on colon cell proliferation. *Prev Medicine* 16:566–571.

52. McKeown-Eyssen, G. 1987. Fiber intake in different populations and colon cancer risk. *Prev Medicine* 16:532–539.

53. McPherson-Kay, R. 1987. Fiber, stool bulk, and bile acid output: Implications for colon cancer risk. *Prev Medicine* 16:540–544.

54. Wynder, E.L., and G.B. Gori. 1977. Contribution of the environment to cancer incidence: An epidemiologic exercise. *J Natl Cancer Inst* 58:825.

55. Wynder, E.L., and B.S. Reddy. 1974. The epidemiology of cancer of the large bowel. *Digestive Diseases* 19:937.

56. *Nutrition and Cancer*, ed. W.D. DeWys.

1983. Seminars in Oncology. 10(3):1–367.

57. Workshop on Nutrition in Cancer Causation and Prevention. *Cancer Research Supplement*. 1983. 43:2386–2519.

58. Willett, W., and B. MacMahon. 1984. Diet and cancer: An overview. *NEJM* 310:633–638, 697–703.

59. Diet and Human Carcinogenesis Proceedings. 1986. *Nutrition and Cancer* 8(1):1–71.

60. Rivlin, et al. 1983. Nutrition and cancer. *Am J Med* 75:843–854.

61. Executive Summary. Diet, Nutrition, and Cancer. 1983. *Cancer Research* 43:3018–3023.

62. Beardshall, et al. 1989. Saturation of fat and pancreatic carcinogenesis. *Lancet* (October 28): 1008–1010.

63. Cohen, L. 1987. Diet and cancer. *Scientific American* 257(5):42–48.

64. Insull, W. 1987. Dietary fats and carcinogenesis. *Prev Medicine* 16:481–484.

65. Reddy, B. 1987. Dietary fat and colon cancer. *Prev Medicine* 16:460–467.

66. Proceeding of a Workshop. 1987. Dietary fat and fiber in carcinogenesis. *Prev Medicine* 16:449–527.

67. National Research Council. 1982. *Diet, Nutrition and Cancer*. Washington, D.C.: National Academy Press.

68. Alcantara, E.N., and E.W. Speckman. 1976. Diet, nutrition, and cancer. *Am J Clin Nutr* 29:1035.

69. Carroll, K.K. 1975. Experimental evidence of dietary factors and hormone dependent cancers. *Cancer Res* 35:3374.

70. Carroll, K.K., E.B. Gammel, and E.R. Plunkett. 1968. Dietary fat and mammary cancer. *Can Med Assoc J* 98:590–594.

71. Drasar, B.S., and D. Irving. 1973. Environmental factors and cancer of the colon and breast. *Br J Cancer* 27:167.

72. Kent, S. 1979. Diet, hormones, and breast cancer. *Geriatrics* 34:83.

73. Paptestas, A.E., D. Panvelliwalla, P. Tartter, S. Miller, D. Pertsemlidis, and A. Aufses. 1982. Fecal steroid metabolites and breast cancer risk. *Cancer* 49:1201.

74. Kolonel, L.N., J.H. Hankin, J. Lee, S.Y. Chu, A.Y. Nomura, and M. Word-Hinds. 1981. Nutrient intakes in relation to cancer incidence in Hawaii. *Br J Cancer* 44:332–339.

75. Gregorio, D.I., L.J. Emrich, S. Graham, J. Marshall, and T. Nemoto. 1985. Dietary fat consumption and survival among women with breast cancer. *JNCI* 75:37–41.

76. Morrison, A.S., C.R. Lowe, B. MacMahon, B.R. Ravnihar, and S. Yuasa. 1977. Incidence, risk factors and survival in breast cancer: Report on five years of follow-up observation. *Europ J Cancer* 13:209–214.

77. Wynder, E.L., T. Kajatani, J. Kuno, J.C. Lucas, Jr., A. DePalo, and J. Farrow. 1963. A comparison of survival rates between American and Japanese patients with breast cancer. *Surg Gynecol Obstet* 117:196–200.

78. Armstrong and Doll. Environmental factors and cancer incidence.

79. Carroll, K.K. Experimental evidence of dietary factors and hormone dependent cancers.

80. Donegan, W.L., A.J. Hartz, and A.A. Rimm. 1978. The association of body weight with recurrent cancer of the breast. *Cancer* 41:1590–1594.

81. Morrison, A.S., C.R. Lowe, B. MacMahon, B. Ravnihar, and S. Yuassa. 1977. Some international differences in treatment and survival in breast cancer. *Int J Cancer* 18:269–273.

82. Tartter, P.I., A.E. Papatestas, J. Ioannovich, M.N. Mulvihill, G. Lesnick, and A.H. Aufses. 1981. Cholesterol and obesity as prognostic factors in breast cancer. *Cancer* 47:2222–2227.

83. Wynder, E.L., F. MacCornack, P. Hill, L.A. Cohen, P.C. Chan, and J.H. Weisburger. 1976. Nutrition and the etiology and prevention of breast cancer. *Cancer Detection and Prevention* 1:293–310.

84. Kolonel, L., J. Hankin, U. Lee, S. Chu, A. Nomura, and M. Word-Hinds. 1981. Nutrient intakes in relation to cancer incidence in Hawaii. *Br J Cancer* 44:332.

85. Nemoto, T., T. Tominago, A. Chamberlain, Z. Iwasa, H. Koyama, M.

Hama, I. Bross, and T. Dao. 1977. Differences in breast cancer between Japan and the United States. *J Natl Cancer Inst* 58:193–197.

86. Wynder and Reddy. The epidemiology of cancer of the large bowel.

87. Abe, R., N. Kumagai, M. Kimura, A. Hirosaki, and T. Nakamura. 1976. Biological characteristics of breast cancer in obesity. *Tohoku J Exp Med* 120:351–359.

88. Ward-Hines, M., L.N. Kolonel, A.M.Y. Nomura, and J. Lee. 1982. Stage-specific breast cancer incidence rates by age among Japanese and Caucasian women in Hawaii, 1960-1979. *Br J Cancer* 45:118–123.

89. Boyd, N.F., J.E. Campbell, T. Germanson, D.B. Thomson, D.J. Sutherland, and J.W. Meakin. 1981. Body weight and prognosis in breast cancer. *J Natl Cancer Inst* 67:785–789.

90. Kwa, H.G., R.D. Bulbrook, F. Cleton, et al. 1978. An abnormal early evening peak of plasma prolactin in nulliparous and obese postmenopausal women. *Int J Cancer* 22:691–693.

91. deWaard and Baanders-van Halewign. A prospective study in general practice on breast cancer risk in postmenopausal women.

92. McDonald, R., J. Grodin, and P. Sitteri. 1969. The utilization of plasma androstenedione for estrone production in women in endocrinology. *Excerpta Med Int Congr Ser* 184:770–776.

93. O'Dea, J., R. Wieland, M. Hallberg, L.A. Llerena, E.M. Zorn, and S.M. Genuth. 1979. Effect of dietary weight loss on sex steriod binding, sex steroids and gonadotropins on obese postmenopausal women. *J Lab Clin Med* 93:1004–1008.

94. Santiago-Delpin, E.A., and J. Szepsenwol. 1977. Prolonged survival of skin and tumor allografts in mice on high-fat diets. *J Natl Cancer Inst* 59:459.

95. Stuart, A.E., and A.E. Davidson. 1976. Effect of simple lipids on antibody formation after ingestion of foreign red cells. *J Pathol Bacteriol* 87:305.

96. Goldin, B.R., H.A. Adlercreutz, S.L. Gorbach, J.H. Warren, J.T. Dwyer, L. Swenson, and M.N. Woods. 1982. Estrogen excretion patterns and plasma levels in vegetarian and omnivorous women. NEJM 307(25):1542–47.

97. Tannenbaum, A. 1940. The initiation and growth of tumors. Introduction I. Effects of underfeeding. *Am J Cancer* 38:335.

98. Armstrong and Doll. Environmental factors and cancer incidence and mortalities in different countries.

99. Tannenbaum, A. Nutrition and cancer.

100. Kolonel, L., V. Hankin, J. Lee, S. Chu, A. Nomura, and M. Word-Hinds. Nutrient intakes in relation to cancer incidence in Hawaii.

101. Knox, E.G. 1977. Foods and diseases. *Br J Prev Soc Med* 31:71–80.

102. Armstrong and Doll. Environmental factors and cancer incidence and mortalities in different countries.

103. Jain, M., et al. A case control study of diet and colo-rectal cancer.

104. Drasar and Irving. Environmental factors and cancer of the colon and breast.

105. Hems, G. 1978. The contribution of diet and childbearing to breast cancer rates. *Br J Cancer* 37:974–982.

106. Domino, E.F., et al. 1993. The nicotine content of common vegetables. *NEJM* 329(6):437.

107. Castro, A., N. Monji. 1986. Dietary nicotine and its significance in studies on tobacco smoking. *Biochem Arch* 2:91–97.

108. Davis, R.A., et al. 1991. Dietary nicotine: a source of urinary cotinine. *J Food Chem Toxicol* 29:821–827.

109. Domino, E.F., et al. 1992. Current experience with HPLC and GC-MS analyses of nicotine and cotinine. *Med Sci Res* 20:859–860.

110. Ames, B.N. 1983. Dietary carcinogens and anticarcinogens. *Science* 221:1256.

111. Ashwood-Smith, M.J., and G.A. Poulton. 1981. *Mutat Res* 85:389.

112. Concon, J.M., D.S. Newburg, and T.W. Swerczek. 1979. Black pepper (piper nigrum):Evidence of carcinogenesis. *Nutr Cancer* 1(3):22.

113. Hirayama, T., and Y. Ito. 1981. Diet and cancer. *Prev Med* 10:614.

114. Tazima, Y. 1982. In *Environmental mutagenesis, carcinogenesis, and plant biology*, Vol. 1, ed. E.J. Klekowski, Jr. New York: Praeger, 68–95.

115. Toth, B. 1979. In *Naturally occurring carcinogens-mutagens and modulators of carcinogenesis*, ed. E.C. Miller. Tokyo and Baltimore: Japan Scientific Societies Press and University Park Press, 57–65.

116. Tomatis, L., C. Agthe, J. Bartsch, J. Huff, Montesano, R. Saracci, E. Walker, and J. Wilbourn. 1978. Evaluation of the carcinogenicity of chemicals: A review of the monograph program of the International Agency for Research on Cancer. *Cancer Res* 38:877.

117. Ames, B.N. Dietary carcinogens and anticarcinogens.

118. Stich, H.F., M.P. Rosin, C.H. Wu, and W.D. Powrie. 1981. A comparative genotoxicity study of chlorogenic acid. *Mutat Res* 90:201.

119. Browner, W.S., et al. 1991. What if Americans ate less fat? *JAMA* 265:3285–3291.

120. Johnson, C., et al. 1993. Declining serum cholesterol levels among U.S. adults. *JAMA* 269(23):3002–3008.

121. Byers, T. 1993. Dietary trends in the U.S.: Relevance to cancer prevention. *Cancer* 72(3):1015–1018.

122. Sempos, C., et al. 1993. Prevalence of high blood cholesterol among U.S. adults. *JAMA* 269(23):3009–3014.

123. Expert Panel on Detection, Evaluation, and Treatment of High Blood Cholesterol. 1993. Summary of second report of National Cholesterol Education Program. *JAMA* 269(23):3015–3023.

124. Burr, et al. 1989. Effects of changes in fat, fish, and fiber intakes on death and heart attack. *Lancet* (Sept 30):757–761.

125. Ferraro, C. 1990. Why is high-fat food marketed? Customers demand it, that's why. *Investor's Daily* (Sept 6):15.

126. Woodbury, R. 1993. The great fast-food pig-out. *Time* (June 28):51.

127. O'Neill, M. 1994. 'Eat, drink, and be merry' may be the next trend. *New York Times* Jan. 2, front page.

128. Eating in America. 1994. *Natural Foods* June:20. (Survey conducted by MRCA information services for the National Livestock and Meat Board.)

Chapter 9
Obesity

1. Hannon, B.M., and T.G. Lohman. 1978. The energy cost of overweight in the United States. *Am J Public Health* 68:8.

2. McCay, C.M., M.F. Crowell, and L.A. Maynard. 1935. The effect of retarded growth upon the length of lifespan and upon the ultimate size. *J Nutr* 10:63.

3. Jose, D.G., and R.A. Good. 1973. Quantitative effects of nutritional protein and caloric deficiency upon the immune response to tumors in mice. *Cancer Res* 33:807.

4. Jose, D.G., O. Stutman, and R.A. Good. 1973. Good, long term effects on immune function of early nutritional deprivation. *Nature* 241:57.

5. Manson, et al. 1987. Body weight and longevity: A review. *JAMA* 257:353–358.

6. Tannenbaum, A. 1959. Nutrition and cancer. In *Physiopathy of Cancer*, 2nd ed., ed. F. Homberger. New York: Hoeber-Harper, 517–62.

7. Kraybill, H.F. 1963. Carcinogenesis associated with foods, food additives, food degradation products and related dietary factors. *Clin Pharmacol Ther* 4:73.

8. Jose and Good. Quantitative effects.

9. Drori, D., and Y. Folman. 1976. Environmental effects on longevity in the male rat: Exercise, mating, castration, and restricted feeding. *Exp Gerontol* 11:25.

10. Ross, M.H., and G. Bras. 1971. Lasting influence of early caloric restriction on prevalence of neoplasms in the rat. *J Natl Cancer Inst* 47:1095.

11. Armstrong, B., and R. Doll. 1975. Environmental factors and cancer incidence and mortalities in different countries with special reference to dietary practices. *Int J Cancer* 15:616.

12. Gaskill, S.P., et al. 1979. Breast cancer

mortality and diet in the United States. *Cancer Res* 39:3628.

13. de Waard, F., and E.A. Baanders-van Halewign. 1974. A prospective study in general practice on breast cancer risk in postmenopausal women. *J Cancer* 14:153–160.

14. Hin, T.M., K.P. Chen, and B. MacMahon. 1971. Epidemiologic characteristics of cancer of the breast in Taiwan. *Cancer* 27:1497–1504.

15. Mirra, A.P., P. Cole, and B. MacMahon. 1971. Breast cancer in an area of high parity—Sao Paolo, Brazil. *Cancer Res* 31:77–83.

16. National Dairy Council. 1975. Nutrition, diet, and cancer. *Dairy Council Digest* 46(5):25.

17. MacDonald, P.C., et al. 1978. Effect of obesity on conversion of plasma andostenedione to estrone in postmenopausal women with and without endometrial cancer. *Am J Obstet Gynecol* 130:448–455.

18. Marshall, E. 1993. Breast cancer research. *Science* 259:618–621.

19. Grodin, et al. 1973. Source of estrogen production in post menopausal women. *J Clin Endocrinol Metab* 36:207–214.

20. Sitteri, et al. 1973. Role of extraglandular estrogen in human endocrinology. In *Handbook of physiology*, ed. Greep, Astwood. Section 7, vol 2, part 1, pp. 15–629. Washington, DC: Am Physiol Soc.

21. Schindler, et al. 1972. Conversion of andostenedione to estrone by human fat tissue. *J Clin Endocrinol Metab* 35:627–630.

22. Wynder and Hill. 1977. Prolactin, estrogens, and lipids in breast fluid. *Lancet* 2:840.

23. Rose, P., et al. 1986. Serum and breast duct fluid prolactin and estrogen levels in healthy Finnish and American women and patients with fibrocystic breast disease. *Cancer* 57:1550–1554.

24. Rose, P., et al. 1985. Low fat diet in fibrocystic disease of the breast with cyclical mastalgia: a feasibility study. *Am J Clin Nutr* 42:856.

25. Lee-Han, et al. 1988. Compliance in a randomized clinical trial of dietary fat reduction in patients with breast dysplasia. *Am J Clin Nutr* 48:575–586.

26. Insuli, et al. 1990. Results of a randomized feasibility study of a low fat diet. *Arch Intern Med* 150:421–427.

27. Heber, et al. 1991. Reduction in serum estradiol in postmenopausal women given free access to a low fat high carbohydrate diet. *Nutrition* 7:137–139.

28. Prentice, et al. 1990. Dietary fat reduction and plasma estradiol concentrations in healthy postmenopausal women. *JNCI* 82:129–134.

29. Zumoff, B. 1982. Relationship of obesity to blood estrogens. *Cancer Res* 42:3289–3294.

30. Abe, et al. 1976. Biological characteristics of breast cancer in obesity. *Tohoku J Exp Med* 120:351–359.

31. Kalish, L. 1984. Relationship of body size with breast cancer. *J Clin Oncol* 2:287–293.

32. Donegan, et al. 1978. The association of body weight with recurrent cancer of the breast. *Cancer* 41:1590–1594.

33. Howson, et al. 1986. Body weight, serum cholesterol, and stage of primary breast cancer. *Cancer* 58:2372–2381.

34. Kampert, et al. 1988. Combined effects of childbearing, menstrual events, and body size on age-specific cancer risk. *Am J Epidemiol* 128:962–979.

35. Albanes, D. 1987. Caloric intake, body weight, and cancer: A review. *Nutr Cancer* 9:199–217.

36. Verreault, et al. 1989. Body weight and prognostic indicators in breast cancer. *Am J Epidemiol* 129:260–268.

37. London, et al. 1989. Prospective study of relative weight, height, and risk of breast cancer. *JAMA* 262:2853–2858.

38. Schapira, et al. 1990. Abdominal obesity and breast cancer risk. *Ann Intern Med* 112:182–186.

39. Ballard-Barbesh, et al. 1990. Body fat distribution and breast cancer in the Framingham study. *JNCI* 82:286–290.

40. Folsom, et al. 1990. Increased incidence of breast cancer associated with abdominal adiposity in postmenopausal women. *Am J Epidemiol* 131:794–803.

41. LeMarchand, et al. 1990. Body size at different periods of life and breast cancer risk. *Am J Epidemiol* 128:137–152.

42. Sellers, et al. 1992. Effect of family history, body-fat distribution, and reproductive factors on the risk of postmenopausal breast cancer. *NEJM* 326:1323–1329.

43. Schapira, et al. 1991. Estimate of breast cancer risk reduction with weight loss. *Cancer* 67:2622–2625.

44. Gaskill, S.P., W.L. McGuire, et al. 1979. Breast cancer mortality and diet in the United States. *Cancer Res* 39:3628.

45. Sylvester, P.W., et al. 1981. Relationship of hormones to inhibition of mammary tumor development by underfeeding during the "critical period" after carcinogen administration. *Cancer Res* 41:1384.

46. Newberne, P.M., and G. Williams. 1979. Nutritional influences on the cause of infection. In *Resistance to Infectious Diseases*, ed. R.H. Dunlop, and H.W. Moon. Saskatoon: Saskatoon Modern Press.

47. Leonard, P.J., and K.M. MacWilliam. 1964. Cortisol binding in the serum in kwashiorkor. *J Endocrinol* 29:273.

48. Hadler and Margolis. 1992. Hepatitis B immunization: vaccine types, efficacy, and indications for immunization. In *Current Clinical Topics in Infectious Diseases*, vol. 12, ed. Remington and Swartzvol. Boston: Blackwell Scientific, pp. 282–308.

49. Manson, et al. 1990. A prospective study of obesity and risk of coronary heart disease in women. *NEJM* 322:882–889.

50. Donahue, et al. 1987. Central obesity and coronary heart disease in men. *Lancet* (April 11):821–823.

51. Harris, et al. 1988. Body mass index and mortality among nonsmoking older persons. *JAMA* 259:1520–1524.

52. Sims, et al. 1982. Obesity and hypertension. *JAMA* 247:49–52.

53. MacMahon, et al. 1986. The effect of weight reduction on left ventricular mass. *NEJM* 314:334–339.

54. Hall, et al. 1986. Smoking cessation and weight gain. *J Consult Clin Psychol* 54:342–346.

54. Perkins, et al. 1989. The effect of nicotine on energy expenditure during light physical activity. *NEJM* 320:898–903.

56. Hamm, P.B., et al. 1989. Large fluctuations in body weight during young adulthood and twenty-five year risk of coronary death in men. *Am J Epidemiol* 129:312–18.

57. Hamm, P.B., et al. Large fluctuations in body weight during young adulthood.

58. Lissner, L., et al. 1989. Body weight variability and mortality in the Gothenburg Prospective Studies of men and women. In *Obesity in Europe 88: Proceedings of the First European Congress on Obesity*, ed. P. Bjorntorp, and S. Rossner. London: Libbey, 55–60.

59. Lissner, L., et al. 1991. Variability of body weight and health outcomes in the Framingham population. *NEJM* 324:1839–1844.

Chapter 10
Food Additives, Contaminants, and Pesticides

1. Resin, A., and H. Ungar. 1957. Malignant tumors in the eyelids and the auricular region of thiourea treated rats. *Cancer Res* 17:302.

2. Nelson, A.A., and G. Woodward. 1953. Tumors of the urinary bladder, gall bladder, and liver in dogs fed o-aminoazotoluene or p-dimethyl-aminoazobenzene. *J Nat Cancer Inst* 13:1497.

3. Witschi, H., D. Williamson, and S. Lock. 1977. Enhancement of urethan tumorigenesis in mouse lung by butylated hydroxytoluene. *J Nat Cancer Inst* 58:301.

4. Wattenberg, L.W. 1978. Inhibition of chemical carcinogenesis. *J Nat Cancer Inst* 60:11.

5. Munro, E.C., C. Moodie, D. Krewski, et al. 1975. A carcinogenicity study of commercial saccharin in the rat. *Toxicol Appl Pharmacol* 32:513.

6. Kessler, I. 1976. Non-nutritive sweeteners and human bladder cancer: Preliminary findings. *J Urol* 115:143.

7. Shubik, P. 1979. Food additives (natural and synthetic). *Cancer* 43:1982.

8. Sen, N.P. 1972. The evidence for the presence of dimethylnitrosamine in meat products. *Food Cosmet Toxicol* 10:219.

9. Newberne, P.M. 1979. Nitrite promotes lymphoma incidence in rats. *Science* 204:1079.

10. Shubik, P. 1980. Food additives, contaminants, and cancer. *Prev Med* 9:197.

11. Toth, B., and D. Nagel. 1978. Tumors induced in mice by N-methyl-N-formylhydrazine of the false moral *Gyromitra esculenta*. *J Nat Cancer Inst* 60:201.

12. Lijinsky, W., and P. Shubik. 1964. Benzo(a)pyrene and other polynuclear hydrocarbons in charcoal broiled meats. *Science* 145:53.

13. Jeyaratnam, J. 1985. Health problems of pesticide usage in the Third World. *Br J Indust Med* 42:505–6.

14. Interagency Pesticide Training Coalition. 1981. Pesticide training: Course syllabus and manual for health personnel. Berkeley, CA: California State Health and Welfare Agency.

15. Pimentel, D., and J. Perkins. 1980. *Pest Control: Cultural and Environmental Aspects*. Boulder, Colorado: Westview Press.

16. Wong, K., et al. 1985. Potent induction of human placental mono-oxygenase activity by previous dietary exposure to polychlorinated biphenyls and their thermal degradation products. *Lancet* (March 30): 721–724.

17. Biscardi, S. 1991. Pesticides linked to breast cancer? *Oncology Times* (February):36.

18. Wolff, M., et al. 1993. Blood levels of organochlorine residues and risk of breast cancer. *JNCI* 85:648–652.

19. Longnecker, M., et al. 1993. Blood levels of organochlorine residues and risk of breast cancer. *JNCI* 85:1696–1697.

20. Milne, D. 1992. Small study implicates PCBs in breast cancer. *JNCI* 84:834–835.

21. Falck, F., et al. 1992. Pesticides and polychlorinated biphenyl residues in human breast lipids and their relation to breast cancer. *Arch Environmental Health* 47:143–146.

22. Mussalo-Rauhamaa, H., et al. 1990. Occurrence of beta-hexachlorocyclohexane in breast cancer patients. *Cancer* 6:2124–2128.

23. Westin, J.B. 1993. Carcinogens in Israeli milk: a study in regulatory failure. *International J Health Services* 23:497–517.

24. Borzsonyi, M., et al. 1984. Agriculturally related carcinogen at risk. International Agency for Research on Cancer. *Science Publication* 56:465–486.

25. National Toxicology Program. 1985. *Fourth Annual Report on Carcinogens: Summary*. U.S. Department of Health and Human Services. Publication NTP 85-002.

26. Vainio, H., et al. 1985. Data on the carcinogenicity of chemicals in the IARC monographs programme. *Carcinogenesis* 6:1653–1665.

27. Environmental Protection Agency. 1986. Carcinogens. *Federal Register* (September 24).

28. Bocchatta, A., and G.U. Corsini. 1986. Parkinson's disease and pesticide. *Lancet* (November 15):1163.

29. Peters, et al. 1987. *JNCI*.

30. Watterson, Andrew. 1988. *Pesticide user's health and safety handbook: An international guide*. New York: Van Nostrand Reinhold, 420.

31. Richards, et al. 1987. *Nature* 327:129.

32. Council on Scientific Affairs. 1982. Health effects of Agent Orange and dioxin contaminants. *JAMA* 248(15, October 15):1895–1897.

33. Sterling, T.D., A.V. Arundel. 1986. Health effects of phenoxy herbicides: A review. *Scand J Work Environ Health* 12:161–173.

34. Advisory Committee on Pesticides. 1980. Further review of the safety of the use of herbicides 2,4,5-T. Washington, D.C.: H.M. Stationary Office.

35. Hardell, L., et al. 1979. Case-control study: Soft-tissue sarcomas and exposure to phenoxyacetic acids or chlorophenols. *Br J Cancer* 39:711–7.

36. Eriksson, M., et al. 1981. Exposure to dioxins as a risk factor for soft tissue

sarcoma: A population-based case-control study. *Br J Ind Med* 38:27–33.

37. Hardell, L., et al. Case-control study: Soft-tissue sarcomas and exposure to phenoxyacetic acids or chlorophenols.

38. Eriksson, M., et al. Exposure to dioxins as a risk factor for soft tissue sarcoma.

39. Hardell, L., et al. 1988. The association between soft tissue sarcomas and exposure to phenoxyacetic acids: A new case-referent study. *Cancer* 62:652–56.

40. Hardell, L., et al. 1983. Epidemiologic study of socioeconomic factors and clinical findings in Hodgkin's disease, and reanalysis of previous data regarding chemical exposure. *Br J Cancer* 48:217–25.

41. Hardell, L., et al. 1981. Malignant lymphoma and exposure to chemicals, especially organic solvents, chlorophenols and phenoxy acids: A case-control study. *Br J Cancer* 43:169–76.

42. Woods, J.S., et al. 1987. Soft tissue sarcoma and non-Hodgkin's lymphoma in relation to phenoxyherbicide and chlorinated phenol exposure in western Washington. *J Natl Cancer Inst* 78:899–910.

43. Persson, B., et al. 1989. Malignant lymphomas and occupational exposures. *Br J Ind Med* 46:516–20.

44. Axelson, O., et al. 1980. Herbicide exposure and tumor mortality: An updated epidemiologic investigation on Swedish railroad car workers. *Scand J Work Environ Health* 6:73–9.

45. Thiess, A.M., et al. 1982. Mortality study of persons exposed to dioxin in a trichlorophenol-process accident that occurred in the BASF AG on November 17, 1953. *Am J Ind Med* 3:179–89.

46. Hardell, L., et al. 1982. Epidemiological study of nasal and nasopharyngeal cancer and their relation to phenoxy acid or chlorophenol exposure. *Am J Ind Med* 3:247–57.

47. Kociba, R., et al. 1982. Results of a two-year chronic toxicity and oncogenicity study of 2, 3, 7, 8-tetrachlorodibenzo-p-dioxin in rats. *Toxicol Appl Pharmacol* 46:279–303.

48. National Toxicology Program (NTP). 1982. Carcinogenesis bioassay of 2, 3, 7, 8-tetrachlorodibenzo-p-dioxin (CAS No. 1746-01-6) in Osborne-Mendel rats and B6C3F1 mice (gavage study) 1982. Washington, D.C.: Government Printing Office, 1982. (DHHS publication no. [NIH] 82-1765.)

49. Smith, A.H., et al. 1984. Soft tissue sarcoma and exposure to phenoxyherbicides and chlorophenols in New Zealand. *J Natl Cancer Inst* 73:1111–17.

50. Wiklund, K., and L. Holm. 1986. Soft tissue sarcoma risk in Swedish agriculture and forestry workers. *J Natl Cancer Inst* 76:229–34.

51. Pearce, N.E., et al. 1987. Non-Hodgkin's lymphoma and farming: An expanded case-control study. *Int J Cancer* 39:155–61.

52. Wilkund K., et al. 1987. Risk of malignant lymphoma in Swedish pesticide appliers. *Br J Cancer* 56:505–8.

53. Olsen, J.H., and O.M. Jensen. 1984. Nasal cancer and chlorophenols. *Lancet* 2:47–8.

54. Hardell, L., et al. 1984. Aetiological aspects on primary liver cancer with special regard to alcohol, organic solvents and acute intermittent porphyria—an epidemiological investigation. *Br J Cancer* 50:389–97.

55. Fingerhut, et al. 1991. Cancer mortality in workers exposed to 2, 3, 7, 8 -tetrachlorodibenzo-p-dioxin. *NEJM* 324(4):212–218.

56. Bailer, J.C. 1991. How dangerous is dioxin? *NEJM* 324(4):260–262.

57. Brand, O. 1990. Pesticide regulation. *Newsweek* (April 23):17.

58. Hopmann, C. 1990. (reporter-no title) *Newsweek* (April 23):17.

59. *Handbook on Pest Management in Agriculture.* 1991. Boca Raton, FL: CRC Press.

Chapter 11
Smoking

1. Conference on Smoking and Health. 1990. *Lancet* (April 28):1026.

2. Conference on Smoking and Health.

3. Public Health Service. 1979. *Smoking and health, a report of the surgeon general.* U.S. Dept. of HEW.

4. Fielding. 1985. Smoking: Health effects and control. *NEJM* 313:491–498.

5. MacMahon, B., et al. 1982. Cigarette smoking and urinary estrogens. *NEJM* 307:1062–1065.

6. Vessey, et al. 1983. Oral contraceptives and breast cancer: Final report of an epidemiological study. *Br J Cancer* 47:455.

7. Rosenberg, et al. 1984. Breast cancer and cigarette smoking. *NEJM* 310:92–94.

8. Schechter, et al. 1985. Cigarette smoking and breast cancer: A case-control study of screening program participants. *Am J Epidemiol* 121:479.

9. Danielson, et al. 1982. Drug monitoring of surgical patients. *NEJM* 248:1482–1485.

10. Jick, H., et al. 1979. Replacement estrogens and endometrial cancer. *NEJM* 300:218–222.

11. Jick, H., et al. 1980. Oral contraceptives and breast cancer. *Am J Epidemiol* 112:577–585.

12. Prentice, R. 1976. Use of the logistic model in retrospective studies. *Biometrics* 32:599–606.

13. Hiatt, et al. 1982. Breast cancer and serum cholesterol. *JNCI* 68:885–889.

14. Vessey, et al. 1983. Oral contraceptives and breast cancer: final report of an epidemiological study. *Br J Cancer* 47:455–462.

15. Garfinkle, L. 1980. Cancer mortality in non-smokers: prospective study by the ACS. *JNCI* 65:1169–1173.

16. Neugut, A., et al. 1993. New warning for breast cancer patients who smoke. *Oncology Times* 15(6):1.

17. Shackney, S.E. 1982. Carcinogenesis and tumor cell biology. Surgeon General's Report.

18. Winn, D.M., W.J. Blot, et al. 1981. Snuff dipping and oral cancer among women in the southern United States. *NEJM* 304:745.

19. Slattery, M., et al. 1989. Cigarette smoking and exposure to passive smoke are risk factors for cervical cancer. *JAMA* 261:1593–1598.

20. Trevathan, E., et al. 1983. Cigarette smoking and dysplasia and carcinoma in situ of the uterine cervix. *JAMA* 250:499–502.

21. Hoff, et al. 1987. Relationship between tobacco smoking and colorectal polyps. *Scand J Gastroenterol* 22:13–16.

22. Kikendall, et al. 1989. Cigarettes and alcohol as independent risk factors for colonic adenomas. *Gastroenterology* 97:660–664.

23. Buntain, et al. 1972. Premalignancy of polyps of the colon. *Surg Gyn Obstet* 134:499–508.

24. Fenoglio, et al. 1982. Colorectal adenomas and cancer. *Cancer* 50:2601–2608.

25. Ricker, et al. 1979. Adenomatous lesions of the large bowel. *Cancer* 43:1847–1857.

26. Zahm, et al. 1991. Tobacco smoking as a risk factor for colon polyps. *Am J Public Health* 81:846–849.

27. Nakayama, T., et al. 1985. Cigarette smoke induces DNA single-stranded breaks in human cells. *Nature* 314:462.

28. Pic, A. 1981. Heavy smoking and exercise can trigger MI. *Int Med News* 14(9):3.

29. Abbott, et al. 1986. Risk of stroke in male cigarette smokers. *NEJM* 315:717–720.

30. Wolf, et al. 1988. Cigarette smoking as a risk factor for stroke. *JAMA* 259:1025–1029.

31. Colditz, et al. 1988. Cigarette smoking and risk of stroke in middle-aged women. *NEJM* 318:937–941.

32. Rogers, et al. 1985. Abstention from cigarette smoking improves cerebral perfusion among the elderly chronic smokers. *JAMA* 253:2970–2974.

33. Baron, J.A. 1984. Smoking and estrogen-related disease. *Am J Epidemiol* 119:9–22.

34. Baird, et al. 1985. Cigarette smoking associated with delayed conception. *JAMA* 253:2979–2983.

35. Stjernfeldt, et al. 1986. Maternal smoking during pregnancy and risk of childhood cancer. *Lancet* (June 14):1350–1352.

36. Hopkin, J.M., and H.J. Evans. 1980. Cigarette smoke induced DNA damage and lung cancer risks. *Nature* 283:388.

37. Evans, H.J., et al. 1981. Sperm abnormalities and cigarette smoking. *Lancet* (March):627.

38. Finch, et al. 1982. Surface morphology and functional studies of human alveolar macrophages from cigarette smokers and nonsmokers. *J Reticuloendothel Soc* 32:1–23.

39. Cantin and Crystal. 1985. Oxidants, antioxidants, and the pathogenesis of emphysema. *Eur J Respir Dis* 139:7–17.

40. Bridges, et al. 1985. Effect of smoking on peripheral blood leukocytes and serum antiproteases. *Eur J Respir Dis* 139:24–33.

41. Ginns, et al. 1982. Alterations in immunoregulatory cells in lung cancer and smoking. *J Clin Immunol 3 Suppl:* 90S–94S.

42. Miller, et al. 1982. Reversible alterations in immunoregulatory T cells in smoking. *Chest* 82:526–529.

43. Nguyen and Keast. 1986. Effects of chronic daily exposure to tobacco smoke on the high leukemic AKR strain of mice. *Cancer Res* 46(7):3334–40.

44. Hersey, et al. 1983. Effects of cigarette smoking on the immune system. *Med J Aust* 2(9):425–9.

45. Burrows, et al. 1983. Interactions of smoking and immunologic factors in relation to airway obstruction. *Chest* 84(6):657–61.

46. Burrows, et al. Interactions of smoking and immunologic factors.

47. McSharry, et al. 1985. Effect of cigarette smoking on antibody response to inhaled antigens. *Clin Allergy* 15:487–94.

48. Fielding and Phenow. 1988. Health effects of involuntary smoking. *NEJM* 319:1452–1460.

49. Department of Health and Human Services. 1984. *Health consequences of smoking: Chronic obstructive lung disease: A report of the surgeon general.* Washington, D.C.: Government Printing Office. PHS: 84-50205.

50. Department of Health and Human Services. 1986. *Health consequences of involuntary smoking: A report of the surgeon general.* Washington, D.C.: GPO. Publication No. 87-8398.

51. National Research Council, Committee on passive smoking. 1986. *Environmental tobacco smoke: Measuring exposures and assessing health effects.* Washington, D.C.: GPO.

52. National Research Council, Committee on passive smoking.

53. Uberla. 1987. Lung cancer from passive smoking: Hypothesis or convincing evidence? *Ant Arch Occupa Environ Health* 59:421–37.

54. Janerich, D., et al. 1990. Lung cancer and exposure to tobacco smoke in the household. *NEJM* 323(10):632–636.

55. Slattery, M., et al. 1989. Cigarette smoking and exposure to passive smoke are risk factors for cervical cancer. *JAMA* 261:1593–1598.

56. Stjernfeldt, et al. Maternal smoking during pregnancy and risk of childhood cancer.

57. Kabat, G.C., et al. 1986. Bladder cancer in non-smokers. *Cancer* 57:362–367.

58. Hermanson, B., et al. 1988. Beneficial six year outcome of smoking cessation in older men and women with coronary heart disease: Results from the CASS registry. *NEJM* 319:1365–9.

59. LaCroix, A., et al. 1991. Smoking and mortality among older men and women in three communities. *NEJM* 324:1619–25.

60. Williamson, D.F., et al. 1991. Smoking cessation and severity of weight gain in a national cohort. *NEJM* 324:739–45.

61. Sharfstein and Sharfstein. 1994. Campaign contributions from the AMA Political Action Committee to members of Congress. *NEJM* 330:32–37.

Chapter 12
Alcohol and Caffeine

1. Adams, et al. 1993. Alcohol-related hospitalizations of elderly people. *JAMA* 270:1222–1225.

2. Rosenberg, L., D. Sloan, S. Shapiro, et al. 1982. Breast cancer and alcoholic consumption. *Lancet* 30:267.

3. Schatzkin, et al. 1987. Alcohol consumption and breast cancer in the epidemiologic follow-up study of the first NHANES. *NEJM* 316:1169–1173.

4. Graham, S. 1987. Alcohol and breast cancer. *NEJM* 316:1211–1212.
5. Longnecker, et al. 1988. A meta-analysis of alcohol consumption in relation to risk of breast cancer. *JAMA* 260:652–656.
6. Editorial. 1985. Does alcohol cause breast cancer? *Lancet* (June 8):1311–12.
7. Webster, et al. 1983. Alcohol consumption and the risk of breast cancer. *Lancet* (Sept 24):724–726.
8. Lindegard, et al. Alcohol and breast cancer. *NEJM* 317:1285–1286.
9. Willett, et al. 1987. Moderate alcohol consumption and the risk of breast cancer. *NEJM* 316:1174–1180.
10. Friend, T. 1992. Alcohol may speed up cancer. Society for Neuroscience meeting. *USA Today*. Oct. 28:1.
11. Stampfer, et al. 1988. A prospective study of moderate alcohol consumption and the risk of coronary heart disease and stroke in women. *NEJM* 319:267–273.
12. Gill, et al. 1986. Stroke and alcohol consumption. *NEJM* 315:1041–1046.
13. Simon, D., S. Yen, and P. Cole. 1975. Coffee drinking and cancer of the lower urinary tract system. *J Natl Cancer Inst* 54(3):587.
14. Mulvihill, J. 1973. Caffeine as teratogen and mutagen. *Teratology* 8:69.
15. Weinstein, D., I. Mauer, and H. Solomon. 1972. The effects of caffeine on chromosomes of human lymphocytes. *Mutat Res* 16:391.
16. Soyka, L.F. 1979. Effects of methylxanthines on the fetus. *Clinics in Perinatol* 6(1):37.
17. Weathersbee, P.S., L.K. Olsen, and J.R. Lodge. 1977. Caffeine and pregnancy. *Postgrad Med* 62(3):64.
18. LaCroix, A., et al. 1986. Coffee consumption and the incidence of coronary heart disease. *NEJM* 315:977–982.
19. Barrett-Connor, E., et al. 1994. Coffee-associated osteoporosis offset by daily milk consumption. *JAMA* 271:280–283.

Chapter 13
Hormonal and Sexual-Social Factors

1. Grossman, C. 1985. Interactions between the gonadal steroids and the immune system. *Science* 227:257–261.
2. Adami, et al. 1990. The effect of female sex hormones on cancer survival. *JAMA* 263:2189–2193.
3. Marshall, E. 1993. Search for a killer: focus on hormones. *Science* 259:618–621.
4. Kvale, et al. 1988. Menstrual factors and breast cancer risk. *Cancer* 62:1625–1631.
5. Hughes and Jones. 1985. Intake of dietary fibre and the age of menarche. *Ann Human Biology* 12:325–332.
6. MacMahon, et al. 1970. Age at first birth and breast cancer risk. *Bull WHO* 42:209–221.
7. Miller, et al. 1986. Multidisciplinary project on breast cancer: the epidemiology, etiology, and prevention of breast cancer. *Int J Cancer* 37:174–177.
8. Kvale and Heuch. 1987. A prospective study of reproductive factors and breast cancer II: age at first and last birth. *Am J Epidemiol* 126:842–850.
9. Arruda, et al. 1987. Pesquisa nacional sobre saude materno-infantil e planejamento familiar. Rio de Janerio: PNSMIPF.
10. Kalache, et al. 1993. Age at last full term pregnancy and risk of breast cancer. *Lancet* 341:32–35.
11. Pike, M., et al. 1981. Oral contraceptive use and early abortion as risk factors for breast cancer in young women. *Br J Cancer* 43:72–76.
12. Dvoirin and Medvedev. 1978. The role of reproductive history in breast cancer causation. *Methods and results of studies of breast cancer epidemiology.* Tallinn, Estonia (in Russian), pp. 53–56.
13. Brinton, et al. 1983. Reproductive factors in the etiology of breast cancer. *Brit J Cancer* 47:757–782.
14. Segi, et al. 1957. An epidemiological study of breast cancer in Japan. *GANN* 48:1.
15. Lin, et al. 1970. Epidemiological characteristics of cancer of the breast in Taiwan. *Cancer* 27:1497–1504.
16. Parazzini, et al. 1991. Menstrual and reproductive factors and breast cancer in women with family history of the disease. *Int J Cancer* 51:677–681.

17. Olsson, et al. 1991. Her-2/neu and INT2 proto-oncogene amplification in malignant breast tumors in relation to reproductive factors and exposure to exogenous hormones. *JNCI* 83:1483–1487.

18. Olsson, et al. 1991. Proliferation and DNA ploidy in malignant breast tumors in relation to early oral contraceptive use and early abortion. *Cancer* 67:1285–1290.

19. Lindefors-Harris, et al. 1989. Risk of cancer of the breast after legal abortion during first trimester: a Swedish register study. *Brit Med J* 299:1430–1432.

20. Howe, et al. 1989. Early abortion and breast cancer risk among women under age 40. *Int J Epidemiol* 18:300–304.

21. Russo, et al. 1980. Susceptibility of the mammary gland to carcinogenesis, II. Pregnancy interruption as a risk factor in tumor incidence. *Am J Pathol* 100:497–509.

22. Brooks and Pauley. 1991. Breast cancer biology. In *Encyclopedia of Human Biology,* ed. R. Dulbecco.

23. Trichopoulos, D. 1990. Hypothesis: does breast cancer originate in utero? *Lancet* 335:939–940.

24. Yen, S.C.C. 1989. Endocrinology of pregnancy. In *Maternal-Fetal Medicine,* ed. Creasy and Resnic. Philadelphia: W.B. Saunders. pp. 375–403.

25. Ekbom, et al. 1992. Evidence of prenatal influences on breast cancer risk. *Lancet* 340:1015–1018.

26. Brinton, et al. 1983. Epidemiology of minimal breast cancer. *JAMA* 249:483–487.

27. Gammon and John. 1993. Recent etiologic hypothesis concerning breast cancer. *Epidemiol Rev* 15:163–168.

28. Wynder, E., et al. 1960. Dietary factors in breast cancer. *Cancer* 13:559–601.

29. MacMahon, B., et al. 1970. Lactation and cancer of the breast: a summary of an international study. *Bull World Health Organ* 42:185–194.

30. Byers, et al. 1985. Lactation and breast cancer: evidence for a negative association in premenopausal women. *Am J Epidemiol* 12:664–674.

31. Newcomb, et al. 1994. Lactation and a reduced risk of premenopausal breast cancer. *NEJM* 330:81–87.

32. McTiernan, et al. 1986. Evidence for a protective effect of lactation on risk of breast cancer in young women: results from a case-control study. *Am J Epidemiol* 124:353–358.

33. Katsouyanni, et al. 1986. Diet and breast cancer: a case control study in Greece. *Int J Cancer* 38:815-820.

34. Rosero-Bixby, et al. 1987. Reproductive history and breast cancer in a population of high fertility: Costa Rica 1984–1985. *Int J Cancer* 40:747–754.

35. Yuan, et al. 1988. Risk factors for breast cancer in Chinese women in Shanghai. *Cancer Res* 48:1949–1953.

36. Siskind, et al. Breast cancer and breast feeding: results from an Australian case-control study. *Am J Epidemiol* 130:229–236.

37. Yoo, et al. 1992. Independent protective effect of lactation against breast cancer: a case-control study in Japan. *Am J Epidemiol* 135:726–733.

38. United Kingdom National Case-Control Study Group. 1993. Breast feeding and risk of breast cancer in young women. *BMJ* 307:17–20.

39. Ing, et al. 1977. Unilateral breast feeding and breast cancer. *Lancet* (July 16):124–127.

40. Henderson, et al. 1982. Endogenous hormones as a major factor in human cancer. *Cancer Res* 42:3232–3239.

41. Petrakis, et al. 1987. Influence of pregnancy and lactation on serum and breast fluid estrogen levels: implications for breast cancer risk. *Int J Cancer* 40:587–591.

42. Avery and Taeusch, eds. 1984. *Shaffer's Diseases of the Newborn.* Fifth edition. Philadelphia: W.B. Saunders.

43. Mannella, et al. 1991. The transfer of alcohol to human milk—effects on flavor and the infant's behavior. *NEJM* 325:981–985.

44. Levine and Ilowite. 1994. Sclerodermalike esophageal disease in children breast-fed by mothers with silicone breast implants. *JAMA* 271:213–216.

45. Donegan, W.L. 1983. Cancer and

pregnancy. *CA-A Cancer J for Clinicians* 33(4):194–214.

46. Orr, J.W., and H.M. Shingleton. 1983. Cancer in pregnancy. *Current problems in cancer.* Yearbook Medical Publishers. 8(1):3–50.

47. Danforth, D. 1991. How subsequent pregnancy affects outcome in women with a prior breast cancer. *Oncology* 5:23–35.

48. Petrek, et al. 1991. Prognosis of pregnancy-associated breast cancer. *Cancer* 67:869–872.

49. Lambe, M., et al. 1994. Transient increase in the risk of breast cancer after giving birth. *NEJM* 331:5–9.

50. Guinee, V.F., et al. 1994. Effect of pregnancy on prognosis for young women with breast cancer. *Lancet* 343:1587–1589.

51. Boyd, N.F., et al. 1988. Effect of low fat, high carbohydrate diet on symptoms of cyclical mastopathy. *Lancet* (July 16): 128–129.

52. Henderson, et al. 1982. Endogenous hormones as a major factor in human cancer. *Cancer Research* 42:3232–3239.

53. Musey, et ¯l. 1987. Long term effect of a first pregnancy on the secretion of prolactin. *NEJM* 316:229–234.

54. Herbst, et al. 1971. Adenocarcinoma of the vagina. *NEJM* 284:878–81.

55. Robboy, S.J., et al. 1984. Increased incidence of cervical and vaginal dysplasia in 3980 diethylstilbesterol exposed young women. *JAMA* 252:2979–2990.

56. Greenberg, et al. 1984. Breast cancer in mothers given DES in pregnancy. *NEJM* 311:1393–1398.

57. Bibbo, et al. 1978. A twenty-five year follow up study of women exposed to DES during pregnancy. *NEJM* 298:763–7.

58. Melnick, et al. 1987. Rates and risk of DES related clear cell adenocarcinoma of the vagina and cervix. *NEJM* 316:514–516.

59. Conley, et al. 1983. Seminoma and epididymal cysts in a young man with known DES exposure in utero. *JAMA* 249:1325–1326.

60. Loizzo, et al. 1984. Italian baby food containing DES: Three years later. *Lancet* (May 5):1013–1014.

61. Centers for Disease Control cancer and steroid hormone study: Long term oral contraceptive use and the risk of breast cancer. 1983. *JAMA* 249:1591–1595.

62. Pike, M.C., et al. 1983. Breast cancer in young women and use of oral contraceptives: Possible modifying effect of formulation and age at use. *Lancet* (October 22): 926–930.

63. McPherson, et al. 1983. Oral contraceptives and breast cancer. *Lancet* ii:1414–1415.

64. Rookus, M., et al. 1994. Oral contraceptives and risk of breast cancer in women aged 20–54 years. *Lancet* 344:844–851.

65. UK National Case Control Study Group. Oral contraceptive use and breast cancer risk in young women. 1989. *Lancet* (May 6):973–982.

66. Rosenberg, L., et al. 1984. Breast cancer and oral contraceptive use. *Am J Epidemiol* 119:167–76.

67. Olsson, et al. 1985. Oral contraceptive use and breast cancer in young women in Sweden. *Lancet* i:748–49.

68. Kalach, et al. 1983. Oral contraceptives and breast cancer. *Br J Hosp Med* 30:278–83.

69. Royal College of General Practitioners. 1981. Breast cancer and oral contraceptives in the royal college of general practitioners study. *Br Med J* 282:2089–93.

70. Vessey, et al. 1983. Neoplasia of the cervix uteri and contraception: A possible adverse effect of the pill. *Lancet* (October 22): 930–934.

71. Neuberger, et al. 1986. Oral contraceptives and hepatocellular carcinoma. *Br Med J* 292:1355–1361.

72. Cancer and steroid hormone study for CDC. 1987. Combination oral contraceptive use and the risk of endometrial cancer. *JAMA* 257:796–800.

73. Cancer and steroid hormone study of the CDC. 1987. Reduction in the risk of ovarian cancer associated with oral contraceptive use. *NEJM* 316:650–655.

74. Liange, et al. 1983. Risk of breast,

uterus, and ovarian cancer in women receiving medroxyprogesterone injections. *JAMA* 249:2909–2912.

75. WHO collaborative study of neoplasia and steroid contraceptives. 1984. Breast cancer, cervical cancer, and depot medroxy progesterone acetate. *Lancet* (Nov. 24): 1207–1208.

76. Nabulsi, et al. 1993. Association of hormone-replacement therapy with various cardiovascular risk factors in postmenopausal women. *NEJM* 328:1069–1075.

77. Schwarz, Barry. 1981. Does estrogen cause adenocarcinoma of the endometrium. *Len Ob Gyn* 24:243–251.

78. Henderson, et al. 1975. Elevated serum levels of estrogen and prolactin in daughters of patients with breast cancer. *NEJM* 293:790–795.

79. Kirk, M.E. 1979. Tumorogenic aspects. *Int J Gyn OBS* 16:473–478.

80. Colditz, et al. 1990. Prospective study of estrogen replacement therapy and risk of breast cancer in postmenopausal women. *JAMA* 264(20): 2648–2653.

81. Orentreich, N., and N.P. Durr. 1974. Mammogenesis in transsexuals. *J Invest Dermatol* 63:142.

82. Symmers, W.S. 1968. Carcinoma of the breast in transsexuals. *Br Med J* 1:83.

83. Treves, N., and A. Holleb. 1955. Cancer of the male breast. *Cancer* 8:1239.

84. Orentreich and Durr. Mammogenesis in transsexuals.

85. Treves and Holleb. Cancer of the male breast.

86. Hoover, R., L.A. Gray, and B. MacMahon. 1976. Menopausal estrogens and breast cancer. *NEJM* 295:401.

87. Casagrande, J., U. Gerkins, et al. 1976. Exogenous estrogens and breast cancer in women with natural menopause. *J Natl Cancer Inst* 56:839.

88. Burch, J., et al. 1975. The effects of long term estrogen therapy, estrogen in the postmenopause. *Front Horm Res* 3:208.

89. Barrett-Conner, et al. 1993. Estrogen replacement therapy and cognitive function in older women. *JAMA* 269:2637–2641.

90. Hulka, B. 1990. Hormone-replacement therapy and the risk of breast cancer. *CA-A Cancer J for Clinicians* 40:289–296.

91. Steinberg, et al. 1991. A meta-analysis of the effect of estrogen replacement therapy on the risk of breast cancer. *JAMA* 265:1985–1990.

92. Marx, J. 1989. Estrogen use linked to breast cancer. *Science* 245:593–595.

93. Pike, et al. 1993. Estrogens, progestogens, normal breast cell proliferation, and breast cancer risk. *Epidemiol Rev* 15:17–35.

94. Bergkvist, et al. 1989. The risk of breast cancer after estrogen and estrogen-progestin replacement. *NEJM* 321:293–297.

95. Spicer, et al. 1990. The question of estrogen replacement therapy in patients with a prior diagnosis of breast cancer. *Oncology* 4:49–54.

96. Hoffman, D., et al. 1984. Breast cancer in hypothyroid women using thyroid supplements. *JAMA* 251:616–619.

Chapter 14
Air and Water

1. Buell, P. 1967. Relative impact of smoking and air pollution on lung cancer. *Arch Environ Health* 15:291–297.

2. Cederlof, R., et al. 1975. The relationship of smoking and social covariables to mortality and cancer mortality, a ten year follow up in a probability sample of 55,000 Swedish subjects age 18–69. Stockholm: Department of Environmental Hygiene, The Karolinska Institute.

3. Dean, G. 1966. Lung cancer and bronchitis in Northern Ireland. *Br Med J* 1:1506.

4. Lee, M.L., N. Novotny, and K.D. Bartle. 1976. Gas chromatography/mass spectometric and nuclear magnetic resonance determination of polynuclear aromatic hydrocarbons in airborne particulates. *Anal Chem* 48:1566.

5. Editorial. 1992. Environmental pollution: it kills trees, but does it kill people? *Lancet* 340:821–822.

6. Editorial. 1993. Tiny particles in air

linked to early death. *The Japan Times* (May 18):18.

7. Dockery, D.W., et al. 1993. An association between air pollution and mortality in six U.S. cities. *NEJM* 329:1753–1759.

8. Editorial. 1993. Air pollution and mortality. *NEJM* 329:1807–1808.

9. Hoffmann, D., I. Schmeltz, S.S. Hecht, et al. 1986. Volatile carcinogens. Occurence, formation, and analysis. In *Prevention and detection of cancer. Part 1. Prevention. Vol. 2. Etiology, prevention methods*, ed. H.E. Nieburgs. New York and Basel: Marcel Dekker, Inc., pps. 1943–1959.

10. National Research Council. 1976. *Vapor-phase organic pollutants*. Committee on medical and biological effects of environmental pollutants. Washington, D.C.: National Academy of Sciences.

11. U.S. Department of Health and Human Services, National Institute for Occupational Safety and Health. 1988. *Carcinogenic effects of exposure to diesel exhaust*. Washington, D.C.: Government Printing Office. (Current intelligence bulletin No. 50. [August]).

12. Committee on the Atmosphere and Biosphere, National Research Council. 1981. *Atmosphere biosphere interactions: Toward a better understanding of the ecological consequences of fossil fuel combustion*. Washington, D.C.: National Academy Press.

13. Luoma, J.R. 1984. *Troubled Skies, Troubled Waters*. New York: Viking Press.

14. Cronan, C.S., et al. 1979. Aluminum leaching response to acid precipitation: Effects on high elevation water sheds in the northeast. *Science* 204:304–306.

15. Perl, D.P., et al. 1982. Intraneuronal aluminum accumulation in amyotrophic lateral sclerosis and parkinsonism in Guam. *Science* 217:1053–1055.

16. Shore, D., et al. 1983. Aluminum and Alzheimer's disease. *J Nerv Ment Dis* 171:553–558.

17. Letters. 1986. *Geophysical research* 13 (November).

18. Isaksen, I. 1986. Ozone perturbations studies in a two dimensional model in a feedback on the stratosphere included UNEP workshop.

19. Hocking, M. 1991. Paper versus polystyrene: A complex choice. *Science* 251:504–505.

20. Blumthaler and Ambach. 1991. How well do sunglasses protect against ultraviolet radiation? *Lancet* 337:1284.

21. World Health Organization. 1983. *Indoor air pollutants: Exposure and health effects assessment*. Report No. 78. Nordlingen Copenhagen: WHO.

22. National Council on Radiation Protection and Measurements. 1984. Exposures from the uranium series with emphasis on radon and its daughters. *NCRP* March 15.

23. Nero, AV. 1983. Indoor radon exposures from radon and its daughters. *Health Physics* 45:277–88.

24. Abelson, P. 1990. Uncertainties about health effects of radon. *Science* 250:353.

25. BEIR IV. 1988. *Health risks of radon and other internally deposited alpha emitters*. Washington, D.C.: National Academy Press.

26. Repace, J.L. 1984. Consistency of research data on passive smoking and lung cancer. *Lancet* i:506.

27. Hueper, W.C. 1960. Cancer hazards from natural and artificial water pollutants. In *Proceedings, Physiological Aspects of Water Quality*, ed. H.A. Farber, and J.L. Bryson. Washington, D.C.: Public Health Service, 181–193.

28. U.S. Environmental Protection Agency. 1975. *Preliminary assessment of suspected carcinogens in drinking water*. Report to Congress. Washington, D.C.: Government Printing Office.

29. Harris, R.H., T. Page, and N.A. Reiches. 1977. Carcinogenic hazards of organic chemicals in drinking water. In *Book A. Incidence of Cancer in Humans*, ed. H.H. Hiatt, J.D. Watson, and J.A. Winsten. Cold Spring Harbor, NY: Cold Spring Harbor Laboratory.

30. Hogan, M.D., et al. 1979. Association between chloroform and various site-specific cancer mortality rates. *J Environ Pathol Toxicol* 2:873.

31. Cantor, K.P., et al. 1978. Associations

of cancer mortality with halomethanes in drinking water. *JNCI* 61:979.

32. National Research Council. 1978. Chloroform, carbon tetrachloride, and other halomethanes—an environmental assessment. Washington, D.C.: National Academy of Sciences.

33. Rafferty, P.J. 1978. Public health aspects of drinking water quality in North Carolina. Master's thesis, Department of Environmental Sciences and Engineering, School of Public Health, University of North Carolina, Chapel Hill, North Carolina.

34. Spivey, G.H., et al. 1977. *Cancer and chlorinated drinking water. Final report.* EPA contract No. CA-6-99-3349-J. Cincinnati, Ohio: U.S. Environmental Protection Agency.

35. Tuthill, R.W., et al. 1978. *Chlorination of public drinking water supplies and subsequent cancer mortality: An ecological-time lag study. Final report.* EPA contract No. EPA-68-03-1200. Cincinnati, Ohio: U.S. Environmental Protection Agency.

36. U.S. Environmental Protection Agency. 1975. Preliminary Assessment.

37. Comstock, G. 1980. The epidemiologic perspective: Water hardness and cardiovascular disease. *J Environ Path Toxicol* 4(2):3–9.

38. Hewitt, D., et al. 1980. Development of the water story: some recent Canadian studies. *J Environ Path Toxicol* 4-2, 3:51.

39. McCarron, et al. 1985. Blood pressure response to oral calcium in persons with mild to moderate hypertension. *Ann Intern Med* 103:825.

40. Garland, et al. 1985. Dietary vitamin D and calcium and risk of colorectal cancer: A 19-year prospective study in man. *Lancet* i:307.

41. Rozen, et al. 1989. Calcium supplements protect against colorectal cancer. *Gut* 30:650–655.

42. U.S. Atomic Energy Commission. 1974. *Plutonium and other transuranium elements; Sources, environmental distribution and biomedical effects.* Washington, D.C.: Government Printing Office.

43. National Research Council, Safe drinking water committee. 1977. *Drinking water and health.* Washington, D.C.: National Academy of Sciences.

44. Kanarek, M.S. 1978. Asbestos in drinking water and cancer incidence in the San Francisco Bay Area. Ph.D. Dissertation, Department of Epidemiology, School of Public Health, University of California, Berkeley, California.

Chapter 15
Electromagnetic Radiation

1. Land, et al. 1980. Breast cancer risk from low dose exposures to ionizing radiation. *JNCI* 65:353–376.

2. Miller, et al. 1989. Mortality for breast cancer after radiation during fluoroscopic examinations in patients being treated for tuberculosis. *NEJM* 321:1285–1289.

3. Feig, S.A. 1984. Radiation risks from mammography: Is it clinically significant? *AJR* 143:469–475.

4. Hall, F.M. 1986. Screening mammography: potential problems on the horizon. *NEJM* 314:53–55.

5. Roberts, T. 1992. Women radiated for Hodgkin's have high breast cancer risk. *Radiology Today* (Sept):12–13.

6. Li, F., et al. 1983. Breast carcinoma after cancer therapy in childhood. *Cancer* 51:521–523.7. Harvey, et al. 1985. Second cancer following cancer of the breast in Connecticut, 1935 to 1982. *NCI Monograph* 68:99–112.

7. Harvey, E., et al. 1985. Second cancer following cancer of the breast in Connecticut, 1935 to 1982. *NCI Monograph* 68:99–112.

8. Storm, H., and O. Jensen. 1986. Risk of contralateral breast cancer in Denmark. *Br J Cancer* 54:483–492.

9. Boice, J., et al. 1992. Cancer in the contralateral breast after radiotherapy for breast cancer. *NEJM* 326:781–785.

10. Fisher, B., et al. 1985. Ten year results of a randomized clinical trial comparing radical mastectomy and total mastectomy with or without radiation. *NEJM* 312:674–681.

11. Basco, V., et al. 1985. Radiation dose and second breast cancer. *Br J Cancer* 52:319–325.

12. McCredie, J., et al. 1975. Consecutive primary carcinomas of the breast. *Cancer* 35:1472–1477.

13. Schell, S., et al. 1982. Bilateral breast cancer in patients with initial stage I and II. *Cancer* 50:1191–1194.

14. Burns, P. 1984. Bilateral breast cancer in northern Alberta. *Can Med Assoc Journal* 130:881–886.

15. Horn, P., and W. Thompson. 1988. Risk of contralateral breast cancer. *Cancer* 62:412–424.

16. Parker, R., et al. 1989. Contralateral breast cancers following treatment for initial breast cancer in women. *Am J Clin Oncol* 12:213–216.

17. Hildreth, N., et al. 1989. The risk of breast cancer after irradiation of the thymus in infancy. *NEJM* 321:1281–1284.

18. Modan, B., et al. 1989. Increased risk of breast cancer after low dose radiation. *Lancet* (March 25):629–631.

19. Land, et al. 1993. *JNCI* (Oct. 20).

20. Bonnell, J.A. 1982. Effects of electric fields near power transmission plant. *J Roy Soc Med* 75:933–44.

21. Pool, Robert. 1990. Electromagnetic fields: The biological evidence. *JAMA* 249:1378–1381.

22. Wertheimer, and Leeper. 1979. Electrical wiring configurations in childhood cancer. *Am J Epidemiol* 109:273–84.

23. Wertheimer, and Leeper. 1982. Adult cancer related to electrical wires near the home. *Int J Epidemiol* 11:354–55.

24. Gauger, J.R. 1985. Household appliance magnetic field survey. IEEE Trans PAS-104, No. 9. In *Epidemiological studies relating human health to electric and magnetic fields; criteria for evaluation, 1988.* International Electricity Research Exchange (June 22): 26.

25. Milham. 1982. Mortality from leukemia in workers exposed to electrical and magnetic fields. *NEJM* 307:249.

26. Wright, et al. 1982. Leukemia in workers exposed to electrical and magnetic fields. *Lancet* ii: 1160–61.

27. McDowall. 1983. Leukemia mortality in electrical workers in England and Wales. *Lancet*, 246.

28. Tynes and Anderson. 1990. Electromagnetic fields and male breast cancer. *Lancet* 336:1596.

29. Demers, P.A., et al. 1991. Occupational exposure to electromagnetic fields and breast cancer in men. *Am J Epidemiol* 134:340–347.

30. University of California News Service. 1988. 63:13.

31. Stevens, R.G., et al. 1992. Electric power, pineal function, and the risk of breast cancer. *Faseb J* 6:853–860.

32. Vena, J.E., et al. 1991. Use of electric blankets and risk of postmenopausal breast cancer. *Am J Epidemiol* 134:180–185.

33. Worries about radiation continue, as do studies. 1990. *The New York Times* (July 8).

34. Worries about radiation continue, as do studies. 1990.

35. *J Electro Anal Chem.* 1986. 211:447–456.

36. *Immunol Lett.* 1986. 13:295–299.

Chapter 16
Sedentary Lifestyle

1. Tomasi, et al. 1982. Immune parameters in athletes before and after strenuous exercise. *J Clin Immunol* 2:173–178.

2. Soppi, et al. 1982. Effect of strenuous physical stress on circulating lymphocyte number and function before and after training. *J Clin Lab Immunol* 8:43–46.

3. Robertson, et al. 1981. The effect of strenuous physical exercise on circulating blood lymphocytes and serum cortisol levels. *J Clin Lab Immunol* 5:53–57.

4. Hanson, et al. 1981. Immunological responses to training in conditioned runners. *Clin Soc* 60:225–228.

5. Green, et al. 1981. Immune function in marathon runners. *Ann Allergy* 47:73–75.

6. Busse, W.W., et al. 1980. The effect of exercise on the granulocyte response to isoproterenol in the trained athlete and unconditioned individual. *J Allergy Clin Immunol* 65:358–364.

7. Eskola, et al. 1978. Effect of sport stress on lymphocyte transformation and antibody formation. *Clin Exp Immunol* 32:339–345.

8. Yu, et al. 1977. Effect of corticosteroid on exercise induced lymphocytosis. *Clin Exp Immunol* 28:326–331.

9. Hedfors, et al. 1976. Variations of blood lymphocytes during work studied by cell surface markers, DNA synthesis and cytotoxicity. *Clin Exp Immunol* 24:328–335.

10. Cannon and Kluger. 1983. Endogenous pyrogen activity in human plasma after exercise. *Science* 220:617–619.

11. Dinarello and Wolff. 1982. Molecular basis of fever in humans. *Am J Med* 72:799–819.

12. Dinarello. 1984. *Rev Infect Dis* 6:51–94.

13. Cannon, V., and C. Dinarello. 1984. Interleukin I activity in human plasma. *Fed Proc* 43:462.

14. Gershbein, L.L., et al. 1974. An influence of stress on lesion growth and on survival of animals bearing parental and intracerebral leukemia. L 1210 and Walker tumors. *Oncology* 30:429.

15. DeRosa, G., and N.R. Suarez. 1980. Effect of exercise on tumor growth and body composition of the host. *Fed Am Soc Exp Biol*, 1118.

16. Frisch, R.E., et al. 1985. Lower prevalence of breast cancer in cancers of the reproductive system among former college athletes compared to non-athletes. *Br J Cancer* 52:885–891.

17. Garabrant, D.H., et al. 1984. Job activity and colon cancer risk. *Am J Epidemiol* 119(6):1005–1014.

18. Vena, J.E., et al. 1985. Lifetime occupational exercise and colon cancer. *Am J Epidemiol* 122(3):357–365.

19. Gerhardsson, M., et al. 1986. Sedentary jobs and colon cancer. *Am J Epidemiol* 123(5):775–780.

20. Paffenbarger, R., et al. 1986. Physical activity, all cause mortality, and longevity of college alumni. *NEJM* 314:605–613.

21. Harris, S.S., et al. 1989. Physical activity counseling for healthy adults as a primary preventive intervention in the clinical setting report for the U.S. Preventive Services Task Force. *JAMA* 261:3590–3598.

22. Mittleman, et al. 1993. Triggering of acute myocardial infarction by heavy physical exertion. *NEJM* 329:1677–1683.

23. Pollack, M.L. 1973. The quantification and endurance training programs. In *Exercise and sport sciences reviews*, vol. I, ed. J.H. Wilmore. New York: Academic Press.

24. Louis Harris and Associates, Inc. 1978. Perrier survey of fitness in America. Study No. S 2813. New York, NY.

25. Blair, et al. 1989. Physical fitness, an all cause mortality. *JAMA* 262:2395–2401.

26. Centers for Disease Control. 1989. Progress toward achieving the 1990 national objectives for physical fitness and exercise. *MMWR* 38:449–453.

27. Duncan, et al. 1991. Women walking for health and fitness. *JAMA* 266:3295–3299.

28. King, et al. 1991. Group- vs. home-based exercise training in healthy older men and women. *JAMA* 266:1535–1542.

29. Somers, V.K., et al. 1991. Effects of endurance training on baroreflex sensitivity and blood pressure in borderline hypertension. *Lancet* 337:1363–68.

30. Rippe, James M., et al. 1988. Walking for health and fitness. *JAMA* 259:2720–2724.

31. Porcari, J., et al. 1987. Is fast walking an adequate aerobic training stimulus for 30-69 year old men and women? *Physician and Sports Medicine* 15(2):119–129.

32. Petty, B.G., et al. 1986. Physical activity and longevity of college alumni, letter. *NEJM* 315(6):399.

33. Winningham, M.L., et al. 1986. Exercise for cancer patients: Guidelines and precautions. *Physician and Sports Medicine* 14(10):125–134.

34. Medical News and Perspectives. 1991. Exercise, health links need hard proof, say researchers studying mechanisms. *JAMA* 265 (22):2928.

35. Horton, E. 1991. Exercise and de-

creased risk of NIDDM. *NEJM* 325(3):196–97.

36. Helmrich, S., et al. 1991. Physical activity and reduced occurrence of non-insulin-dependent diabetes mellitus. *NEJM* 325(3):147–52.

Chapter 17
Stress

1. LeShan, L.L. 1959. Psychological states as factors in the development of malignant disease: A critical review. *JNCI* 22:1–18.
2. Ader, R., ed. 1981. *Psychoneuroimmunology.* New York: Academic Press.
3. Angeletti, R., W. Hickey. 1985. A neuroendocrine marker in tissues of the immune system. *Science* 230:89–90.
4. Bulloch, K. 1985. *Neuralmodulation of Immunity.* New York: Raven Press, 111.
5. Riley, V. 1981. Psychoneuroendocrine influences on immunocompetence and neoplasia. *Science* 212:1100–1109.
6. Bartrop, R., et al. 1977. Depressed lymphocyte function after bereavement. *Lancet* i:834–836.
7. Schleifer, S.␣., et al. 1983. Suppression of lymphocyte stimulation following bereavement. *JAMA* 250:374–377.
8. Kronfol, Z., et al. 1983. Impaired lymphocyte function in depressive illness. *Life Science* 33:241–247.
9. Schleifer, S.J., et al. 1984. Lymphocyte function in major depressive disorder. *Arch J Psychiatry* 41:484–486.
10. Schleifer, S.J., et al. 1985. Lymphocyte function in ambulatory depressed patients, hospitalized schizophrenic patients, and patients hospitalized for herniorrhaphy. *Arch Jen Psychiatry* 42:129–133.
11. Locke, S., et al. 1984. Life change stress, psychiatric symptoms, and natural killer cell activity. *Psychosomatic Med* 46:441–453.
12. Heisel, J.S., et al. 1984. Natural killer cell activity and MMPI scores of a cohort of college students. *Am J Psychiatry* 143:1382–86.
13. Jemmott, J.B., et al. 1983. Academic stress, power motivation and decrease

in secretion rate of salivary secretory immunoglobulin A. *Lancet* ii:1400–1402.
14. Ader, R., N. Cohen. 1975. Behaviorally conditioned immunosuppressant. *Psychosomatic Medicine* 37:333–340.
15. Black, S., et al. 1963. Inhibition of mantoux reaction by direct suggestion under hypnosis. *Br Med J* 1:1649–1652.
16. Smith, G.R., et al. 1985. Psychological modulation of human immune response to varicella zoster. *Arch Intern Med* 145:2110–2112.
17. Horne, R.L. and R.S. Picard. 1979. Psychosocial risk factors for lung cancer. *Psychosomatic Medicine* 41:503–514.
18. Jacobs, T.J., and E. Charles. 1980. Life events and the occurrence of cancer in children. *Psychosomatic Medicine* 42:11–24.
19. Bloom, B.L., et al. 1978. Marital disruption as a stressor: A review and analysis. *Psychological Bulletin* 85:867–894.
20. Fox, B.H. 1978. Premorbid psychological factors as related to cancer incidence. *Journal of Behavioral Medicine* 1:45–133.
21. Bloom, B.L., et al. 1978. Marital disruption as a stressor: A review and analysis. *Psychological Bulletin* 85:867–894.
22. LeShan, L.L. 1966. An emotional life history pattern associated with neoplastic disease. *Ann NY Acad Sci* 125:780–793.
23. Ernster, B.L., et al. 1979. Cancer incidence by marital status: U.S. third national cancer survey. *J Natl Cancer Inst* 63:567–585.
24. Mastrovito, R.C., et al. 1979. Personality characteristics of women with gynecological cancer. *Cancer Detection and Prevention* 2:281–287.
25. Stavraky, K.C., et al. 1968. Psychological factors in the outcome of human cancer. *Journal of Psychosomatic Research* 12:251–259.
26. Bacon, C.L., et al. 1952. A psychosomatic survey of cancer of the breast. *Psychosomatic Medicine* 14:453–560.
27. Greer, S., and T. Morris. 1975. Psychological attributes of women who de-

velop breast cancer: A controlled study. *Journal of Psychosomatic Research* 19:147–153.

28. Horne, R.L., and R.S. Picard. 1979. Psychosocial risk factors for lung cancer. *Psychosomatic Medicine* 41:503–514.

29. Paykel, E.S. 1979. Recent life events in the development of depressive disorders. In *The Psychobiology of the Depressive Disorders,* ed. R.A. Depue. New York: Academic Press.

30. Schmale, A., et al. 1966. The psychological setting of the uterine cervical cancer. *Ann NY Acad Sci* 125:807–813.

31. Rogentine, G., et al. 1979. Psychological factors in the prognosis of malignant melanoma. *Psychosomatic Medicine* 41:647–655.

32. Derogatis, L., et al. 1979. Psychological coping mechanisms and survival time in metastatic breast cancer. *JAMA* 242:1504–1508.

33. Greer, S., et al. 1979. Psychological response to breast cancer: Effect on outcome. *Lancet* ii:785–787.

34. Greer, S., and T. Morris. 1975. Psychological attributes of women who develop breast cancer. *Journal of Psychosomatic Research* 19:147–153.

35. Thomas, C.B., et al. Family attitudes reported in youth as potential predictors of cancer. *Psychosomatic Medicine* 41:287–302.

36. Editorial. 1993. Stress and colorectal cancer. *Epidemiol* Sept.

37. *Impact of psychoendocrine systems in cancer and immunity,* ed. Fox, Newberry. 1984. Lewiston, New York: C.J. Hogrefe.

38. Bahnson. 1981. Stress and cancer: The state of the art. *Psychosomatics* 22(3):207–220.

39. Visintainer, et al. 1982. Tumor rejection in rats after inescapable or escapable shock. *Science* 216:437–439.

40. Sklar and Anisman. 1979. Stress and coping factors influence tumor growth. *Science* 205:513–515.

41. Morris, T., et al. 1981. Patterns of expression of age and their psychological correlates in women with breast cancer. *J Psychosom Res* 25:111–117.

42. Grassi, L., et al. 1986. Eventi stressanti supporto sociale e caratteristiche psicologiche in pazienti affecte da carcinoma della mammella. *Revista di Psichiatria* 21:315–328.

43. Watson, M., et al. 1984. Emotional control and automatic arousal in breast cancer patients. *J Psychosom Res* 28:467–474.

44. Gross, J. 1989. Emotional suppression in cancer onset and progression. *Soc Sci Med* 12:1239–1248.

45. Jasmin, et al. 1990. Evidence for a link between certain psychological factors and the risk of breast cancer in a case controlled study. *Ann Oncol* 1:22–29.

46. Watson, M., et al. 1991. Relationships between emotional control, adjustment to cancer, and depression and anxiety in breast cancer patients. *Psycholog Med* 21:51–57.

47. Maunsell, E. 1993. Better survival in patients with confidants. *Oncology News International.* December:16.

48. Levy, S., et al. 1991. Immunological and psychosocial predictors of disease recurrence in patients with early stage breast cancer. *Behavioral Medicine.* Summer. pp. 67–75.

49. House, J., et al. 1988. Social relationships and health. *Science* 241:540–545.

50. Spiegel, E., et al. 1989. Effect of psychosocial treatment on survival of patients with metastatic breast cancer. *Lancet* ii:888–891.

51. Greer, S., et al. 1990. Psychological response to breast cancer and 15-year outcome. *Lancet* 335:49–50.

52. Phillips, et al. 1993. Psychology and survival. *Lancet* 342:1142–1145.

Chapter 18
Genetics and Breast Implants

1. Easton, D.F., et al. 1993. Genetic linkage analysis in familial breast and ovarian cancer: results from 214 families. *Am J Hum Genet* 52:678–701.

2. Ferguson-Smith, et al. 1990. Genomic imprinting and cancer. *Cancer Survive* 9:487–503.

3. Reik, W. 1989. Genomic imprinting and genetic disorders in man. *Trends Genet* 5:331–336.

4. Karp, J., et al. 1993. Oncology. *JAMA* 270:237–239.
5. Hall, J., et al. 1990. Linkage of early onset familial breast cancer to chromosome 17q21. *Science* 250:1684.
6. Coles, C., et al. 1990. Evidence implicating that at least two genes on chromosome 17p in a breast carcinogenesis. *Lancet* 336:761–763.
7. Weber, B. 1994. Susceptibility genes for breast cancer. *NEJM* 331:1523–1524.
8. Narod, et al. 1991. Familial breast ovarian cancer locus on chromosome 17q12-23. *Lancet* 338:82.
9. Arason, A., et al. 1993. Linkage analysis of chromosome 17q markers and breast-ovarian cancer in Icelandic families and possible relationship to prostatic cancer. *Am J Hum Genet* 52:711.
10. Ford, D., et al. 1993. The risks of cancer in BRCA1 mutation carriers. *Am J Hum Genetics* 53:298.
11. Ford, D., et al. 1994. Risks of cancer in BRCA1 - mutation carriers. *Lancet* 343:692–695.
12. Hollstein, M., et al. 1991. p53 mutations in human cancers. *Science* 253:49–52.
13. Harris, C. 1993. p53: at the crossroads of molecular carcinogenesis and risk assessment. *Science* 262:1980–1981.
14. Culotta, E., and D. Koshland. 1994. p53 sweeps through cancer research. *Science* 262:1958–1961.
15. Li, F., and J. Fraumeni. 1969. Soft tissue sarcomas, breast cancer, and other neoplasms: a familial syndrome? *Ann Intern Med* 71:747–751.
16. Skolnick, M., et al. 1990. Inheritance of proliferative breast disease in breast cancer kindreds. *Science* 250:1715–1720.
17. Biesecker, B., et al. 1993. Genetic counseling for families with inherited susceptibility to breast and ovarian cancer. *JAMA* 269:1970–1974.
18. King, M., et al. 1993. Inherited breast and ovarian cancer. *JAMA* 269:1975–1980.
19. Smith, H., et al. 1991. Allelic loss correlated with primary breast cancer. *PNAS* 88:3847–3851.
20. Eng, C., et al. 1994. Familial cancer syndromes. *Lancet* 343:709–713.
21. Eklund, G., et al. 1988. Improved imaging of the augmented breast. *AJR* 151:469–473.
22. Moffat, S. 1991. Breast implant industry. *Los Angeles Times* (Nov. 15): D1.
23. Hayes-Macaluso, M., et al. 1993. Imaging the augmented breast. *Applied Radiology* (Dec.):21–26.
24. Press, R., et al. 1992. Antinuclear autoantibodies in women with silicone breast implants. *Lancet* 340:1304–1307.
25. Levine, J., and N. Ilowite. 1994. Scleroderma-like esophageal disease in children breast fed by mothers with silicone implants. *JAMA* 271:213–216.
26. Flick, V. 1994. Silicone implants and esophageal dysmotility. *JAMA* 271:240–241.
27. Berkel, H., et al. 1992. Breast augmentation: a risk factor for breast cancer? *NEJM* 326:1649–1653.
28. Levin, M., and B. Modan. 1993. Breast augmentation and the risk of subsequent breast cancer. Institute for Cancer and Blood Related Diseases, National Center for Health Statistics. *NEJM* 328:661–664.
29. Weiss, R. 1991. Implants: How big a risk? *Science* 252:1059p1060.
30. Council on Scientific Affairs, AMA. 1993. Silicone gel breast implants. *JAMA* 270:2602–2606.

Chapter 19
Breast Cancer Detection and Diagnosis

1. Morrison, A.S. 1991. Is self-examination effective in screening for breast cancer? *JNCI* 83:226–227.
2. Semiglazov, et al. 1987. Current evaluation of the contribution of self-examination to secondary prevention of breast cancer. *Eur J Epidemiol* 3:78–83.
3. Phillips, et al. 1984. Breast self-examination: Clinical results from a population based prospective study. *Br J Cancer* 50:7–12.
4. Mant, et al. 1987. Breast self-examination and breast cancer at diagnosis. *Br J Cancer* 55:207–211.
5. Frank and Mai. 1985. Breast self-exami-

nation in young women: More harm than good? *Lancet* (Sept 21):654–658.

6. Taylor, et al. 1984. Breast self-examination among diagnosed breast cancer patients. *Cancer* 54:2528–2532.

7. Fletcher, et al. 1985. Physicians' abilities to detect lumps in silicone breast models. *JAMA* 253:2224–2228.

8. Breslow, et al. 1977. Final report of the NCI ad hoc working groups on mammography in screening for breast cancer and summary report. *JNCI* 59:467–541.

9. Bailar, J.C. 1976. Mammography: A contrary view. *Ann Intern Med.* 84:77–84.

10. Mittra, I. 1994. Breast screening: the case for physical examination without mammography. *Lancet* 343:342–344.

11. Seidman, et al. 1987. Survival experience in the Breast Cancer Detection Demonstration Project. *Cancer* 37:258–290.

12. Sener, et al. 1977. Potential accuracy of Xeroradiographic examination of the breast with respect to menopausal status and location of pathological findings. *Breast* 3:39–47.

13. Hermansen, et al. 1987. Diagnostic reliability of combined physical examination, mammography, and fine needle puncture in breast tumors. *Cancer* 60:1866–1871.

14. Testimony of Samuel Broder, M.D., Director of National Cancer Institute, National Institutes of Health, Dept. HHS, before Subcommittee on Aging, Senate Committee on Labor and Human Resources, March 9, 1994.

15. Eastman, P. 1994. ACS vigorously defends mammography screening for women in their forties. *Oncology Times* (January):28–30.

16. Marwick, C. 1993. NCI Board votes to keep mammography guidelines. *JAMA* 270:2783.

17. Shapiro, S. 1994. The call for change in breast cancer screening guidelines. *Am J Public Health* 84:10–12.

18. Guidelines for Screening Mammography. *Oncology Bulletin* (February 1994):7.

19. Shapiro, S., et al. 1971. Periodic breast cancer screening in reducing mortality from breast cancer. *JAMA* 215:1777–1785.

20. Beahrs, O., et al. 1979. Report of the working group to review the National Cancer Institute—American Cancer Society Breast Cancer Detection Demonstration Projects. *JNCI* 62:640–709.

21. UICC Multidisciplinary Project on Breast Cancer. *UICC Tech Rep Ser* 1982:69.

22. Tabar, L., et al. 1981. Screening for breast cancer - the Swedish trial. *Radiology* 138:219–222.

23. Miller, A., et al. 1981. The National Study of Breast Cancer Screening. Protocol for a Canadian randomized controlled trial of screening for breast cancer in women. *Clin Invest Med* 4:277–258.

24. Roberts, M., et al. 1984. The Edinburgh randomized trial of screening for breast cancer. *Br J Cancer* 50:77–84.

25. UK Trial of Early Detection of Breast Cancer Group. 1981. Trial of early detection of breast cancer: Description of method. *Br J Cancer* 44:618–627.

26. Verbeek, A., et al. 1984. Reduction of breast cancer mortality through mass screening with modern mammography. *Lancet* (June 2):1222–1224.

27. Collette, J.H., et al. 1984. Evaluation of screening for breast cancer in a nonrandomized study by means of a case control study. *Lancet* i:1224–1226.

28. Shapiro, S., et al. 1982. Ten to fourteen year effects of breast cancer screening on mortality. *JNCI* 69:349–355.

29. Gad, A., et al. 1984. Screening for breast cancer in Europe: achievements, problems, and future. *Rec Results Cancer Res* 90:179–194.

30. Eddy, D., et al. 1988. The value of mammography screening in women under age 50 years. *JAMA* 259:1512–1519.

31. Palli, et al. 1986. A case controlled study of the efficacy of a non-randomized breast cancer screening program in Florence, Italy. *Int J Cancer* 38:501–504.

32. Bailar, John C. 1988. Mammography before age 50 years? *JAMA* 259:1548–1549.

33. Baines, C.J., et al. 1990. Canadian National Breast Screening Study: Assessment of technical quality by external review. *A J R* 153:23–32.

34. Baines, C.J. 1989. Evaluation of mammography and physical examination has independent screening modalities in the Canadian National Breast Screening Study. In *Practical Modalities of an Efficient Screening for Breast Cancer in the European Community*, ed. G. Ziant. Amsterdam: Elsevier. pp. 3–9.

35. Miller, A., et al. 1990. Report on a workshop of the UICC project on evaluation of screening for cancer. *Int J Cancer* 46:761–769.

36. Kopans, D.B. 1990. The Canadian Screening Program: A different perspective. *A J R* 155:748–749.

37. Miller, A.B. 1991. Breast screening in women under 50. *Lancet* 338:113.

38. Stacey-Clear, et al. 1992. Breast cancer survival among women under age 50: Is mammography detrimental? *Lancet* 340:991–994.

39. Elwood, et al. 1993. The effectiveness of breast cancer screening in young women. *Curr Clin Trials* 2:227.

40. Haagensen, C.D. 1986. The relation of age to the frequency of breast carcinoma. In *Diseases of the Breast*. Philadelphia: Saunders. pp. 402–407.

41. Tabar, L., et al. 1989. The Swedish two county trial of mammographic screening for breast cancer: Recent results and calculations of benefit. *J Epidemiol Commun Health* 43:107–114.

42. Frisell, J., et al. 1991. Randomized study of mammography screening: Preliminary report on mortality in the Stockholm trial. *Breast Cancer Res Treat* 18:49–56.

43. Tabar, L., et al. 1992. Update of the Swedish two-county program of mammographic screening for breast cancer. *Radiol Clin N Am* 30:187–210.

44. Spratt, et al. 1986. Geometry, growth rates, and duration of cancer and carcinoma *in situ* of the breast before detection by screening. *Cancer Res* 46:970–974.

45. Nystrom, L., et al. 1993. Breast screening with mammography: Overview of Swedish randomized trials. *Lancet* 341:973–978.

46. Kerilkowske, K., et al. 1995. Efficacy of screening mammography. *JAMA* 273:149–154.

47. Thomas, B.A. 1995. Population breast cancer screening: theory, practice, and service implications. *Lancet* 345:205–206.

48. Kattlove, H., et al. 1995. Benefits and costs of screening and treatment for early breast cancer. *JAMA* 273:142–148.

49. Kerlikowske, K., et al. 1993. Positive, predictive value of screening mammography by age and family history of breast cancer. *JAMA* 270:2444–2450.

50. Kaplan, et al. 1989. Breast cancer risk and participation in mammographic screening. *Am J Public Health* 79:1494–1498.

51. Zapka, J.G., et al. 1993. Breast screening by mammography: Utilization and associated factors. *Am J Public Health* 79:1499–1501.

52. Harris, R.P., et al. 1991. Mammography and age: Are we targeting the wrong women? A community survey of women and physicians. *Cancer* 67:2010–2014.

53. Devitt, J.E. 1989. False alarms of breast cancer. *Lancet* (November 25): 1257–1258.

54. Lee, J.M. 1993. Screening and informed consent. *NEJM* 328:438–439.

55. Frisell, J., et al. 1991. Randomized study of mammography screening: Preliminary report on mortality in the Stockholm trial. *Breast Cancer Res Treat* 18:49–56.

56. Mammography and breast examination for older women—results from Behavioral Risk Factor Surveillance System, 1992. 1993. *Oncology* 7(12):48–53.

57. Dodd, G.D. 1987. The major issues in screening mammography: the history and present status of radiographic screening for breast cancer. *C A* 60:1669–1702.

58. Eddy, D.M. The value of mammography screening in women under age 50 years.

59. Eddy, D.M. 1989. Screening for Breast Cancer. *Ann Intern Med* 111:389–399.
60. Council on Scientific Affairs. 1989. Mammographic screening in asymptomatic women aged 40 years and older. *JAMA* 261:2535–2542.
61. Spiera, H. 1988. Scleraderma after silicone augmentation mammoplasty. *JAMA* 260:236.
62. Hayes, et al. 1988. Mammography and breast implants. *Plast Reconstr Surg* 82:1–6.
63. Eklund, G., et al. 1988. Improved imaging of the augmented breast. *A J R* 151:469–473.
64. Leibman, J., et al. 1989. Modified mammography detects breast cancer in women with breast implants. *Oncology* 3:89.
65. Leibman, J., et al. 1990. Imaging of the augmented breast. *Oncology* 4:71.
66. Watmough, D.J. 1992. X-ray mammography and breast compression. *Lancet* 340:122.
67. Smatchio, K., et al. 1979. Ultrasonic treatment of tumours: absence of metastases following treatment of a hamster fibrosarcoma. *Ultrasound Med Biol* 5:45–49.
68. Egan, R.L. 1980. Mammographic patterns and breast cancer risk. *JAMA* 244:287.
69. Clark, D., et al. 1990. Pressure measurements during automatic breast compression in mammography.
70. Andersson, I., et al. 1988. Mammographic screening and mortality from breast cancer: the Malmo mammographic screening trial. *BMJ* 297:943–948.
71. Brawley, O. 1994. NCI abandons mammography guidelines. *Oncology* (March):9.

Chapter 20
Establishing the Diagnosis and Stage

1. Herman, J.B. 1971. Mammary cancer subsequent to aspiration of cyst in the breast. *Ann Surg* 173:40.
2. Harrington and Lesnick. 1981. The association between gross cysts of the breast and breast cancer. *Breast* 7:13.
3. Haagensen, C.D. 1986. In *Diseases of the Breast*. Philadelphia: W.B. Saunders Company. p. 253.
4. Ciatto, S., et al. 1987. The value of routine cytological examination of breast cyst fluids. *Acta Cytol* 31:301–304.
5. Wolberg, W.H., et al. 1989. Fine needle aspiration for breast mass diagnosis. *Arch Surg* 124:814–818.
6. Miller, T.R., et al. 1992. *Cancer Detection and Prevention.*
7. Rosemond, G.P., et al. 1969. Needle aspiration of breast cysts. *Surg Gynecol Obstet* 128:351–354.
8. Schwartz, G.F., and S.A. Feig. 1991. Management of patients with non-palpable breast lesions. *Oncology* 5:39–44.
9. Schwartz, G.F. 1994. The role of excision and surveillance alone in subclinical DCIS of the breast. *Oncology* 8:21–35.
10. Freund, et al. 1976. Breast cancer arising in surgical scars. *J Surg Oncology* 8:477–480.
11. Brenner, R.J., and E.A. Sickles. 1989. Acceptability of periodic follow-up as an alternative to biopsy for mammographically detected lesions interpreted as probably benign. *Radiology* 171:645–646.
12. Meyer, J., et al. 1990. Biopsy of occult breast lesions. *JAMA* 253:2341–2343.

Chapter 21
"Conventional" Localized Treatment Options for Breast Cancer

1. Harris, R.P., et al. 1985. Current status of conservative surgery and radiotherapy as primary local treatment for early carcinoma of the breast. *Breast Cancer Research and Treatment* 5:245.
2. Cancer Research Campaign Working Party. 1980. Cancer research campaign trial for early breast cancer: a detailed update at the tenth year. *Lancet* 2:55–60.
3. Fisher, B., et al. 1985. Ten year results of a randomized clinical trial comparing radical mastectomy and total mastectomy with or without radiation. *NEJM* 312:674–681.

4. Fisher, B., et al. 1989. Eight year results of a randomized clinical trial comparing total mastectomy and lumptctomy with or without irradiation in the treatment of breast cancer. *NEJM* 320:822–828.

5. Veronesi, U., et al. 1990. Breast conservation is the treatment of choice in small breast cancer: long term results of a randomized trial. *Eur J Cancer* 26:668–670.

6. Sarrazin, D., et al. 1989. Ten year results of a randomized trial comparing a conservative treatment to mastectomy in early breast cancer. *Radiother Oncol* 14:177–184.

7. von Dongen, J., et al. 1992. Randomized clinical trial to assess the value of breast conserving therapy in stage I and II breast cancer, EORTC 10801 trial. In *Consensus Development Conference on the Treatment of Early Stage Breast Cancer. JNCI Monograph No. 11.* Washington, D.C.: Government Printing Office, pps. 15–18.

8. Straus, K., et al. 1992. Results of the National Cancer Institute Early Breast Cancer Trial. *JNCI Monograph No. 11.* Washington, D.C.: Govt Printing Office, pp. 27–32.

9. Blichert-Toft, M., et al. 1992. Danish randomized trial comparing breast conservation therapy with mastectomy: six years of life table analysis. *JNCI Monograph No. 11.* Washington, D.C.: Government Printing Office, pps. 19–25. (NIH publication 90-3187.)

10. Vicini, F., et al. 1992. Recurrence in the breast following conservative surgery and radiation therapy for early stage breast cancer. *JNCI Monograph No. 11.* Washington, D.C.: Govt Printing Office, pps. 33–39. (NIH publication 90-3187.)

11. Clark, R., et al. 1987. Breast cancer: experiences with conservation therapy. *Am J Clin Oncol* 10:461–468.

12. Spitalier, J., et al. 1986. Breast conserving surgery with radiation therapy for operable mammary carcinoma: a 25 year experience. *World J Surg* 10:1014–1020.

13. Fourquet, A., et al. 1989. Prognostic factors of breast recurrence in conservative management of early breast cancer: A 25 year follow-up. *Int J Radiat Oncol Biol Phys* 17:719–725.

14. Treatment of early stage breast cancer. 1991. *JAMA* 256:391–395.

15. Veronesi, U., et al. 1990. Quadrantectomy versus lumpectomy for small size breast cancer. *Eur J Cancer* 26:671–673.

16. Fisher, B., et al. 1991. Significance of ipsilateral breast tumor recurrence after lumpectomy. *Lancet* 338:327–331.

17. Uppsala-Orebro Breast Cancer Study Group. 1990. Sector resection with or without postoperative radiation therapy for stage I breast cancer: A randomized trial. *JNCI* 82:277–282.

18. Weidner, N., et al. 1991. Tumor angiogenesis and metastases—correlation in invasive breast carcinoma. *NEJM* 324:1–8.

19. Goldie, J.H., et al. 1979. A mathematical model for relating the drug sensitivity of tumors to their spontaneous mutation rate. *Cancer Treat Rep* 63:1727–1733.

20. DeWyss, W.D. 1972. Studies correlating the growth rate of a tumor and its metastases and providing evidence for tumor-related systemic growth retarding factors. *Cancer Res* 32:374–379.

21. Fisher, B., et al. 1983. Influence of the interval between primary tumor removal and chemotherapy on kinetics and growth of metastases. *Cancer Res* 43:1488–1492.

22. Bonadonna, G., et al. 1990. Primary chemotherapy to avoid mastectomy in tumors with diameters of 3 cm or more. *JNCI* 82:1539–1545.

23. Mauriac, L., et al. 1991. Effects of primary chemotherapy in conservative treatment of breast cancer patients with operable tumors larger than 3 cm: results of a randomized trial in a single center. *Ann Oncol* 2:347–354.

24. Hrushesky, W.J.M., et al. 1989. Menstrual influence on surgical cure of breast cancer. *Lancet* 2:949–952.

25. Badwe, R.A., et al. 1991. Timing of surgery during menstrual cycle and survival of premenopausal women

with operable breast cancer. *Lancet* 337:1261–1264.

26. Badwe, R.A., et al. 1991. Surgical procedures, menstrual cycle phase, and prognosis in operable breast cancer. *Lancet* 338:815–816.

27. Senie, R.T., et al. 1991. Timing of breast cancer excision during the menstrual cycle influences duration of disease-free survival. *Ann Intern Med* 115:337–342.

28. McGuire, W.L. 1991. The optimal timing of mastectomy: low tide or high tide? *Ann Intern Med* 115:401–403.

29. Fisher, B., et al. 1985. Five year results of a randomized clinical trial comparing total mastectomy and segmental mastectomy with or without radiation in the treatment of breast cancer. *NEJM* 312:665–673.

30. Farrow, D.C., et al. 1992. Geographic variation in the treatment of localized breast cancer. *NEJM* 326:1097–1101.

31. Nattinger, A.B., et al. 1992. Geographic variation in the use of breast conserving treatment for breast cancer. *NEJM* 326:1102–1107.

32. Lazovich, D., et al. 1991. Underutilization of breast conserving surgery and radiation therapy among women with stage I or II breast cancer. *JAMA* 266:3433–3438.

33. Silliman, R.A., et al. 1989. Age as predictor of diagnostic and initial treatment intensity in newly diagnosed breast cancer patients. *J Gerontol* 44:M46–M50.

34. Kiebert, G.M., et al. 1991. The impact of breast conserving treatment and mastectomy on the quality of life of early stage breast cancer patients: a review. *J Clin Oncol* 9:1059–1070.

35. Average charges for modified radical mastectomies. 1991. *Oncology* 5:51–58.

36. Krishnan, et al. 1990. Role for adjuvant radiation therapy after modified radical mastectomy. *Applied Radiology* (May):16–23.

37. Osborne, M., et al. 1988. We would very rarely recommend prophylactic mastectomy. *Primary Care and Cancer* (January):25–31.

38. Pressman, P. 1988. When we would recommend prophylactic mastectomy. *Primary Care and Cancer.* pps. 11–16.

39. Physicians often fail to recognize post-mastectomy pain syndrome. 1993. *Oncology News International* November: 20.

Chapter 22
"Conventional" Systemic Treatment for Breast Cancer

1. Fisher, B. 1978. *The surgical dilemma in the primary therapy of invasive breast cancer: A critical appraisal.* Chicago: Yearbook.

2. Kennedy, B.J. 1965. Hormone therapy for advanced breast cancer. *Cancer* 18:1551–1557.

3. Legha, S.S., et al. 1978. Hormonal therapy of breast cancer: New approaches and concepts. *Ann Intern Med* 88:69–77.

4. DeVita, Hellman, Rosenberg. 1985. In *Cancer Principles and Practice of Oncology.* Second edition. Philadelphia: Lippincott Co., pg. 1154.

5. Goldhirsh, A., et al. 1994. Effect of systemic adjuvant treatment on first sites of breast cancer relapse. *Lancet* 343:377–381.

6. Pritchard, K. 1994. Adjuvant systemic therapy for breast cancer: a tale of relapse and survival. *Lancet* 343:370–371.

7. Dodwell, D.J. 1993. Cytotoxic drugs: A search for dose response. *Lancet* 341:614–616.

8. Pfeiffer, N. 1991. DeVita: shorter, more intensive chemo works best in adjuvant therapy. *Oncology Times* (Sept): 3.

9. Stewart, et al. 1994. Dose response in the treatment of breast cancer. *Lancet* 343:402–404.

10. Fisher, B., et al. 1975. Ten year follow-up results of patients with carcinoma of the breast in a co-operative clinical trial evaluating surgical adjuvant chemotherapy. *Surg Gynecol Obstet* 140:528–534.

11. Nissen-Meyer, R., et al. 1978. Surgical adjuvant chemotherapy: results with one short course with cyclophosphamisde after mastectomy for breast cancer. *Cancer* 41:2088–2098.

12. Nissen-Meyer, R., et al. 1988. Short perioperative versus long-term adjuvant chemotherapy. *Recent Results Cancer Res* 98:91–98.
13. CRC Adjuvant Breast Trial Working Party. 1988. Cyclophosphamide and tamoxifen as adjuvant therapies in the management of breast cancer. *Br J Cancer* 57:604–607.
14. Bonadonna, G., et al. 1987. Milan adjuvant trials for Stage I-II breast cancer. In *Adjuvant Therapy of Cancer V*, ed. S.E. Salmon. Orlando, FL: Grune & Stratton, pps. 211–221.
15. Senn, H.J., et al. 1986. Swiss adjuvant trial (OSAKO 06/74) with chlorambucil, methotrexate, and 5-fluorouracil plus BCG in node-negative breast cancer patients: nine-year results. *NCI Monogr* (1):129–134.
16. Morrison, J.H., et al. 1987. The West Midlands Oncology Association Trials of adjuvant chemotherapy for operable breast cancer. In *Adjuvant Therapy of Cancer V*, ed. S.E. Salmon. Orlando, FL: Grune & Stratton, pp. 311–318.
17. Caffier, H., et al. 1984. Adjuvant chemotherapy versus postoperative irradiation in node negative breast cancer. In *Adjuvant Therapy of Cancer IV*, ed. S.E. Hones and S.E. Salmon. Orlando, FL: Grune & Stratton, pp. 417–424.
18. Jakesz, R., et al. 1987. Adjuvant chemotherapy in node-negative breast cancer patients. In *Adjuvant Therapy of Cancer V*, ed. S.E. Salmon. Orlando, FL: Grune & Stratton, pp. 223–231.
19. Williams, C.J., et al. 1987. Adjuvant chemotherapy for T1-2, N0, M0 estrogen receptor negative breast cancer: preliminary results of a randomized trial. In *Adjuvant Therapy of Cancer V*, ed. E. Salmon. Orlando, FL: Grune & Stratton, pp. 233–241.
20. Treatment alert issued for node-negative breast cancer. 1988. *JNCI* 80:550–551.
21. The Ludwig Breast Cancer Study Group. 1988. On the safety of perioperative adjuvant chemotherapy with cyclophosphamide, methotrexate, and 5-fluorouracil in breast cancer. *Eur J Cancer Clin Oncol* 24:1305–1308.
22. The Ludwig Breast Cancer Study Group. 1989. Prolonged disease-free survival after one course of perioperative adjuvant chemotherapy for node negative breast cancer. *NEJM* 320:491–496.
23. Ramot, B., et al. 1976. Blood leucocyte enzymes. Diurnal rhythm of activity in isolated lymphocytes of normal subjects and chronic lymphocytic leukemic patients. *Br J Hematol* 34:79–85.
24. Kachergene, N.B., et al. 1972. Circadian rhythm of dehydrogenase activity in blood cells during acute leukemia in patients. *Pediatrics* 51:81–85.
25. Hrushesky, W.J. 1983. The clinical application of chronobiology to oncology. *Am J Anat* 168:519–542.
26. Haus, E., et al. 1983. Chronobiology in hematology and immunology. *Am J Anat* 168:467–517.
27. Rivard, G.E., et al. 1985. Maintenance chemotherapy for childhood acute lymphoblastic leukemia: better in the evening. *Lancet* (Dec 7) 1264–1266.
28. Early Breast Cancer Trialists' Collaborative Group. 1992. Systemic treatment of early breast cancer by hormonal, cytotoxic, or immune therapy. *Lancet* 339:1–15; 71–85.
29. Editorial. Adjuvant systemic therapy for early breast cancer. 1992. *Lancet* 339:27.
30. Ravdin, R.G., et al. 1970. Results of a clinical trial concerning the worth of prophylactic oophorectomy for breast carcinoma. *Surg Gynecol Obstet* 31:1055–1064.
31. Nevinny, H.V., et al. 1969. Prophylactic oophorectomy in breast cancer therapy: a preliminary report. *Am J Surg* 117:531–536.
32. Cole, M.F. 1968. Suppression of ovarian function in primary breast cancer. In *Prognostic Factors in Breast Cancer*, ed. A.P.M. Forrest, and P.B. Kunkler. Edinburgh: Livingstone, pp. 146–156.
33. Tengrup, I., et al. 1986. Prophylactic oophorectomy in the treatment of carcinoma of the breast. *Surg Gynecol Obstet* 152:209–214.
34. Nissen-Meyer, R. 1968. Suppression

of ovarian function in primary breast cancer. In *Prognostic Factors in Breast Cancer*, ed. A.P.M. Forrest, and P.B. Kunkler. Edinburgh: Livingstone, pp. 139–145.

35. International Breast Cancer Study Group. 1990. Late effects of adjuvant oophorectomy and chemotherapy upon premenopausal breast cancer patients. *Ann Oncol* 1:30–35.

36. Bryant, A.J.S., et al. 1981. Prophylactic oophorectomy in operable instances of carcinoma of the breast. *Surg Gynecol Obstet* 153:660–664.

37. Meakin, et al. 1979. Ovarian irradiation and prednisone therapy following surgery and radiotherapy for carcinoma of the breast. *Can Med Assoc J* 120:1221–1238.

38. Brincker, H., et al. 1985. Evidence of castration mediated effect of adjuvant chemotherapy (CT) in a randomized trial of cyclophosphamide monotherapy versus CMF in premenopausal stage II breast cancer. *Proc Am Soc Clin Oncol* 4:56.

39. Tormey, D.C. 1984. Adjuvant systemic therapy in postoperative node positive patients with breast carcinoma: The CALGB trial and ECOG premenopausal trial. *Rec Res Cancer Res* 96:155–165.

40. Padmanabhan, N., et al. 1986. Mechanism of action of adjuvant chemotherapy in early breast cancer. *Lancet* II:411–414.

41. Ahmann, G., et al. 1977. An evaluation of early or delayed adjuvant chemotherapy in premenopausal patients with advanced breast cancer undergoing oophorectomy. *NEJM* 297:356–360.

42. Scottish Cancer Trials Breast Group. 1993. Adjuvant ovarian ablation versus CMF chemotherapy in premenopausal women with Stage II breast cancer, the Scottish Trial. *Lancet* 341:1293–1298.

43. Tengrup, I., et al. 1986. Prophylactic oophorectomy in breast cancer patients. *Surg Gynecol Obstet* 162:209.

44. Brunner, et al. 1977. Combined chemo and hormonal therapy in advanced breast cancer. *Cancer* 39:2923–2933.

45. Bonadonna, G., et al. 1992. Treating early breast cancer. *Lancet* 339:675.

46. Glick, J.H. 1988. Adjuvant therapy of node negative breast cancer: another point of view. *JNCI* 80:1076.

47. The Ludwig Cancer Study Group. 1989. Prolonged disease-free interval after one course of perioperative adjunctive chemotherapy for node negative breast cancer. *NEJM* 320:491–496.

48. Fisher, B., et al. 1989. A randomized clinical trial evaluating sequential methotrexate and fluorouracil in the treatment of patients with node negative breast cancer who have estrogen receptor negative tumors. *NEJM* 320:473–478.

49. Fisher, B., et al. 1989. A randomized clinical trial evaluating tamoxifen in the treatment of patients with node negative breast cancer who have estrogen receptor positive tumors. *NEJM* 320:479–484.

50. Mansour, E.G., et al. 1989. Efficacy of adjuvant chemotherapy in high risk node negative breast cancer: an intergroup study. *NEJM* 320:485–490.

51. McGuire, W.L. 1989. Adjuvant therapy of node negative breast cancer. *NEJM* 320:525–527.

52. NIH Consensus Conference. 1991. Treatment of early stage breast cancer. *JAMA* 265:391–395.

53. McGuire, W.L., et al. 1990. How to use prognostic factors in axillary node negative breast cancer patients. *JNCI* 82:1006–1015.

54. McGuire, W.L., and G.M. Clark. 1992. Prognostic factors and treatment decisions in axillary node negative breast cancer. *NEJM* 326:1756–1761.

55. Hillner and Smith. 1991. Efficacy and cost effectiveness of adjuvant chemotherapy in women with node negative breast cancer. *NEJM* 324:160–168.

56. Kramer, B.S. 1991. Breast cancer control: weighing cost versus effect. *Contemporary Oncology* (Nov–Dec):43–50.

57. Bagenal, F.S., et al. 1990. Survival of patients with breast cancer attending Bristol Cancer Help Center. *Lancet* 336:606–610.

58. Duggan, D. 1991. Local therapy of

locally advanced breast cancer. *Oncology* 5:67–82.

59. Swain, S., and M. Lippman. 1989. Systemic therapy of locally advanced breast cancer: review and guidelines. *Oncology* 3:21–30.

60. Eddy, D.M. 1992. High-dose chemotherapy with autotransplantation for the treatment of metastatic breast cancer. *J Clin Oncol* 4:657.

61. Peters, W., et al. 1986. High-dose combination alkylating agents with bone marrow support as initial treatment for metastatic breast cancer. *J Clin Oncol* 6:1368.

62. Dunphy, F., et al. 1990. Treatment of estrogen receptor negative or hormonally refractory breast cancer with double high-dose chemotherapy intensification and bone marrow support. *J Clin Oncol* 8:1207.

63. Williams, S.F., et al. 1992. High-dose consolidation therapy with autologous stem cell rescue in stage IV breast cancer: follow-up report. *J Clin Oncol* 10:1743.

64. Wallerstein, R., et al. 1990. A Phase II study of mitoxantrone, etoposide, and thiotepa with autologous marrow support for patients with relapsed breast cancer. *J Clin Oncol* 8:1782.

65. Eder, J.P., et al. 1986. High-dose combination alkylating agent chemotherapy with autologous bone marrow support for metastatic breast cancer. *J Clin Oncol* 4:1592.

66. Antman, K., et al. A Phase II study of high-dose cyclophosphamide, theotepa, and carboplatin with autologous marrow support in women with measurable advanced breast cancer responding to standard-dose therapy. *J Clin Oncol* 10:102.

67. Kennedy, M.J., et al. 1991. High-dose chemotherapy with reinfusion of purged autologous bone marrow following dose-intense induction as initial therapy for metastatic breast cancer. *J Natl Cancer Inst* 83:920.

68. Tallman, M., et al. 1992. High-dose chemotherapy (HDC), autologous bone marrow transplant (ABMT), and post-transplant *in vivo* purging che-

motherapy for patients with advanced breast cancer. *Proc Am Soc Clin Oncol* 11:84.

69. Peters, W.P. 1991. High-dose chemotherapy and autologous bone marrow support for breast cancer. In *Important Advances in Oncology*, eds. V.T. De Vita, S. Hellman, S.A. Rosenberg. Philadelphia, PA: J.B. Lippincott.

70. Peters, W.P., et al. 1993. High-dose chemotherapy and autologous bone marrow support as consolidation after standard-dose adjuvant therapy for high-risk primary breast cancer. *J Clin Oncol* 11:1132.

71. Gianni, A.M., et al. 1992. Growth factor-supported high-dose sequential (HDS) adjuvant chemotherapy in breast cancer with more than 10 positive modes. *Proc Am Soc Clin Oncol* 11:60.

72. Jahnke, L. and J. Winter. 1993. High-dose therapy's role in breast cancer management. *Contemporary Oncology* (Dec):38–49.

73. Mangan, K. 1994. Progress in peripheral blood stem cell transplantation. *Hem/Onc Annals* 2(1):14–18.

74. Stadtmauer, E. 1994. Peripheral blood stem cell transplantation in breast cancer. *Hem/Onc Annals* 2(1):61–68.

75. Rochefordiere, et al. 1993. Age as prognostic factor in premenopausal breast cancer. *Lancet* 341:1039–1043.

76. Adami, H.O., et al. 1985. Age as a prognostic factor in breast cancer. *Cancer* 56:898–902.

77. Adami, H.O., et al. 1986. The relation between survival and age at diagnosis in breast cancer. *NEJM* 315:559–563.

78. Muss, H. 1993. How to treat the older woman with breast cancer. *Contemporary Oncology* (May):27–38.

79. Goldhirsch, A., et al. 1990. Treatment of breast cancer in elderly patients. *Lancet* 336:564–565.

80. Christman, K., et al. 1992. Chemotherapy of metastatic breast cancer in the elderly. *JAMA* 268:57–62.

81. DiSaia, D., et al. 1993. Hormone replacement therapy in breast cancer. *Lancet* 342:1232.

82. Cobleigh, M., et al. 1994. Estrogen

replacement therapy in breast survivors. *JAMA* 272:540–545.

83. Schapira, et al. 1991. A minimalist policy for breast cancer surveillance. *JAMA* 265:380–382.

84. Holland, J.F. 1983. Karnofsky Memorial Lecture: Breaking the cure barrier. *J Clin Oncol* 1:74–90.

85. Legha, S.S., et al. 1979. Complete remissions in metastatic breast cancer treated with combination drug therapy. *Ann Intern Med* 91:847–852.

86. Blumenschein, et al. 1983. Seven year follow-up of stage IV patients entering complete remission from FAC presented at the Third European Oncology Research and Treatment Conference, April 19, 1983. Amsterdam, the Netherlands.

87. Lippman, M., et al. 1988. *Diagnosis and Management of Breast Cancer.* Philadelphia, PA: W.B. Saunders Company, pp. 375–406.

88. Zwaveling, et al. 1987. An evaluation of routine follow-up for detection of breast cancer recurrences. *J Surg Oncol* 34:194–197.

89. Broyn, and Froyen. 1982. Evaluation of routine follow-up after surgery for breast cancer. *ACTA Chir Scand* 148:401–404.

90. The GIVIO Investigators. 1994. Impact of follow-up testing on survival and health-related quality of life in breast cancer patients. *JAMA.* 271:1587–1592.

91. Rosselli, M., et al. 1994. Intensive diagnostic follow-up after treatment of primary breast cancer. *JAMA* 271:1593–1597.

92. Fisher, B., et al. 1994. Endometrial cancer in tamoxifen-treated breast cancer patients: Findings from NSABP B-14. *JNCI* 86:527–537.

93. Barakat, R. 1995. The effect of tamoxifen on the endometrium. *Oncology* 9(2):129–139.

94. Bissett, R., et al. 1994. Gynaecological follow-up of breast cancer patients on tamoxifen. *Lancet* 343:1244–1246.

95. Amy, J.J., et al. 1995. Gynaecological monitoring during tamoxifen therapy. *Lancet* 345:253–254.

96. Kedar, R.P., et al. 1994. Effects of tamoxifen on uterus and ovaries of postmenopausal women in a randomized breast cancer prevention trial. *Lancet* 343:1318–1321.

97. Makris, A., et al. 1995. Study suggests schedule for gyn exams in women on tamoxifen. *Onçology News International* 4(2):6.

98. Rowinsky, E.K., and W. McGuire. 1992. Taxol: present status and future prospects. *Contemporary Oncology* (March):29–36.

99. Curtis, R.E., et al. 1992. Risk of leukemia after chemotherapy and radiation therapy for breast cancer. *NEJM* 326:1745–1751.

100. Haas, J.F., et al. 1987. Risk of leukemia in ovarian tumor and breast cancer patients following treatment by cyclophosphamide. *Br J Cancer* 55:213–218.

101. Andersson, M., et al. 1991. Adjuvant chemotherapy and subsequent malignant disease. *Lancet* 338:885–886.

102. Reizenstein, P., et al., editors. 1988. *Managing Minimal Residual Malignancy in Man.* Oxford: Pergamon Press.

103. Arriagada, R., and L.E. Rutqvist. 1991. Adjuvant chemotherapy in early breast cancer and incidence of new primary malignancies. *Lancet* 338:535–538.

104. Evans, R.A. 1992. A letter. *NEJM* 327:1317–1318.

105. Adler, A., et al. 1980. Immunocompetence, immunosuppression, and human breast cancer. *Cancer* 45:2061–2083.

106. Mandeville, R., et al. 1982. Biological markers and breast cancer. Multiparametric study. II. Depressed immunocompetence. *Cancer* 50:1280–1288.

107. Greenspan, E.M. 1985. Prior tuberculosis in long term survivors of breast and ovarian cancer from a New York oncology practice (1954–1974). *Mount Sinai Journal Medicine* 52:465–468.

108. Greenspan, E.M. 1986. Is BCG an orphan drug suffering from chemotherapists' overkill? *Cancer Invest* 4:81–92.

109. Simone, C.B. 1992. *Cancer and Nutrition: A Ten-Point Plan to Reduce Your Risk of Getting Cancer.* Garden City Park, NY: Avery Publishing Group.

110. House Select Committee on Aging. 1984. *Quackery: A $10 billion scandal.* 98th Congress, 2nd sess, S. Doc. 98-435.

111. Cassileth, B., et al. 1991. Survival and quality of life among patients receiving unproven as compared with conventional cancer therapy. *NEJM* 324:1180–1185.

112. Muss, H., et al. 1991. Interrupted versus continuous chemotherapy in patients with metastatic breast cancer. *NEJM* 325:1342–1348.

113. Hudis, C. 1994. Is there an alternative to alternating adjuvant therapy for breast cancer? *Cancer Investigation.* 12(3):329-335.

114. Editorial. 1993. Breast Cancer: have we lost our way? *Lancet* 341:343–344.

115. Lancet Conference Summary. 1994. The challenge of breast cancer. *Lancet* 343:1085–1086.

Chapter 23
Male Breast Cancer

1. Adami, H.O., et al. 1989. The survival pattern in male breast cancer: an analysis of 1429 patients from the Nordic countries. *Cancer* 64:1177–1182.

2. Bagley, C.S., et al. 1987. Adjuvant chemotherapy in males with cancer of the breast. *Am J Clin Oncol* 10:55–60.

3. Eldar, S., et al. 1989. Radiation carcinogenesis in the male breast. *Eur J Surg Oncol* 15:274–278.

4. Orentreich, et al. 1974. Mammogenesis in transsexuals. *J Invest Dermatol* 63:142.

5. Symmers, W.C. 1968. Carcinoma of the breast in transsexuals. *Br Med J* 1:83.

6. Treves and Holleb. 1955. Cancer of the male breast. *Cancer* 8:1239.

7. Fodor. 1989. Breast cancer in a patient with gynecomastia. *Plast Reconstruct Surg* 84:976–979.

8. Olsson, H., et al. 1988. Head trauma and exposure to prolactin elevating drugs as risk factors for male breast cancer. *JNCI* 80:679–683.

9. Mabuchi, K., et al. 1985. Risk factors for male breast cancer. *JNCI* 74:371–375.

10. Lin, R.S. 1980. Epidemiological findings in male breast cancer. *Proc Am Assoc Cancer Res* 21:72.

11. Fisher, B., et al. 1989. Eight year results of a randomized clinical trial comparing total mastectomy and lumpectomy with or without irradiation in the treatment of breast cancer. *NEJM* 320:822–828.

12. Veronesi, U., et al. 1986. Comparison of Halsted mastectomy with quadrantectomy, axillary dissection, and radiotherapy in early breast cancer: Long-term results. *Eur J Cancer Clin Oncol* 22:1085–1089.

13. Friedman, M.A., et al. 1981. Estrogen receptors in male breast cancer: clinical and pathological correlations. *Cancer* 47:134–137.

14. Gupta, N., et al. 1980. Estrogen receptors in male breast cancer. *Cancer* 46:1781–1784.

15. Everson, R.B., et al. 1980. Clinical correlations of steroid receptors and male breast cancer. *Cancer Res* 40:991–997.

16. Donegan, W.L., et al. 1973. Carcinoma of the male breast. A 30 year review of 28 cases. *Arch Surg* 106:273–279.

17. Horn, B., and Roof, Y. 1976. Male breast cancer: 2 cases with objective regressions from caluster-one (7 alpha, 17 beta- dimethyl testosterone) after failure of orchiectomy. *Oncology* 33:188–191.

18. Ribeiro, G. 1983. Tamoxifen in the treatment of male breast carcinoma. *Clin Radiol* 34:625–628.

19. Donegan, W. 1991. Cancer of the breast in men. *CA-A Cancer Journal for Clinicians* 41:339–354.

20. Kinne, D. 1991. Management of male breast cancer. *Oncology* (March):45–48.

Chapter 24
Quality of Life and Ethics

1. *Cancer Treat Rep.* 1985. 69:1155–1157.

2. Gelber, R.D., et al. 1991. Quality of life adjusted evaluation of adjuvant therapies for operable breast cancer. *Ann Int Med* 114:621–628.

3. Hurny, C., et al. 1992. Quality of life studies in international groups. *Eur J Cancer* 28:118–124.

4. Cassileth, B., et al. 1991. Survival quality of life among patients receiving unproven or conventional cancer therapy. *NEJM* 324:1180–1185.
5. Winer, E.R., and L.M. Sutton. 1994. Quality of life after bone marrow transplantation. *Oncology* 8:19–26.
6. Andrykowski, M.A., et al. 1990. Cognitive dysfunction in adult survivors of allogeneic marrow transplantation. *Bone Marrow Transplant* 6:269–276.
7. Kurtzman, S.H., et al. 1988. Rehabilitation of the cancer patient. *Am J Surg* 155:791–803.
8. Bullard, D.G., et al. 1980. Sexual health care and cancer. *Front Radiat Ther Oncol* 14:55‡58.
9. Silberfarb, P.M., et al. 1980. Psychosocial aspects of neoplastic disease. Functional status of breast cancer patients. *Am J Psychiatry* 137:450–455.
10. Jamison, K.R., et al. 1978. Psychosocial aspects of mastectomy. *Am J Psychiatry* 135:432–436.
11. Battersby, C., et al. 1978. Mastectomy in a large public hospital. *Aust N Z J Surg* 48:401–404.
12. Schover, L.R., 1991. The impact of breast cancer on sexuality, body image, and intimate relationships. *CA-A Cancer J for Clinicians* 41:112–120.
13. Psychological Aspects of Breast Cancer Study Group: Psychological response to mastectomy. 1987. *Cancer* 59:189–196.
14. Vinokur, A.D., et al. 1989. Physical and psychosocial functioning in adjustment to breast cancer. *Cancer* 63:394–405.
15. Taylor, S.E., et al. 1984. Attributions, beliefs about control and adjustment to breast cancer. *J Person Soc Psychol* 46:489–502.
16. Steinberg, M.D., et al. 1985. Psychological outcome of lumpectomy versus mastectomy in the treatment of breast cancer. *Am J Psychiatry* 142:34–39.
17. Margolis, G., et al. 1990. Psychological effects of breast conserving cancer treatment and mastectomy. *Psychosom Med* 31:33–39.
18. Dean, C., et al. 1983. Affects of immediate breast reconstruction on psychosocial morbidity after mastectomy. *Lancet* 1:459–462.
19. Noone, R.B., et al. 1982. Patient acceptance of immediate reconstruction following mastectomy. *Plast Reconstruct Surg* 69:632–640.
20. Schain, W.S., et al. 1985. The sooner the better: a study of psychological factors in women undergoing immediate versus delayed breast reconstruction. *Am J Psychiatry* 142:40–46.
21. Masters and Johnson. 1966. *Human Sexual Response*. Boston: Little, Brown.
22. Kaiser, F. 1992. Sexual function and the older cancer patient. *Oncology* 6:112–118.
23. McGinnis, S. 1986. How can nurses improve the quality of life of the hospice client and family? In *Nursing in Hospice and Terminal Care*, ed. J. Petrosino. New York: The Hayworth Press, pp. 23–36.
24. President's Commission for the Study of Ethical Problems in Medicine and Biomedical and Behavioral Research. 1982. *Making Health Care Decisions*. Vol. 2. Appendices. Washington, D.C.: Government Printing Office. pp. 245–246.
25. Arato v. Avedon, 5 Cal. 4th 1172, 23 Cal Rptr. 2D. 131, 858 P. 2D 598 (1993).
26. Moertel, C.G. 1991. Off-label drug use for cancer therapy and National Health Care Priorities. *JAMA* 266:3031–3032.

Chapter 25
Untreated Breast Cancer: Its Natural History

1. Bloom, H.J.G., et al. 1962. Natural history of untreated breast cancer (1805–1933). Comparison of untreated and treated cases according to histological grade of malignancy. *Br Med J* ii:213–221.
2. Buchanan, J.B., et al. 1983. Tumor growth, doubling times, and inability of the radiologist to diagnosis certain cancers. *Radiol Clin N Am* 21:115–126.
3. Heuser, L., et al. 1979. Relation between mammary cancer growth kinetics and the interval between screenings. *Cancer* 43:857–862.

4. Bauer, W.C., et al. 1980. Cronologie du cancer mammaire utilisant un modele de croissance de Gompertz. *Ann Anat Pathol Paris* 25:39–56.

5. Haagensen, C.D., et al. 1981. *Breast Carcinoma-Risk and Detection*. Philadelphia: W.B. Saunders.

6. Spratt, J.S., et al. 1982. Variations and associations in histopathology, clinical factors, mammographic patterns, and growth rates among breast cancers confirmed in a population. In *Issues in Cancer Screening and Communication*, ed. C. Metlin, and G.P. Murphy. New York: A. Liss, pg. 295.

7. Fournier, D., et al. 1980. Growth rate of 147 mammary carcinomas. *Cancer* 45:2198–2207.

8. Kramer, W.M., and B.F. Rush. 1973. Mammary duct proliferation in the elderly. *Cancer* 31:130–137.

9. Nielsen, M., et al. 1984. Precancerous and cancerous breast lesions during lifetime and at autopsy. *Cancer* 54:612–615.

10. Baum, M. 1976. The curability of breast cancer. *Br Med J* i:439–442.

11. Fox, M.S. 1979. On diagnosis and treatment of breast cancer. *JAMA* 241:489–494.

12. Brinkley, D., and J.L. Haybittle. 1984. Long term survival of women with breast cancer. *Lancet* i:1118.

13. Le, M.G., et al. 1984. Long term survival of women with breast cancer. *Lancet* ii:922.

14. Rutqvist, L.F., and A. Wallgren. 1985. Long term survival of 458 young breast cancer patients. *Cancer* 55:658–665.

15. Adair, et al. 1974. Long term follow-up of breast cancer patients: the 30 year report. *Cancer* 33:1145–1150.

16. Jackson, A. 1888. On carcinoma of the breast and its treatment. *Med Press* i:552–553.

17. Bruce, J. 1969. The enigma of breast cancer. *Cancer* 24:1314–1318.

18. Feinstein, A.R., et al. 1969. The epidemiology of cancer therapy. Clinical problems of statistical surveys. *Arch Intern Med* 123:171–186.

19. Edelstyn, G. 1969. Surgery and radiotherapy for breast cancer. *Br J Hosp Med* 3:1861–1872.

20. Lewison, E.F., and A.C.W. Montague, eds. 1981. *Diagnosis and Treatment of Breast Cancer*. Baltimore: Williams and Wilkins, pg. 3.

21. Skrabanek, P. 1985. False premises and false promises of breast cancer screening. *Lancet* (August):316–319.

22. Fisher, B. 1980. Laboratory and clinical research in breast cancer: a personal adventure: the David A. Karnofsky Memorial Lecture. *Cancer Res* 40:3863–3874.

23. Fisher, E.R. 1988. Pathobiological considerations in the treatment of breast cancer. In *Controversies in Breast Disease*, ed. Grundfest-Broniatowski and Esselstyn. New York: Marcel Dekker, pp. 151–180.

24. Chargaff, E. 1976. Triviality in science: a brief meditation on fashions. *Perspect Biol Med* 19:324–333.

25. Fisher, B., et al. 1985. Five year results of a randomized clinical trial comparing total mastectomy and segmental mastectomy with or without radiation in the treatment of breast cancer. *NEJM* 312:665–673.

26. Fisher, B., et al. 1985. Ten year results of a randomized clinical trial comparing radical mastectomy and total mastectomy with or without radiation. *NEJM* 312:674–681.

27. Cady, B. 1984. Lymph node metastases. Indicators, but not governors of survival. *Arch Surg* 119:1067–1072.

28. Dunken, W., and G.R. Kerr. 1976. The curability of breast cancer. *Br Med J* ii:781–783.

Glossary of Medical Terms

Adjuvant treatment. Treatment given in addition to the primary treatment.

Aspiration. Removal of liquids or solids from a lump using a needle and syringe.

Autosomal dominant trait. A single gene, acting alone, to produce an outcome.

Axilla. Armpit.

Benign. A noncancer, nonmalignant growth.

Biopsy. The gross and microscopic examination of tissues removed from the body to make a medical diagnosis; excisional biopsy is the removal of the entire breast lump, whereas incisional biopsy is the removal of a small piece of the breast mass.

Brachytherapy. *See* Implant radiation.

Cancer. A malignant uncontrollable growth that invades surrounding tissues and spreads to other organs as well.

Carcinoma. A cancer that begins in the lining or coverings of organs.

Chemotherapy. Chemical drugs used to treat an illness.

Computed tomography (CT). A computerized X-ray study that details the cross-sectional anatomy of a part of a body.

Cyst. An abnormal sac in an organ filled with fluid, gas, or semisolid material.

Diagnostic mammography. An X-ray picture of the breast done for a woman who has symptoms. *See also* Mammogram; Screening mammography.

Duct. Tubes in breast from lobes to the nipple through which milk is delivered.

Estrogen. A steroid hormone produced mainly in the ovaries responsible for the development of female characteristics and the menstrual cycle.

Executive physical examination. Combines a complete history with a scalp-to-toes examination.

External radiation. Radiation from a machine outside the body delivered to a cancer in the body. *See also* Implant radiation; Radiation therapy.

Genotype. The hereditary make-up of an individual as determined by her/his genes.

Gynecologist. Physician who treats diseases of the female reproductive organs.

Hormone therapy. Adding or removing hormones to treat cancer.

Hormones. Steroid chemicals produced by various organs for different purposes.

Implant radiation (also known as brachytherapy). A radioactive substance is placed directly into the tissue in the body that needs treatment. *See also* External radiation; Radiation therapy.

Lobe. A section of the breast.

Lobule. A division of the lobe in the breast.

Local-regional therapy. Treatment directed to the tumor bed and its adjacent surrounding tissues.

Lumpectomy. Removal of only the breast lump; excisional biopsy is sometimes used synonymously.

Lymph nodes. Oval or round bodies located along the lymphatic vessels that remove bacteria or foreign particles from the lymph. Cancers can spread to lymph nodes, and their growth will increase the size of those nodes.

Lymphedema. Fluid that *sometimes* collects in the tissues of extremities as a result of removing lymph vessels or lymph nodes.

Malignant. Describing a cancerous tumor that is growing and spreading.

Mammogram. *See* Diagnostic mammography, Screening mammography.

Mastectomy. Surgical removal of the breast.

Mendelian inheritance. Classical genetics that has two genes operating to produce a single outcome.

Menopause. The time when menstrual cycles stop permanently.

Metastasis. The spread of cancer from the primary organ, like breast, to another more distant organ, like bone. In this particular case, the patient has breast cancer that has spread to her bones; she does not have breast cancer *and* bone cancer.

Oncologist. Physician who treats cancer.

Palpation. A technique of examining organs by feeling them to detect abnormalities.

Pathologist. Physician who reads prepared microscopic slides containing biopsied tissue in order to determine a diagnosis.

Pathology. The study and classification of tissue specimens with the use of a microscope.

Progesterone. A female hormone secreted by the ovaries.

Prosthesis. The artificial replacement of a body part, as with a breast that is worn underneath clothing.

Radiation therapy. Treatment of cancer using high energy radiation from X-ray or other sources. *See also* External radiation; Implant radiation.

Screening. Tests used to find disease when a person has no symptoms of an illness.

Screening mammography. An X-ray picture of the breast done for a woman with no symptoms. *See also* Diagnostic mammography; Mammogram.

Staging. Determining where the cancer is located in all parts of the body.

Systemic therapy. Treatment that travels to all parts of the body, usually by way of the bloodstream.

Tumor. The Latin word that means growth or swelling; today's usage refers to an abnormal growth of tissue; it does not imply, however, that the mass is a cancer.

Tumor marker. Something detectable in the body that may suggest a cancer is growing.

Ultrasound. A diagnostic test that bounces harmless sound waves off body tissues, a process that can differentiate solid from liquid. This is most useful to distinguish the contents of a mass in a breast. A solid mass needs further investigation, but a liquid-filled mass usually needs no further work-up.

Sources of
Information

You can contact the following organizations/agencies for more information:

- **National Cancer Institute, Cancer Information Service**

Call 1–800–4–CANCER and you can speak with someone who can answer your questions.

The Cancer Information Service can also send you free booklets:

> *After Breast Cancer: A Guide to Follow-up Care.*
> *Breast Biopsy: What You Should Know.*
> *Breast Cancer: Understanding Treatment Options.*
> *Breast Exams: What You Should Know.*
> *Mastectomy: A Treatment for Breast Cancer.*
> *What You Need to Know About Breast Cancer.*
> *What You Need to Know About Cancer.*
> *Chemotherapy and You.*
> *Radiation Therapy and You.*
> *Eating Hints: Recipes and Tips for Better Nutrition During Cancer Treatment.*
> *Taking Time: Support for People With Cancer and the People Who Care About Them.*
> *What Are Clinical Trials All About?*
> *Advanced Cancer: Living Each Day.*
> *When Cancer Recurs: Meeting the Challenge Again.*
> *Research Report: Bone Marrow Transplantation.*

You can also write to the National Cancer Institute at this address:

> National Cancer Institute
> Building 31, Room 10A24
> 9000 Rockville Pike
> Bethesda, MD 20892

- **FDA**

For more information on breast implants, you can write to the FDA at this address:

> Breast Implants
> Food and Drug Administration
> HFE-88
> Rockville, MD 20857

The FDA also has a hotline to answer questions about silicone-gel-filled breast implants. Call 1–800–532–4440, Monday through Friday, 9 A.M. to 7 P.M. Eastern Standard Time.

- **NABCO**

> National Alliance of Breast Cancer Organizations
> 1180 Avenue of the Americas, 2nd floor
> New York, NY 10036
> 212–719–0154

- **The American Cancer Society (ACS)**

> National Office
> Tower Place
> 3340 Peachtree Road, NE
> Atlanta, GA 30026
> (404) 320–3333
> (800) ACS–2345

The ACS has chartered divisions in every state in the country from which you can obtain information and services including names of doctors and approved hospital programs.

- **The American College of Radiology (ACR)**

> 1891 Preston White Drive
> Reston, VA 22091

> ACR will refer you to approved mammogram sites.

- **The American Society of Plastic and Reconstructive Surgeons**

> 444 East Algonquin Road
> Arlington Heights, IL 60005
> (312) 2289900
> (800) 635–0635

- **The Health Insurance Association of America (HIAA)**

    Fulfillment Department
    PO Box 41455
    Washington, DC 20018
    (202) 866–6244

HIAA will answer your questions concerning insurance coverage.

- **The YWCA Encore Program**

    National Headquarters
    726 Broadway
    New York, NY 10003
    (212) 614–2827

This program provides support for breast cancer patients.

- **PDQ (Physicians Data Query)**

The cancer treatment database of the NCI provides prognostic, stage, and treatment information and more than 1000 protocol summaries. A computer modem is needed for access to PDQ. For more information, call the NCI at (310) 496–7403.

- **National Cancer Institute supported Comprehensive and Clinical Cancer Centers**

The National Cancer Institute supports a number of cancer centers throughout the country. Call (301) 496–4000 to find the designated NCI supported Cancer Center near you.

National Organizations for Breast Cancer Patients

4-Cancer
800-4-CANCER
A service of the National Cancer Institute. Supplies information about cancer prevention, symptoms, kinds of cancer, clinical trials, and second opinions. Will provide referrals to local support groups.

National Alliance of Breast Cancer Organizations
212-719-0154
An answering machine records your inquiry, which will be answered on the next business day. In an emergency, call 212-889-0606.

Share
212-382-2111
Provides emotional support and references for information. Will place callers' names on mailing list for educational seminars.

Y-Me
800-221-2141
All counselors are breast-cancer survivors. Provides information on early detection, accredited mammography facilities and cancer centers, and referrals to physicians and support groups.

About the Author

Dr. Charles B. Simone is a nationally renowned medical oncologist, immunologist, and radiation oncologist with a practice in Princeton, New Jersey. He graduated from Rutgers College of Medicine with both a Master's of Medical Science (M.MS.), and a Medical Degree (M.D.). After training in internal medicine at the Cleveland Clinic, Dr. Simone was offered a position as clinical associate in the Immunology Branch and Medicine Branch of the National Cancer Institute (NCI) in Bethesda, MD. Later, he became an investigator in the Pharmacology Branch and Medicine Branch of the NCI. While at the NCI, he trained in medical oncology (chemotherapy) and clinical immunology.

In 1982, he accepted a position in the Department of Radiation Therapy at the University of Pennsylvania, Philadelphia; and in 1985, he became an associate professor in the Department of Radiation Therapy and Nuclear Medicine at Thomas Jefferson University, Philadelphia. Since 1989, he has worked to establish the Simone Protective Cancer Center, a multifunctional facility dedicated to comprehensive patient care.

In addition, Dr. Simone has served as a consultant to major corporations and foreign countries, and has advised many prominent figures, including former President Ronald Reagan, on the principles of cancer prevention.

Index

Acid rain, 160–162
Acquired immunodeficiency syndrome.
    See AIDS.
Actinic keratosis, 93
Adrenal hormone, 18
Adriamycin. *See* Doxorubicin.
AFIP. *See* Armed Forces Institute of
    Pathology.
Aflatoxin, 31, 122
Agent Orange. *See* Dioxin.
AIDS, 39, 157
Air pollution
    indoor, 166–167
    outdoor, 158–160
Alcohol
    as disease risk factor, 141
    breast cancer and, 142–143
    cancer and disease and, 143
    immunity and, 141–143
    nutrition and, 141
    Simone Ten-Point-Plan recommen-
        dations on, 327
    statistics, 140–141
Alcholism
    immunity and, 142
    nutrition and, 141
Aldrin, 122
Alpha-BHC, 125
Alzheimer's disease, 66
Amcide, 129
American Academy of Family Practice, 217
American Alliance for Health, Physical
    Education, Recreation and Dance, 184
American Association for Cancer Research,
    4
American Association of Family Practitio-
    ners, 217
American Cancer Society, 2, 3, 97, 114
American College of Physicians, 217
American Dietetic Association, 111
American Lung Association, 137, 158, 327
American Medical Association, House of
    Delegates of, 204
Ames, B. N., 109
Aminogluthethimide, 260, 262

Androgens
    as cancer risk factor, 156–157
    as hormone for breast cancer treatment,
        260
Aneuploidy, 241
Angina, 65
Antibodies, 49, 50
Antioxidants
    cancer studies involving, 59–63
    disease and, 65–66, 94, 96
    effects on cancer, 57–59
    individual, descriptions of, 59–71
    See also Nutritional supplements.
Apocrine cells, 20
Apoptosis, 200
Arato v. Avedon, 307–310
Armed Forces Institute of Pathology
    (AFIP), 231
Asbestos, 33, 159–160
Aspiration, needle, of a breast mass,
    226–227
Atherosclerosis, 68
    cancer and, 37–38
Axillary node dissection, 246, 247, 250
    chemotherapy prior to, 250–251
    combined with radiation therapy,
        248–249
    menstrual cycle's influence on, 251
    side effects of, 255–256

B cells, 50, 182
B lymphocytes. *See* B cells.
Bacilli Calmette-guerin (BCG), 290
Bacillus thuringiensis, 129
BaP. *See* Benzopyrene.
Battell Pacific Northwest Laboratory, 176
BCG. *See* Bacilli Calmette-guerin.
Benign breast disease, 151–152, 328
Benzopyrine (BaP), 71, 78, 101, 159
Beta-carotene, 67, 83, 84
Betahexachlorocyclohexane. *See* HCH.
Bioflavonoids, 69
Biopsy
    excisional, 227–228
    incisional, 227